# BASIC NUTRITION AND
# DIET THERAPY

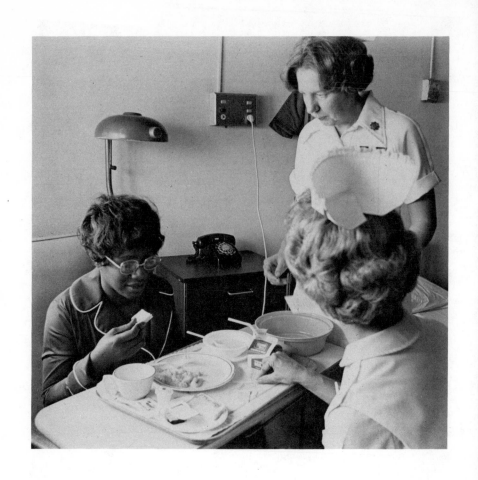

THIRD EDITION

# BASIC NUTRITION
# AND
# DIET THERAPY

## CORINNE H. ROBINSON, M.S., R.D.

Nutrition Consultant and Professor of Nutrition Emeritus.
Formerly, Head, Department of Nutrition and Food, Drexel University,
and Instructor, Normal and Therapeutic Nutrition,
School of Nursing, Thomas Jefferson University, Philadelphia

MACMILLAN PUBLISHING CO., INC.
NEW YORK
Collier Macmillan Publishers
LONDON

MACMILLAN PUBLISHING CO., INC.
866 Third Avenue, New York, New York 10022

COLLIER-MACMILLAN CANADA, LTD.

Figures 5-1, 8-2, 9-2, 9-3, 11-1, 12-2, 12-3, 12-4, and 12-5 herein are reproduced from the fifth printing (1974) of C. H. Robinson, *Normal and Therapeutic Nutrition*, 14th ed. (New York: Macmillan Publishing Co., Inc., 1972). Frontispiece courtesy of Department of Nursing, Delaware County Community College, Media, Pennsylvania.

---

*Library of Congress Cataloging in Publication Data*

Robinson, Corinne Hogden.
  Basic nutrition and diet therapy.

  Includes bibliographies and index.
   1. Diet in disease. 2. Nutrition. I. Title.
[DNLM: 1. Diet therapy—Nutrition. WB100 R655b]
RM216.R652   1975              641.1              74-11751
ISBN 0-02-402400-7

---

Printing:   2 3 4 5 6 7 8                Year:   5 6 7 8 9 0

# PREFACE TO THE THIRD EDITION

The aim of the third edition of this textbook is to present basic information on nutrition and diet therapy to students of practical and vocational nursing, associate-degree nursing, dietetic technology, and other health-related fields. It is intended for use in basic courses that prepare students to apply principles of nutrition in relatively simple situations. Some of the more complex problems of nutritional care are briefly described so that the bedside nurse and dietetic technician will be able to assist other members of the health team.

An important concept herein is that the basis for all nutritional planning depends upon a full understanding of the principles of normal nutrition. The study of nutrition is viewed as applicable to the student's own daily living and in her/his associations within the community as well as to the use of modified diets for patient care. Repeated emphasis is given to the team approach in providing nutritional care.

The book is organized into four units. Unit I, "Introduction to Food and Nutrition—Individual and Community Goals," enables the student to develop personal and professional goals for study. The unit presents an overview of the meanings of nutrition, the problems of nutrition in the community, a discussion of digestive processes, and practical guides for nutritional planning, including the 1974 Recommended Dietary Allowances and the four food groups. Metric measures are introduced and are used throughout the text, although English measures are indicated in parentheses. For modified diets and for tables of food values household measures in English units have been retained.

v

Unit II, "The Nutrients," includes information on nutrient functions, utilization, food sources, Recommended Dietary Allowances, and effects of deficiencies. An important change is the presentation of mineral elements in two chapters with greater emphasis upon fluid and electrolyte balance (Chapter 10). Food fallacies and facts are included at the end of each chapter so that the reader can relate the knowledge of a specific nutrient to refute a given fallacy. Summary tables of minerals and vitamins appear at the end of Chapters 10 and 12.

Unit III, "Practical Planning for Good Nutrition," includes many revisions and additions. Among these are the 1970 recommendations of the Committee on Maternal Nutrition of the Food and Nutrition Board for diet during pregnancy, emphasis upon the special needs of the teen-age pregnant girl, community programs for feeding the elderly, and some fallacies and facts relating to diet in pregnancy and for the aging (Chapter 13). The use of premodified formulas and supplementary feeding for infants, dietary planning for preschool, school, and teen-age children, and some suggestions for the improvement of food habits are presented in Chapter 14. The dietary pattern typical of black Americans in the southeastern United States has been added to the discussion of cultural food patterns (Chapter 15). "Safeguarding the Food Supply" (Chapter 16) pertains to foodborne infections and intoxications, natural toxicants in foods, food preservation, and food additives. New federal regulations on labeling for nutritional information are important for all consumers, but especially for those who must assist patients in the selection of modified diets. These regulations are fully described in Chapter 17, "Food Legislation, Labeling, and Selection."

Unit IV, "Diet Therapy," has been completely reorganized, rewritten, and enlarged. Each chapter may be correlated with study in medical-surgical nursing of pathologic conditions affecting the body systems. Each chapter includes a full description of the appropriate dietary modification with specific attention to some of the problems the nurse is likely to encounter with patients. Each dietary regimen is based upon modification of the normal diet. Since a given diet may have uses in a number of conditions, many cross references are included.

The dietary modification for diabetes mellitus (Chapter 22) incorporates the recent recommendations of the American Diabetes Association with respect to proportions of protein, fat, and carbohydrate, and considerations for kind of fat and cholesterol. Dietary modifications in hyperthyroidism, hypoglycemia, phenylketonuria, galactosemia, gout, arthritis, and osteoporosis are described in Chapter 23, "Various Metabolic Disorders."

The discussion of diets in cardiovascular and renal diseases (Chapters 24 to 26) has been considerably amplified since these problems are so frequently encountered in nursing practice. Detailed patterns are given for fat- and cholesterol-controlled diets for five types of hyperlipidemia, sodium-restricted diets in congestive failure, and protein-, sodium-, and potassium-restricted diets for renal failure.

Other revisions and additions to this unit include the liberal approach to nutritional therapy for peptic ulcer (Chapter 27); dietary management in ulcerative colitis, sprue, and lactose intolerance (Chapter 28); food allergies (Chapter 30); and dietary planning in surgical conditions, including diets following gastrectomy, burns, and the use of hyperalimentation, chemically defined low-residue diets, and tube feedings (Chapter 31).

Five tables are presented in Appendix A: nutritive values of foods; the food exchange lists; heights and weights for men and women in metric as well as English measures; Recommended Daily Nutrients—Canada, 1974; and metric conversions. An addition to Appendix B is a list of films, film-strips, and slides for correlation with chapters throughout the text. Appendix C presents a glossary of frequently used terms.

Many additions and revisions in this text have resulted from the valuable suggestions given by instructors in nursing and allied health programs who returned a questionnaire submitted by the publisher. These contributions are gratefully acknowledged.

For the many new illustrations of clinical situations the author especially appreciates the assistance of Mrs. Carolyn McGuigan, R.D., Chief, Dietetic Service, Veterans Administration Hospital, Coatesville, Pennsylvania, and Mr. Joseph A. Josephs, photographer; Mrs. Donna Mansfield, R.D., Nutritionist, Handicapped Children's Unit, St. Christopher's Hospital for Children, Philadelphia, and Mr. Douglas G. Baird, photographer; Mrs. Gilberta A. Trani, R.N., Coordinator, Allied Health Programs, Delaware County Community College, Media, Pennsylvania, and Miss B. A. Flynn, photographer; and the patients, students, and staff whose photographs appear in the text. Appreciation is also expressed to governmental agencies and trade organizations for a number of illustrations.

Once again, as in the earlier editions of this text, it has been a pleasure to work with Miss Joan C. Zulch, Medical Editor, Macmillan Publishing Co., Inc. She has generously given her assessments, ideas, and encouragement.

C. H. R.

# CONTENTS

## UNIT III
PRACTICAL PLANNING FOR GOOD NUTRITION

## UNIT IV
DIET THERAPY

# APPENDIXES

# INTRODUCTION TO FOOD AND NUTRITION — INDIVIDUAL AND COMMUNITY GOALS

**1**

# FOOD, NUTRITION, AND HEALTH

## THE STAFF OF LIFE

From birth to death food is a dominant factor in our lives. In a single year, on a three-meal-a-day basis, most of us eat well over 1000 meals. We know that the food we eat is necessary for our very being—we know it provides the energy for the quiet breathing at night and the full activity of the day—we know too that it builds, maintains, and regulates muscles and bones, nerves and brain, eyes, hair, and all our physical being.

But food does much more than nourish, for most of us enjoy eating. Food makes us feel secure and happy; we use food as a link in our friendships, as an expression of pleasure during our holidays, and as a symbol of our religious life.

Food is the world's biggest business. A large part of the world's work is concerned with the growing, processing, and preparation of food. In the United States one farm worker produces enough food for 25 persons, but think of all the people who work in the factories that process the food, in the markets that sell the food, or in restaurants, institutions, and homes that serve the food. We spend an important amount of our income for food. We have food in abundance and in variety.

Most of the world's people spend the greater part of their working days and most of their income for food. In some countries of the world three fourths or more of the working population is directly concerned with growing food; yet it seldom manages to grow quite enough. Tonight millions of the world's people will go to bed more or less hungry. Is it any

3

surprise that these people are discontented, diseased, and die an early death?

From this brief introduction you can see that good nutrition depends upon the understanding, knowledge, and cooperation of many people. Good nutrition alone cannot guarantee good health, but without good nutrition health cannot be at its best.

## SOME DEFINITIONS

Before we can begin the study of nutrition, some definitions need to be made.

*Food* is that which nourishes the body. No two foods are alike in their ability to nourish, because no two foods contain identical amounts of nutrients.

*Nutrients* are those 50 or more chemical substances in food that are needed by the body. They are divided into six classes: proteins and amino acids; fats and fatty acids; carbohydrates; mineral elements; vitamins; and water.

*Nutrition* refers to the processes in the body for making use of food. It includes eating the correct foods for the body's needs; digestion of foods so that the body can use the nutrients; absorption of the nutrients into the bloodstream; use of the individual nutrients by the cells in the body for the production of energy, the maintenance and growth of cells, tissues, and organs; and elimination of wastes.

*Nutritional care* is the application of the art and science of nutrition to the feeding of people. It deals with the assessment of nutritional status; the planning of meals according to physiologic and psychologic needs at any stage in the life cycle; the implementation of the plan through the preparation and service of meals; the education that is necessary so that individuals may apply the principles of nutrition to their daily needs; and the continuous evaluation so that changes can be made as situations require. Nutritional care is personalized for each individual, but the concepts of nutritional care also involve everyone in a group situation.

## GOOD AND POOR NUTRITION

*Nutritional status* is the condition of health as it is related to the use of food by the body. It is evident in some very obvious ways we can all see, such as changes in weight. However, an accurate measure of nutritional status can be made only by the expert examination that a physician can give and through a variety of blood and urine tests. Some contrasts in good and poor nutrition are listed in Table 1–1. You should remember that other reasons for poor health might be lack of sleep, poor sanitation, poor housing, and so on.

TABLE 1–1   SOME CONTRASTS IN NUTRITION

| Good Nutrition | Poor Nutrition |
| --- | --- |
| Normal weight for height, body frame, and age | Overweight; underweight; failure to grow; sudden loss of weight |
| Erect posture; arms and legs straight; abdomen in; chest up; chin in | Poor posture: chest forward; rounded shoulders; protruding abdomen |
| Firm, strong muscles; moderate padding of fat | Thin, flabby muscles; lack of padding of fat, or excessive fat |
| Firm, clear skin with good color; healthy, pink mucous membranes | Dry, scaly, pale skin; pale mucous membranes |
| Well-formed jaw and even teeth | Poorly formed jaw with teeth poorly aligned |
| Soft, glossy hair | Dull, dry hair |
| Clear, bright eyes, not unduly sensitive to light | Dull eyes, sensitive to light; burning, itching; circles and puffiness under eyes |
| Good appetite and digestion | Poor appetite; complaints of indigestion |
| Abundance of energy and endurance | Listlessness, fatigue, and lack of endurance |
| Resistance to disease | Many infections; longer convalescence from disease |
| Ability to concentrate | Short attention span |
| Cooperative, interested, agreeable, cheerful | Irritable, apathetic, worried, depressed |

## NUTRITION AS A SCIENCE

Throughout all of history man has written about food and its effects on the body. Ancient Egyptian writings on tablets of stone record the use of food for the treatment of numerous diseases. In the Old Testament of the Bible we can learn much about the foods available to the Jewish people, the religious symbolism of food, and the laws governing the use of food. Hippocrates, the famous Greek physician who lived several hundred years before Christ, wrote of the proper foods for treating disease. He observed, "Persons who are naturally very fat are apt to die earlier than those who are slender." [1] The thinking of Hippocrates, Galen, and other philosophers governed the whole practice of medicine down through the Middle Ages.

People have learned through the ages that some foods were more nourishing than others, and that some plants were, in fact, poisonous and could not be eaten. Along with this experience a great deal of superstition about

[1] G. Lusk, *Nutrition* (New York: Paul B. Hoeber, Inc., 1933), p. 8.

foods also arose. Some of these false notions are believed even today by many people.

The science of nutrition developed only after the groundwork had been laid for the sciences of chemistry and physiology, and had its beginnings in the late eighteenth century—just about the time of the American Revolution. Most of the understanding of the functions of the nutrients in the body, the nutritive values of foods, the body's requirements for nutrients, and the role of nutrition in health and disease belongs to the last 60 or 70 years. It must be emphasized that nutrition is indeed one of the youngest of sciences, and that much still remains to be learned.

Scientists learn about nutrition through laboratory studies on experimental animals, using rats, mice, guinea pigs, hamsters, chickens, dogs, cattle, and even microorganisms. Many studies have likewise been conducted on healthy human volunteers, since not all of the results obtained on animals can be applied directly to humans.

Studies conducted on animals and on humans usually measure certain physical changes; for example, growth in height and weight, skin condition, and many other conditions that the researcher can note. The amount of nutrients in the food intake and the amount of specific substances excreted in the urine and feces are measured in balance experiments. Thus, if the intake and excretions are equal, the subject is said to be in *balance,* or in *equilibrium.* Many constituents may also be measured in the blood and tissues, for changes in diet will, sooner or later, bring about changes in the level of certain substances in the blood. The techniques of the physician, biologist, physiologist, chemist, and nutritionist are required in nutrition research.

To summarize, when you study nutrition, you will become aware that this is a well-organized science with a tremendous body of knowledge. There is no room for the food faddist or the quack who tries to substitute oratory, unrealistic promises, and emotional appeal for sound knowledge and wise applications to the healthful feeding of people.

### TEAMWORK IN NUTRITION

As a nurse you are part of the professional team that cares for the sick. The physician is the captain of this team, and many people with varying skills work under his direction: nurses, dietitians, dietetic technicians, social workers, physical therapists, occupational therapists, laboratory technicians, and others. You are also a member of the nursing team that includes professional nurses, practical or vocational nurses, nurse's aides, and orderlies. (See Fig. 1–1.)

Nutrition teamwork means that the physician prescribes the diet; the dietitian supervises the planning of menus and the purchase and preparation of food for all patients and personnel; the nurse helps the patient

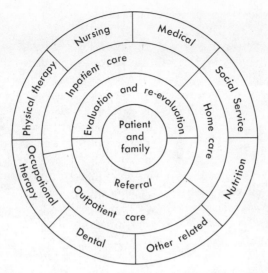

**FIGURE 1–1** The concentric circles of comprehensive care radiate out from the patient and his family. (*Courtesy Miss Geraldine Piper, and the* Journal of the American Dietetic Association, *Chicago.*)

at mealtime and records the acceptance of the meal. The nurse and dietitian may consult with the physician concerning any nutritional problems presented by the patient. The dietitian and nurse may work together in planning the modified diet for the patient and in the various stages of education of the patient. (See Fig. 1–2.)

## YOUR RESPONSIBILITY IN NUTRITION

First of all, you have a responsibility to *yourself.* You will personally benefit from good nutrition, for you will look and feel better; you will be better able to meet the demands of your profession; and you will set an example for others.

You have a responsibility to your *family.* Perhaps this lies in planning and preparing better meals for the family, in helping a child to develop good food habits, or in guiding an elderly person in making adjustments in his diet according to a doctor's prescription. Perhaps this is a responsibility you will assume more fully at some later time.

You have a responsibility as a *nurse* or *other health worker.* Nutrition is an essential part of the total care of a patient. You will need an appreciation of what food means to the patient, how illness changes his feelings about food, and how to help him with his day-to-day meals. See Chapter 18 for specific details on the nutritional care of patients.

You have a responsibility as a *citizen.* Because you are a health worker, many people look to you for an example and for advice. You will need to

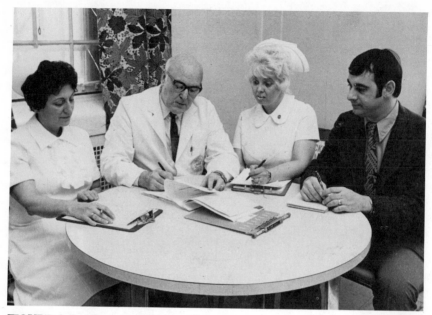

FIGURE 1–2 The nurse, physician, dietitian, and social worker discuss the patient's progress and make plans for his continuing care. (*Courtesy, Veterans Administration Hospital, Coatesville, Pennsylvania.*)

know how to answer simple questions. But you will also need to know when to refer people to physicians if questions concerning diagnosis and treatment are asked. You can give your support to the school lunch program and other activities that improve the nutrition of people. You can take a positive stand for any action by the community government aimed toward better nutrition.

### GOALS FOR NUTRITION STUDY

If you accept seriously the responsibilities outlined, you will find the following goals to be helpful in the study of nutrition:

Understanding and appreciation of:
    the relation of food and nutrition to health, happiness, efficiency, and long life for yourself as well as for others
    the meanings of food to people—religious, cultural, social, psychologic, and economic; respect for individual differences
    the importance of having the right attitude toward food
    the opportunities to help people in the selection of a good diet
    the difficulties involved in changing food habits
    the importance of nutrition to the recovery of the patient

the need for teamwork in the improvement of nutrition of people
your responsibility for the nutritional care of patients
Knowledge concerning:
basic principles of nutrition
functions of the nutrients
requirements for nutrients by various age groups
foods as sources of nutrients
cultural food patterns
techniques for development of good food habits
principles for modifying diets for disease conditions
reliable sources of information on nutrition

*Behavioral outcomes.* Having achieved the understandings, appreciation, and knowledge outlined above, the student should expect to be able to act in the following ways:

Selects own diet for good nutrition
Uses tables of food composition to learn values of foods
Interprets labeling and advertising of food products
Makes adjustments in meal plans for cultural, psychologic, and economic factors
Helps patients use a selective menu
Helps patients at mealtime
Encourages and reassures patient; explains importance of diet
Observes food intake of patients and reports to nursing supervisor or dietitian
Answers simple questions posed by patient; or refers questions to the dietitian
Works with the supervising nurse, dietitian, and physician
Makes use of community resources in helping the patient to care for himself.

## REVIEW QUESTIONS AND PROBLEMS

1. Define nutrient, nutrition, nutritional status, nutritional care.

2. List some signs of good nutrition.

3. In addition to poor diet what factors might be responsible for poor health?

4. Look for advertisements on food in magazines and newspapers. Discuss the good features of the advertisements. What are some of the bad features?

5. Start a file for articles on food and nutrition from current newspapers and magazines. From time to time compare the content of these articles with what you learn in your study of nutrition.

6. Examine the list of goals for nutrition. As you proceed in the study of nutrition, evaluate yourself against these goals. Are there other aims you should include?

**2**

Nutrition in the United States | CHANGING PATTERNS OF LIVING |
NUTRITIONAL PROBLEMS | FAULTY FOOD HABITS | FOOD FADDISM
AND QUACKERY | IDENTIFYING THE FOOD QUACK | RELIABLE
SOURCES OF INFORMATION · Nutrition, a World Concern |
INTERNATIONAL NUTRITION PROBLEMS | INTERNATIONAL
ORGANIZATIONS

# NUTRITION IN THE COMMUNITY

## Nutrition in the United States

The patterns of American diet have resulted from a bountiful and varied food supply and from the cultural impact of many nationality backgrounds. The creativity of the food technologist, the skill of the food engineer, and the speed of transportation from east to west and from north to south have all contributed to the variety of readily available foods.

### CHANGING PATTERNS OF LIVING

Dietitians and nurses must take changes in the patterns of living into account when they try to help people toward better food habits. Most Americans today have more money, more education, more leisure, and more opportunity to travel both here and abroad. Women make up about 40 percent of the work force; some of these are second wage earners in the family, and many others are the sole wage earners. With so many women working, the purchase of food and the meal preparation are often shared with other family members. There is much greater reliance upon convenience foods. Children have lunches at school and sometimes breakfasts as well, and working members of the family eat in restaurants or at quick-lunch counters or carry their own lunches. Business and social obligations and the school activities of children often interfere with families having dinner together. People are eating much more frequently, partly because of the many attractive snacks that are available. Numerous new foods are

10

introduced in the markets each year. Since there is a limit to the amount of food a person can eat, each new food that is adopted replaces another. Is the new food a good replacement or not? Obviously the food patterns of individuals as well as families differ widely and must be taken into account when counseling is provided.

## NUTRITIONAL PROBLEMS

The quality of health is affected when there is too much food, too little food, or the wrong kind of food. Obesity is widely recognized as a public health problem because it is associated with diabetes, gallbladder disease, and heart disease. Moreover, diets high in saturated fat, high in cholesterol, or too high in calories are among the factors leading to coronary disease as the principal cause of death in the United States.

Dental decay is almost universally present, even in young children, and leads in early life to considerable loss of teeth as well as expensive dental repair work. Somewhat later in life many people lose their teeth because of faulty gum structures. Those who lose their teeth often are unable to chew satisfactorily, and they may not eat the foods necessary for good health.

Iron deficiency anemia occurs in a relatively high proportion of infants and preschool children in low-income populations. It is also seen in many pregnant women, especially those who have had more than one baby. (See Fig. 2–1.)

The extent of malnutrition in the United States is not known. The severe deficiencies caused by very low intakes of vitamins, protein, and calories do not occur very often. Occasionally pediatricians see children who have kwashiorkor or marasmus (see Chap. 5) or scurvy (see Chap. 12); such cases are sometimes the result of child neglect and sometimes of ignorance concerning the child's nutritional needs. Rickets and goiter occur occasionally. (See Chaps. 9 and 11.)

## FAULTY FOOD HABITS

Every ten years the U.S. Department of Agriculture conducts a survey of family food consumption. A "good" diet is one that provides the Recommended Dietary Allowances (see Table 4–1, p. 32) for seven nutrients. The last survey in 1965 showed a decline in the quality of diets. Only 50 per cent of the families had diets that could be classified as "good," as compared with 60 per cent in 1955.

Calcium and iron were the nutrients most frequently below the Recommended Dietary Allowances. For infants and young children the average intake of iron was 30 per cent or more below the recommended allowances, while the average intakes of calcium were satisfactory. For females from

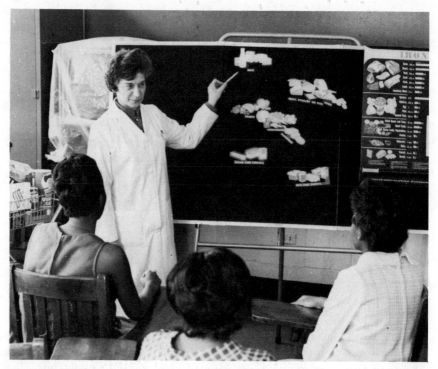

FIGURE 2–1 The importance of iron in the diet is explained to a group of pregnant women by a nutritionist. The sources of iron are related to the food groups. (*Courtesy, School of Nursing, Thomas Jefferson University Hospital, Philadelphia.*)

age 9 years and on the calcium and iron intakes were 20 to 30 per cent or more below the recommended levels. Males of all ages had more adequate intakes of calcium and iron.

The quality of the American diet is directly related to income. People at the lowest income level had poor diets four times as often as those at the highest income level. (See Fig. 2–2.) But the fact that some people at higher income levels also had poor diets indicates that adequate nutrition education has not reached as many people as it should.

Insufficient money, ignorance of the essential foods for an adequate diet, poor facilities for preparing food, and lack of skills must share the blame for the malnutrition seen in this country. The following points need to be recognized in setting up programs for improved nutrition.

1. Infants, preschool children, adolescent girls, and pregnant women are the most vulnerable to the effects of poor food habits.

2. Milk, deep-green and yellow vegetables, and citrus fruits require greater emphasis in dietary planning. The trend among Americans today seems to be away from milk as a beverage, substituting coffee, tea, soft drinks, and fruitades.

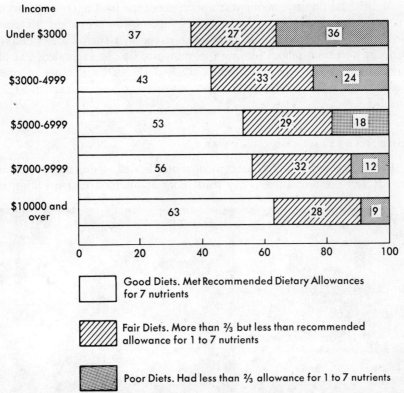

**Income**

| Under $3000 | 37 | 27 | 36 |
| $3000-4999 | 43 | 33 | 24 |
| $5000-6999 | 53 | 29 | 18 |
| $7000-9999 | 56 | 32 | 12 |
| $10000 and over | 63 | 28 | 9 |

☐ Good Diets. Met Recommended Dietary Allowances for 7 nutrients

▨ Fair Diets. More than ⅔ but less than recommended allowance for 1 to 7 nutrients

▨ Poor Diets. Had less than ⅔ allowance for 1 to 7 nutrients

**FIGURE 2–2** As income goes down, the percentage of people having a good diet also goes down. Lack of income is not the sole reason for inadequate diets, however. Note that only 63 per cent of people at the highest income level had good diets. (*Data from family dietary survey, 1965; courtesy Agricultural Research Service, U.S. Department of Agriculture, Washington, D.C.*)

3. The use of convenience foods has greatly increased and no doubt will continue to do so. Homemakers need much more assistance in making the best choices for the money they can spend because the products are so numerous.

4. Snacks are too often made up of foods high in starches, sugars, and fats but providing little by way of other nutrients. These snacks may lead to excessive weight gain, they may replace nutritionally essential foods, or they may destroy the appetite for meals. Teen-agers especially need to learn to control the quality and the amounts of snack foods they consume.

5. Breakfast is often skipped. Lack of time, uninteresting foods, and poor appetite are usually given as reasons. It is hard to make up in the rest of the day for the nutrients that a good breakfast can provide.

6. Lunch is likely to be skimpy, or may consist of high-calorie foods low in nutrients.

7. Too many meals are eaten in a hurry with little enjoyment of them.

Nutritional improvement means public concern for the poor. It means much greater emphasis on nutrition education for people of all ages. Elementary and secondary schools must strengthen their classroom programs in nutrition; school feeding programs need to be expanded; and all segments of the population must be reached through wider use of mass media such as television, radio, and newspapers and magazines. (See Fig. 2–3.)

### FOOD FADDISM AND QUACKERY

People today are more concerned about health, food, and nutrition than at any previous time. They read more about food and nutrition in

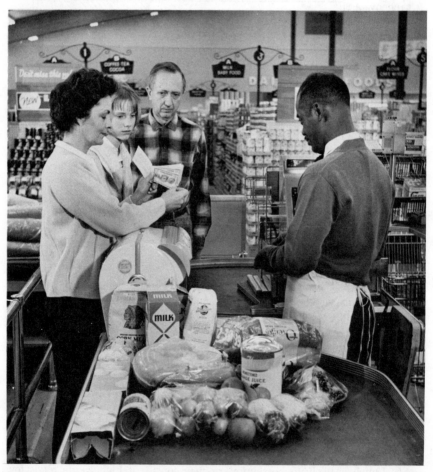

FIGURE 2–3 With the high cost of food, families who have a limited income must choose carefully to meet nutritional needs. The food stamp program enables people with low incomes to purchase more food in greater variety. (*USDA photo.*)

magazines and books and hear much on radio and television. Young people especially have been concerned about the environment and their food supply. Some groups restrict their selection to foods that are "natural" or "organically grown." Some have become strict vegetarians, and others will eat no flesh of animals, although they do eat eggs and drink milk and eat milk products. Other people, especially the elderly, often look to foods as a way to health, but they are often misled into believing that a particular food possesses some miracle properties and that it can cure such specific diseases as diabetes, cancer, arthritis, and many others.

People who accept the claims made for "health foods" or for the nutritional superiority of "organically grown foods" have not been educated in the science of nutrition. They readily accept the false claims of someone who is an enthusiast for a particular product or for a way of life without inquiring about the professional qualifications of the one who makes the claims. The rights of individuals must, of course, be respected; each person has a right to choose his own diet, and to spend his money for food as he wishes. It is tragic, however, when someone is misled into thinking that his health problems can be solved by eating some "wonder" food. When a person substitutes such self-therapy for the advice of a physician, he may be delaying effective treatment until it is too late.

## IDENTIFYING THE FOOD QUACK

It is not always easy to determine who is a food quack. Often he is handsome, a good speaker, very clever, and sounds convincing. But you should become suspicious if he talks about specific foods or supplements as "wonder foods," "miracle foods," "health foods," "nature's own foods," "food cures," or a "secret formula." The faddist and quack claim special virtues for foods such as yogurt, blackstrap molasses, raw sugar, honey, sea salt, stone-ground flour, vegetable juices, wheat germ oil, and foods grown without chemical fertilizers.

No single food possesses unique qualities for health. Rather, good nutrition is served by any combination of foods that will provide the necessary nutrients. The Food and Drug Administration considers a food to be misbranded if it is called a "health" food. (See also Chap. 17.)

The food quack appeals to the emotions and makes extravagant claims for his product: youth, beauty, glamour, long life, cure of disease. He is out to sell something, whether it be a book, an appliance, or a food product. Many of his products are sold from door to door, often with "money back" guarantees to cure some disease in a matter of weeks or months. The product is usually more expensive than similar products sold in food markets.

The food quack may tell you that the food in grocery stores is robbed of its nutritional values because it has been grown on depleted soil or because processes such as canning or dehydration have removed most of the nutrients. He accuses the medical profession of not giving the full facts to the public, and he claims that he is being persecuted by scientists and the government. He quotes frequently from the scientific literature and sounds very learned. A careful search of his sources will often show that he has lifted sentences out of books and journals and is placing his own interpretation upon them.

### RELIABLE SOURCES OF INFORMATION

The best defense against food misinformation and faddism is through sound nutrition education at all levels—in the elementary and high school, in industry, through health agencies in the community. A number of individuals who work in a community may be especially helpful in providing sound information:

Nutritionists from city, county, and state offices of health
Dietitians who are members of the American Dietetic Association
Nutritionists in county and state extension offices
Professors of nutrition in colleges and universities
Physicians

Much sound nutrition information is published by professional organizations, government agencies, and industry groups. A partial list of groups that distribute inexpensive or free materials will be found in Appendix B.

## Nutrition, a World Concern

### INTERNATIONAL NUTRITION PROBLEMS

The central problem in nutrition today is that millions of people in underdeveloped countries of the world do not have enough to eat. Yet, each day approximately 200,000 persons are added to the world's population, and they, too, must somehow be fed. Asia contains one third of the earth's land surface, but it must feed two thirds of the world's people. Thus, supplying more food to keep up with the increase in population as well as trying to improve the state of nutrition is truly a staggering problem.

Infants and young children suffer most from the lack of food. The death rate among infants in many countries is appallingly high. Of infants who survive the first year, many will die before the age of five. The infants and children fail to grow, they are quite susceptible to infection, and many of them die of protein malnutrition known as *kwashiorkor.* Even though these severely malnourished children live, their mental development may have been permanently retarded.

Other deficiency diseases are still quite prevalent in many parts of the world. Anemias caused by lack of iron and of the B-complex vitamins are frequent. Goiter is widespread in areas where there is a lack of iodine. Beriberi occurs because of lack of thiamine; pellagra from lack of niacin; xerophthalmia and blindness from lack of vitamin A; and rickets from lack of vitamin D. As you study nutrition, the characteristics of some of these diseases will become more familiar.

### INTERNATIONAL ORGANIZATIONS

Various agencies of our government and numerous charitable organizations are pledged to providing aid in many ways: direct food supplies; technical assistance in the development of agriculture and industry; education of youth; education of homemakers in food preparation, child care, and sanitation; and many other ways. Several organizations of the United Nations illustrate the humanitarian efforts of that great international body. (See Fig. 2–4.)

The *Food and Agriculture Organization* (FAO) aims especially to improve the growth, distribution, and storage of food. To carry out its aims it might be involved in such widely different activities as irrigation for crops; development of varieties of grain that will grow in a given climate; sponsoring home economics programs to show people how to prepare their foods and to better feed their families; and setting up a food processing plant.

The *World Health Organization* (WHO) aims to eliminate diseases of all kinds, including those that relate to nutrition. It works closely with FAO. Diseases such as malaria and others keep millions from working. When people are treated for these diseases they are able to work and produce food for themselves and their families. WHO works closely with communities to improve the sanitation through insect control, water supplies, housing, and waste disposal.

The *United Nations Children's Fund* (UNICEF) is concerned with all aspects of the health and welfare of children everywhere. We are probably most familiar with the work of this group through the distribution of nonfat dry milk to prevent and treat the protein deficiency disease kwashiorkor.

The *United Nations Education, Scientific, and Cultural Organization* (UNESCO) aims to eliminate illiteracy and thus to help people through education to use science and to understand cultural forces for the improvement of their lives.

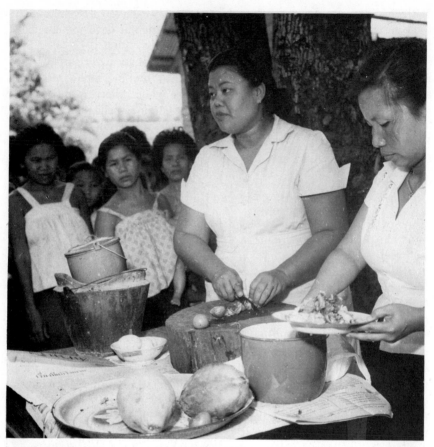

**FIGURE 2–4** A nurse in Thailand gives a cooking demonstration using local foods. (*Courtesy, UNICEF.*)

## REVIEW QUESTIONS AND PROBLEMS

**1.** Prepare a list of false ideas about foods that you have heard. What is your basis for saying that each is false?

**2.** What are some ways by which you can identify a quack?

**3.** What nutritional problems do you know of in your community?

**4.** List some food habits of people you know that could be improved. What are some ways you would use to try to help them?

**5.** Find five examples of materials prepared by food manufacturers that are useful in obtaining a better diet.

**6.** What organizations in your community include nutrition as part of their work?

**7.** Prepare a report for your class on a state, national, or international organization that has the major goal of promoting good nutrition.

**REFERENCES**

Bengoa, J. M.: "Nutrition Activities of the World Health Organization," *J. Am. Diet. Assoc.*, **55**:228–32, 1969.

Goldsmith, G. A.: "More Food for More People," *Am. J. Public Health*, **59**:694–704, 1969.

Livingston, S. K.: "What Influences Malnutrition?" *J. Nutr. Educ.*, **3**:18–27, Summer 1971.

"Highlights from the Ten-State Nutrition Survey," *Nutr. Today*, **7**:4–11, July 1972.

Kamil, A.: "How Natural Are Those 'Natural' Vitamins?" *J. Nutr. Educ.*, **4**:92, Summer 1972.

Sherlock, P., and Rothschild, E. O.: "Scurvy Produced by a Zen Macrobiotic Diet," *JAMA*, **199**:794–98, 1967.

Stare, F. J., *et al.*: " 'Health' Foods: Definitions and Nutrient Values," *J. Nutr. Educ.*, **4**:94–97, Summer 1972.

Williams, C. D.: "Grassroots Nutrition—or Consumer Participation," *J. Am. Diet. Assoc.*, **63**:125–29, 1973.

# THE NUTRIENTS AND THEIR UTILIZATION

## NUTRIENTS AND BODY COMPOSITION

Whatever you eat turns into you. It is quite reasonable to suppose that there is a relationship between the substances present in the body and the kinds of nutrients present in food. Also it is quite reasonable to suppose that the body can be properly built and maintained only if the correct materials are available.

The cell is the unit of body structure. Cells in different body tissues carry out specific kinds of functions; thus liver, bone, muscle, and blood cells differ from each other. Likewise, the kinds and amounts of nutrients that make up cells vary from one type of cell to another. At least 50 nutrients are required by the cells of the body.

Four chemical elements account for 96 per cent of the body weight. They are carbon, hydrogen, oxygen, and nitrogen. Water is by far the most abundant compound in the body; it accounts for about two thirds of the body weight. Protein represents roughly one fifth of the body weight, and fat constitutes one fifth, more or less, of the body weight. The proportions of these major body constituents will vary widely from individual to individual. Obviously, a lean person will have a much lower proportion of fat than an overweight person. A baby has a higher proportion of body water than an adult.

Carbohydrate, so important in the diet for its energy value, actually is present only in limited amounts in body tissues. Somewhat less than 500 gm occurs in the adult body in the forms of liver and muscle glycogen and the blood sugar.

Mineral matter accounts for about 4 per cent of the body weight, but a wide variety of mineral elements is needed for the structure of the tissues. The total store of vitamins in the body would add up to only a few grams.

## FUNCTIONS OF FOOD

Some nutrients function in three categories, whereas others are restricted to one or two classes of functions.

*Nutrients that furnish energy:* carbohydrates, fats, proteins
*Nutrients that build and maintain body tissues:* water, proteins, fats, carbohydrates, mineral elements
*Nutrients that regulate body functions:* water, mineral elements, vitamins, proteins, fats, carbohydrates

## DIGESTION

Digestion includes the mechanical and chemical processes by which foods are broken down to their nutrients so that they may be absorbed into the circulation. Mechanical and chemical changes take place simultaneously on the carbohydrates, fats, and proteins in foods. (See Fig. 3–1.)

The mechanical processes include the chewing of food, the churning actions in the stomach, and the muscular contractions of the intestinal tract. The rhythmic contractions, known as *peristalsis,* break up food into smaller and smaller particles, mix them intimately with the digestive juices, and continually move the food mass along the intestinal tract.

The chemical reactions in digestion involve the addition of water to the protein, fat, and carbohydrate molecules and their splitting up into nutrients that the tissues can use. This process is known as *hydrolysis.* The final end products of digestion are:

Carbohydrates to the simple sugars—glucose, fructose, galactose
Fats to fatty acids and glycerol
Proteins to amino acids

*Enzymes.* The chemical reactions require helpers called *enzymes.* Sometimes enzymes are called living catalysts. A catalyst is any substance that hastens a chemical reaction but does not itself become a part of the compounds that are formed.

Enzymes are composed of specific proteins. They are named for the substance upon which they act; for example, *protease* is an enzyme that digests protein, and *oxidase* is involved in the addition of oxygen. Each enzyme is highly individual in its action. An enzyme that digests fat will

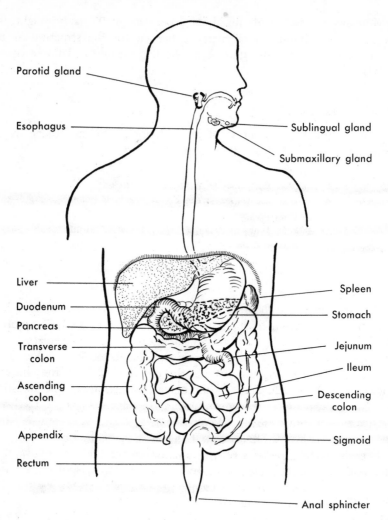

**FIGURE 3–1** The digestive tract. (*Adapted from Youmans, W.B., Human Physiology, 2nd ed. New York: Macmillan Publishing Co., Inc., 1962.*)

not digest starch. Some enzymes act only in an acid medium, such as pepsin in the stomach, whereas others act only in an alkaline medium, such as trypsin in the small intestine. See Table 3–1 for a summary of enzyme activity.

**Digestion in the mouth.** The digestion of food begins in the mouth with the chewing of food and its mixing with saliva. Chewing is important because it increases the surface area of the food particles for later digestive action. Saliva contains *amylase*, a starch-splitting enzyme, but food remains in the mouth for such a short time that only a small amount of starch can be broken down to dextrins and maltose.

TABLE 3–1  SUMMARY OF CHEMICAL REACTIONS IN DIGESTION

| Site of Activity | Enzyme | Substrate | Products of Enzyme Activity |
|---|---|---|---|
| Mouth | Salivary amylase (ptyalin) | Cooked starch | Dextrins, maltose |
| Stomach | Protease (pepsin) | Proteins | Proteoses, peptones, polypeptides |
| | Rennin | Milk casein | Calcium caseinate |
| | Lipase | Emulsified fats | Fatty acids, glycerol |
| Small intestine | Pancreatic juice | | |
| | Protease (trypsin) | Proteins | Proteoses, peptones, polypeptides, some amino acids |
| | Lipase (steapsin) | Fats | Di- and monoglycerides, fatty acids, glycerol |
| | Amylase (amylopsin) | Starch | Maltose |
| | Intestinal juice | | |
| | Peptidases (erepsin) | Peptones, poly-peptides | Amino acids |
| | Sucrase | Sucrose | Glucose, fructose |
| | Maltase | Maltose | Glucose (2 molecules) |
| | Lactase | Lactose | Glucose, galactose |

**Digestion in the stomach.** The stomach serves as a temporary store-house for food, brings about partial digestion of protein, and prepares food for further digestion in the small intestine. The food is con-tinually churned and mixed with gastric juice until it reaches a liquid consistency know as *chyme*. Rhythmic contractions move the chyme toward the pylorus where small portions are gradually released through the pyloric sphincter into the duodenum.

Gastric juice contains hydrochloric acid, pepsin, rennin, mucin, and other substances. Hydrochloric acid has several important functions: (1) it swells the proteins so as to make them more easily attacked by the enzymes; (2) it provides the acid medium necessary for the action of pepsin; (3) it increases the solubility of calcium and iron salts so that they are more readily absorbed; and (4) it reduces the activity of harmful bacteria that may have been present in the food.

Pepsin, a protease, splits proteins into smaller molecules called pro-teoses and polypeptides. Very little digestion of carbohydrates and fats occurs in the stomach. In the upper (cardiac) portion of the stomach the salivary amylase continues to act upon starch to change it to dextrins and maltose. As soon as the food mass is mixed with hydrochloric acid this action ceases. Lipase in the stomach has some effect on emulsified fats as in milk, cream, butter, and egg yolk, but most of the hydrolysis of fats takes place in the small intestine.

*Digestion in the small intestine.* Most of the digestive activity takes place in the small intestine, which includes the duodenum, the jejunum, and the ileum. Bile, manufactured by the liver and stored in the gall-bladder, is essential for fat digestion. As soon as fats enter the duodenum the secretion of a hormone, *cholecystokinin,* is stimulated. Cholecystokinin causes the gallbladder to contract and to release bile into the duodenum. Bile emulsifies the fats, that is, breaks them down into tiny globules so that the fat-splitting enzymes have greater contact with the fat molecules. Bile, being highly alkaline, neutralizes the acid chyme and provides the alkaline reaction necessary for the action of the intestinal enzymes.

As soon as acid chyme enters the duodenum another hormone, *secretin,* is produced. This is carried by the bloodstream to the pancreas where it stimulates the secretion of pancreatic juice. The pancreas also pours its secretion into the duodenum. Pancreatic amylase splits starch to maltose; a protease, *trypsin,* breaks down proteins and polypeptides to much smaller molecules; and lipase, *steapsin,* completes the digestion of fats to fatty acids and glycerol.

Intestinal juice produced by the walls of the intestines contains protein- and sugar-splitting enzymes. Lactase splits lactose to the simple sugars glucose and galactose; maltase acts on the maltose molecule to yield glucose; and sucrase brings about the hydrolysis of sucrose to glucose and fructose. A group of enzymes known as *peptidases* completes the break-down of proteins and polypeptides to amino acids.

*Function of the large intestine.* The large intestine includes the cecum, colon, rectum, and anal canal. Digestion and the absorption of nutrients have been essentially completed by the time the food mass reaches the large intestine, but much water and digestive juices are re-absorbed so that the intestinal contents gradually take on a solid consistency. The feces contain the fibers of food, small amounts of undigested food, mucus, bacteria, and broken-down cellular wastes.

## DIGESTIBILITY OF FOOD

By digestibility is meant the completeness of digestion and also the ease or speed of digestion. The efficiency of digestion is remarkably high. Based upon the typical American diet, 98 per cent of the carbohydrate, 95 per cent of the fat, and 92 per cent of the protein in the food eaten is digested and absorbed.

Fibers and seeds are not digested. Therefore, a diet made up of many fruits, vegetables, and whole-grain products could have a digestibility of carbohydrate of only 85 per cent. The completeness of digestion is greatly reduced in some disorders of the gastorintestinal tract such as severe diarrhea. In some hereditary diseases such as celiac disease, cystic fibrosis of the pancreas, and lactose intolerance, the enzymes for the digestion of fats and carbohydrates may be missing, so that much fat or starch is eliminated in the feces.

The speed of digestion varies widely according to the size of the meal and the composition of the diet and also depends upon certain psychologic factors. As little as 9 hours or as much as 48 hours may elapse from the time food is eaten until the wastes are eliminated. Small meals will remain in the stomach for a far shorter time than will large meals. Foods that are poorly chewed are likely to require a longer time for digestion.

Foods are sometimes said to "stick to the ribs." In other words, they stay in the stomach longer, so that they delay hunger contractions and are therefore more satisfying. They are said to have high *satiety* value. A breakfast of juice and dry toast, being chiefly carbohydrate, has little satiety value. But a breakfast of juice, toast, eggs, and bacon also contains proteins and fats. Because the digestion takes somewhat longer in the stomach, this meal would be more satisfying. An excessive amount of fat, especially in the form of fried foods, slows up digestion so much that discomfort sometimes results.

Extractives in meat increase the flow of digestive juices. A cup of broth or bouillon is sometimes used at the beginning of a meal to stimulate the appetite and to increase the digestive action. The secretion of digestive juices is also increased by the pleasant sight, smell, and taste of food. On the other hand, the secretion is likely to be decreased when foods are unattractively served or when the surroundings are unpleasant. An individual who is excessively tired or who is under emotional stress such as fear, grief, or anger often experiences digestive upsets or may be unable to take food.

## ABSORPTION

Absorption is the process whereby the nutrients released from food by digestion are transferred from the intestinal lumen into the blood and lymph circulation. The intestinal wall is lined with 4 to 5 million tiny fingerlike projections called *villi*. (See Fig. 3–2.) Each villus is a complex organ with a surface layer of epithelium over a layer of connective tissue (lamina propria) that is supplied with capillaries and lacteals. The nutrients are carried across the epithelium by several complex processes, one of which acts like a pump. From the lamina propria the fatty acids, some molecules of fat, and fat-soluble vitamins enter the lacteals and enter into the lymph circulation. Glucose, amino acids, mineral salts, and water-soluble vitamins enter into the blood capillaries and are carried by the portal circulation to the liver.

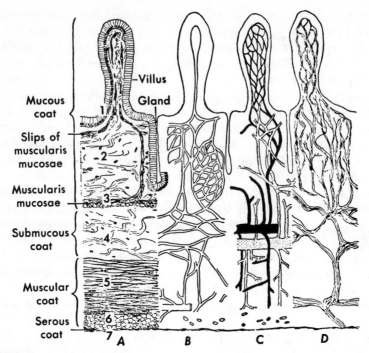

Mucous coat
Villus
Gland
Slips of muscularis mucosae
Muscularis mucosae
Submucous coat
Muscular coat
Serous coat

A  B  C  D

FIGURE 3–2  Diagram of a cross section of small intestine. A shows coats of intestinal wall and tissues of coats: (1) columnar epithelium, (2) areolar connective tissue, (3) muscularis mucosae, (4) areolar connective tissue, (5) circular layer of smooth muscle, (6) longitudinal layer of smooth muscle, (7) areolar connective tissue and endothelium. B shows arrangement of central lacteal, lymph nodes, and lymph tubes. C shows blood supply; arteries and capillaries *black*, veins *stippled*. D shows nerve fibers, the submucous plexus lying in the submucosa, the myenteric plexus lying between the circular and longitudinal layers of the muscular coat. (*From Miller, M. A., and Leavell, L. C.,* Kimber-Gray-Stackpole's Anatomy and Physiology, 16th ed. New York: Macmillan Publishing Co., Inc., 1972.)

## METABOLISM

*Metabolism* is an inclusive term that describes all the changes that take place in the body. *Anabolism* is a more specific term that is used to indicate the building up of complex substances from simpler substances. Building new bone, or hemoglobin, or muscle tissue would be examples of anabolism. *Catabolism*, by contrast, refers to the breaking down of complex substances into simpler substances. The breakdown of glucose or fatty acids to yield energy is an example of catabolism.

The term "dynamic equilibrium" is sometimes used to indicate that the processes of anabolism and of catabolism are continuously taking place and that the one is equal to the other. In growing children, during pregnancy, and during recovery from illness the processes of anabolism are greater than those of catabolism. On the other hand, excessive catabolism takes place with high fever, during acute illness, following surgery, fractures, and burns, or when certain hormones are produced in excessive amounts by the body.

The innumerable reactions in metabolism require the activity of enzymes. Many of these enzymes require another substance called a *coenzyme* in addition to the protein. One of the important functions of vitamins and certain mineral elements is to act as coenzymes.

*Hormones* are substances produced by glands of the body. They maintain a system of checks and balances on metabolism. To name just a few: thyroxine, produced by the thyroid gland, regulates energy metabolism; insulin, produced in the pancreas, controls the level of the blood sugar; an adrenal hormone controls the amount of sodium retained or excreted.

In addition to (1) ingestion, (2) digestion, and (3) absorption, metabolism includes these categories.

4. Transportation of the nutrients to the cells where they are needed and of the wastes to the organs of excretion is the function of the blood circulation.

5. Respiration. In the lungs oxygen is taken into the blood so that the nutrients may be combined with oxygen (oxidized). Through the lungs carbon dioxide is given off as a waste.

6. Utilization. Within every cell are found hundreds of enzymes that bring about the appropriate functions in terms of energy, building or maintenance, and regulation. In a complex series of steps glucose combines with oxygen to release the energy for the body's work. Fats, likewise, are oxidized for energy. Carbohydrates and fats are also stored as potential energy in the form of adipose tissue. Amino acids are used to build new cells, to form hormones, or enzymes, or as a source of energy. Mineral elements enter into the structure of the cell or into any one of many regulatory activities. An important aspect of the study in the chapters to follow will be concerned with more detail of the functions of the nutrients.

7. Excretion of wastes is accomplished by the kidney, which removes nitrogenous wastes, water, mineral salts, and excess water-soluble vitamins; by the bowel, which eliminates indigestible fiber, bile pigments, cholesterol and other products of metabolism, and bacterial wastes; by the skin, through which water, mineral salts, and some nitrogenous wastes are removed; and by the lungs, which remove carbon dioxide and water.

## REVIEW QUESTIONS AND PROBLEMS

1. Name the three functions of food in the body. What functions are performed by fats, by carbohydrates, by mineral elements, by proteins, by vitamins?

**2.** Define metabolism, anabolism, catabolism, enzyme, hormone.

**3.** Name three enzymes in the digestion of foods, and tell what they do.

**4.** What percentage of food eaten is digested under normal circumstances?

**5.** What products result from the complete digestion of proteins, fats, carbohydrates?

**6.** List five factors that may determine the speed with which a meal is digested.

**7.** What relation exists between the oxygen you breathe in and the food you eat?

**8.** How could you explain the fact that your output of urine may be less on a very warm day when you are exercising vigorously?

**9.** What kinds of waste products are excreted in the urine? Refer to a table of constituents in the urine.

## REFERENCES

Rasmussen, S.: *Foundations of Practical and Vocational Nursing.* New York: Macmillan Publishing Co., Inc., 1967, Chap. 34.

Robinson, C. H.: *Normal and Therapeutic Nutrition,* 14th ed. New York: Macmillan Publishing Co., Inc., 1972, Chap. 2.

**4**

STANDARDS OF BODY WEIGHT | USING METRIC MEASURES |
RECOMMENDED DAILY DIETARY ALLOWANCES | TABLES OF FOOD
COMPOSITION | FOUR FOOD GROUPS | A BASIC DIET

# GUIDES FOR NUTRITIONAL PLANNING

Do you weigh what you should? Are you getting enough protein? Is a small glass of tomato juice a good substitute for a small glass of orange juice? How much milk should you drink each day?

Almost everything we do is according to some design. We use recipes for cooking, patterns for sewing, and rules for behavior. Likewise, we have certain guides to answer questions such as the above and to help us in the maintenance of good nutrition and health. Let us examine more closely some of the guides that can be especially useful.

## STANDARDS OF BODY WEIGHT

Probably no aspect of one's health is more often discussed than one's weight. Some people are trying to take off weight, others are trying to put on weight, and still others are fortunate in weighing just what they should. How do you measure up according to the standards of height and weight?

During the teen years boys and girls reach their full height, but in the early twenties they continue to mature somewhat in their body frame and muscle development. The adult is at the peak of his physical development between 20 and 30 years of age. Many people, however, continue to gain somewhat throughout life, so that the average weights for men and women at 35, 45, and 55 years are steadily increased.

Medical and insurance authorities have shown that it is not desirable for men and women to continue to gain throughout their lives. Height

29

and weight tables are, therefore, set up on the basis of weight at age 25 to 30 years. (See Table A–3, p. 333.) One should aim to keep the desirable weight for one's height and body frame at age 25 years for the rest of one's life.

In using this table, some differences are allowed for body frame. Some people with small bones—small wrists, narrow shoulders, and narrow hips—would be classified as "low." Other people of a generally stocky build—large wrists, broad shoulders, wide hips—would have a desirable weight range between "medium" and "high." You should note that the heights indicated in this table are without shoes and that the weights are without clothing.

At best, height-weight tables are only an approximate guide to body fatness. Many athletes could be considered overweight by these standards, but the excess weight results from well-developed muscles, and not fat. On the other hand, some inactive people appear to be of normal weight but have little muscular development and much body fat. Many physicians use the thickness of fat layers under the skin as an estimate of fatness. They use the skin-fold pinch test, or obtain a more precise measurement by using a caliper.

If your weight is less than 10 per cent over or under the desirable weight for your body frame, your weight is about what it should be. If you are between 10 and 20 per cent overweight, you should correct the situation before it gets more severe. If you weigh more than 20 per cent over or under your desirable weight, it would be a good idea to consult your physician about bringing your weight more nearly in line.

## USING METRIC MEASURES

Scientists and health workers have long used metric measures: micrograms, milligrams, grams, kilograms; milliliters, liters; millimeters, centimeters, meters; degrees Centigrade. The United States is the only large country in the world that has not been using the metric system for all of its weights and measures. It appears inevitable that the system will be officially adopted within the next few years. Children are becoming familiar with these measures in school, but older persons will find the transition a little more difficult.

To use the metric system you will need to learn what relationships exist between it and our present system. For example, if you now weigh 120 pounds, what is your weight in kilograms? If you buy 5 pounds of potatoes, how many kilograms would you buy? Some conversion factors are shown in Table A–4. In this text weights and measures are expressed in metric terms, with the present system of measures placed in parenthesis. The following relationships are important to remember:

1 kilogram (kg) = 1000 grams
1 gram (gm) = 1000 milligrams
1 milligram (mg) = 1000 micrograms (mcg or μg)
1 liter = 1000 milliliters (ml); this is used for fluid measures

## RECOMMENDED DAILY DIETARY ALLOWANCES

The Food and Nutrition Board of the National Research Council is the recognized authority for setting standards of nutrition in the United States. This board has set up a table of Recommended Daily Dietary Allowances, which is revised from time to time as new research becomes available. (See Table 4–1.)

If you examine this table carefully, you will find recommendations listed for infants, preschool and school children, older boys and girls, men and women of varying ages, and for pregnancy and lactation. Thus the table is intended to be used as a guide for the entire healthy population.

For each age an individual of given size has been used as a standard. For example, the "reference woman" is 162 cm (65 in.) tall and weighs 58 kg (128 lb) and is assumed to be normally active and to live in a temperate climate. Using this guide, one can estimate what allowances might be suitable for a woman who is larger or smaller, who is younger or older, who lives in a warmer or colder climate, or who is more or less active.

For each age category specific allowances are listed for kilocalories, protein, six minerals, and ten vitamins. The body requires other nutrients that are not listed, but the average well-planned diet will furnish sufficient amounts of these.

The correct interpretation of this table is important. Each person differs from all other individuals in his exact nutritional requirements. There is no practical way to determine which persons use nutrients more or less efficiently than the average. To ensure that these differences are taken into account, the recommended allowances provide a "margin of safety."

An individual who fails to get the full allowances in his diet is not necessarily poorly nourished, since he may be one of those persons whose needs are lower. Nutritional status can be determined only by a thorough physical examination, laboratory tests, and a dietary history. Your goal in dietary planning for yourself and others should be toward obtaining the full allowances each day. If you were catching a plane at a particular time, you would surely allow a little extra time to get to the airport in the event of a traffic tie-up. Why not allow yourself the margin of safety in your nutrition by meeting fully the recommended allowances each day?

## TABLE 4-1 FOOD AND NUTRITION BOARD, NATIONAL ACADEMY OF SCIENCES-NATIONAL RESEARCH COUNCIL
### Recommended Daily Dietary Allowances,[1] Revised 1974
Designed for the maintenance of good nutrition of practically all healthy people in the U.S.A.

| | Age (years) From Up to | Weight (kg) | Weight (lb) | Height (cm) | Height (in) | Energy (kcal)[2] | Protein (gm) | Fat-Soluble Vitamins — Vitamin A Activity (RE)[3] | (IU) | Vitamin D (IU) | Vitamin E Activity[5] (IU) | Water-Soluble Vitamins — Ascorbic Acid (mg) | Folacin[6] (μg) | Niacin[7] (mg) | Riboflavin (mg) | Thiamin (mg) | Vitamin B6 (mg) | Vitamin B12 (μg) | Minerals — Calcium (mg) | Phosphorus (mg) | Iodine (μg) | Iron (mg) | Magnesium (mg) | Zinc (mg) |
|---|---|---|---|---|---|---|---|---|---|---|---|---|---|---|---|---|---|---|---|---|---|---|---|---|
| Infants | 0.0–0.5 | 6 | 14 | 60 | 24 | kg × 117 | kg × 2.2 | 420[4] | 1,400 | 400 | 4 | 35 | 50 | 5 | 0.4 | 0.3 | 0.3 | 0.3 | 360 | 240 | 35 | 10 | 60 | 3 |
| | 0.5–1.0 | 9 | 20 | 71 | 28 | kg × 108 | kg × 2.0 | 400 | 2,000 | 400 | 5 | 35 | 50 | 8 | 0.6 | 0.5 | 0.4 | 0.3 | 540 | 400 | 45 | 15 | 70 | 5 |
| Children | 1–3 | 13 | 28 | 86 | 34 | 1300 | 23 | 400 | 2,000 | 400 | 7 | 40 | 100 | 9 | 0.8 | 0.7 | 0.6 | 1.0 | 800 | 800 | 60 | 15 | 150 | 10 |
| | 4–6 | 20 | 44 | 110 | 44 | 1800 | 30 | 500 | 2,500 | 400 | 9 | 40 | 200 | 12 | 1.1 | 0.9 | 0.9 | 1.5 | 800 | 800 | 80 | 10 | 200 | 10 |
| | 7–10 | 30 | 66 | 135 | 54 | 2400 | 36 | 700 | 3,300 | 400 | 10 | 40 | 300 | 16 | 1.2 | 1.2 | 1.2 | 2.0 | 800 | 800 | 110 | 10 | 250 | 10 |
| Males | 11–14 | 44 | 97 | 158 | 63 | 2800 | 44 | 1,000 | 5,000 | 400 | 12 | 45 | 400 | 18 | 1.5 | 1.4 | 1.6 | 3.0 | 1200 | 1200 | 130 | 18 | 350 | 15 |
| | 15–18 | 61 | 134 | 172 | 69 | 3000 | 54 | 1,000 | 5,000 | 400 | 15 | 45 | 400 | 20 | 1.8 | 1.5 | 1.8 | 3.0 | 1200 | 1200 | 150 | 18 | 400 | 15 |
| | 19–22 | 67 | 147 | 172 | 69 | 3000 | 54 | 1,000 | 5,000 | 400 | 15 | 45 | 400 | 20 | 1.8 | 1.5 | 2.0 | 3.0 | 800 | 800 | 140 | 10 | 350 | 15 |
| | 23–50 | 70 | 154 | 172 | 69 | 2700 | 56 | 1,000 | 5,000 | | 15 | 45 | 400 | 18 | 1.6 | 1.4 | 2.0 | 3.0 | 800 | 800 | 130 | 10 | 350 | 15 |
| | 51+ | 70 | 154 | 172 | 69 | 2400 | 56 | 1,000 | 5,000 | | 15 | 45 | 400 | 16 | 1.5 | 1.2 | 2.0 | 3.0 | 800 | 800 | 110 | 10 | 350 | 15 |
| Females | 11–14 | 44 | 97 | 155 | 62 | 2400 | 44 | 800 | 4,000 | 400 | 12 | 45 | 400 | 16 | 1.3 | 1.2 | 1.6 | 3.0 | 1200 | 1200 | 115 | 18 | 300 | 15 |
| | 15–18 | 54 | 119 | 162 | 65 | 2100 | 48 | 800 | 4,000 | 400 | 12 | 45 | 400 | 14 | 1.4 | 1.1 | 2.0 | 3.0 | 1200 | 1200 | 115 | 18 | 300 | 15 |
| | 19–22 | 58 | 128 | 162 | 65 | 2100 | 46 | 800 | 4,000 | 400 | 12 | 45 | 400 | 14 | 1.4 | 1.1 | 2.0 | 3.0 | 800 | 800 | 100 | 18 | 300 | 15 |
| | 23–50 | 58 | 128 | 162 | 65 | 2000 | 46 | 800 | 4,000 | | 12 | 45 | 400 | 13 | 1.2 | 1.0 | 2.0 | 3.0 | 800 | 800 | 100 | 18 | 300 | 15 |
| | 51+ | 58 | 128 | 162 | 65 | 1800 | 46 | 800 | 4,000 | | 12 | 45 | 400 | 12 | 1.1 | 1.0 | 2.0 | 3.0 | 800 | 800 | 80 | 10 | 300 | 15 |
| Pregnant | | | | | | +300 | +30 | 1,000 | 5,000 | 400 | 15 | 60 | 800 | +2 | +0.3 | +0.3 | 2.5 | 4.0 | 1200 | 1200 | 125 | 18+[8] | 450 | 20 |
| Lactating | | | | | | +500 | +20 | 1,200 | 6,000 | 400 | 15 | 80 | 600 | +4 | +0.5 | +0.3 | 2.5 | 4.0 | 1200 | 1200 | 150 | 18 | 450 | 25 |

[1] The allowances are intended to provide for individual variations among most normal persons as they live in the United States under usual environmental stresses. Diets should be based on a variety of common foods in order to provide other nutrients for which human requirements have been less well defined. See text for more-detailed discussion of allowances and of nutrients not tabulated.

[2] Kilojoules (KJ) = 4.2 × kcal.

[3] Retinol equivalents.

[4] Assumed to be all as retinol in milk during the first six months of life. All subsequent intakes are assumed to be one-half as retinol and one-half as β-carotene when calculated from international units. As retinol equivalents, three-fourths are as retinol and one-fourth as β-carotene.

[5] Total vitamin E activity, estimated to be 80 percent as α-tocopherol and 20 percent other tocopherols. See text for variation in allowances.

[6] The folacin allowances refer to dietary sources as determined by Lactobacillus casei assay. Pure forms of folacin may be effective in doses less than one-fourth of the RDA.

[7] Although allowances are expressed as niacin, it is recognized that on the average 1 mg of niacin is derived from each 60 mg of dietary tryptophan.

[8] This increased requirement cannot be met by ordinary diets, therefore, the use of supplemental iron is recommended.

## TABLES OF FOOD COMPOSITION

In order to use the table of recommended allowances you need to know the nutritive values of the foods you eat. Table A–1, Appendix A, lists numerous foods and the values for many of the nutrients recommended in the table of allowances. The nutritive values are averages of many samples of food analyzed in laboratories. Many factors determine the nutritive values of the foods we eat: the conditions of growing; the handling from farm to market to consumer; the care given to food in the home; and the manner in which food is cooked. The study of the individual nutrients in the chapters that follow will point out some of the effects of food preparation.

Generally speaking, the values listed in Table A–1 are for household measures of food. Some measures are greater than the usual serving portions—for example, a cupful of vegetables. Note that the foods in this table are grouped by classes such as Milk, Cream, Cheese; Meat, Poultry, Fish; Vegetables; and so on. This arrangement makes it easy to compare the nutritive value of one food in a group with another food in that same group.

Suppose you were going to calculate the nutritive value of your own diet for one day. You would need to list each meal in terms of the kinds and amounts of every food, not forgetting the sugar, butter, jelly, coffee, cream, and other incidentals. You should also record the kinds and amounts of every food that you eat between meals. For example, your breakfast might have included juice, toast, cereal, milk, and coffee. In order to look up the nutritive value you would need to have an exact record such as the following:

| | |
|---|---|
| Grapefruit juice | 1 small glass (120 gm) |
| Cornflakes | 1 cup (28 gm) |
| Milk, whole | ½ cup (120 gm) |
| Sugar on cereal | 1 teaspoon (5 gm) |
| Raisin toast | 1½ slices (38 gm) |
| Butter | 2 pats (10 gm) |
| Cream for coffee | 2 tablespoons (30 gm) |

When your day's record is complete, it is a good idea to add up the daily total for all foods that are the same, such as milk, butter, sugar. You may wish to calculate the value of your diet for all nutrients listed in the table; or you might look up the values for only one nutrient at the time. As you study each of the chapters on the nutrients it is a good idea to calculate your own intake of that nutrient. In this way you begin to know the good and poor sources of the nutrients and you also learn how to improve your own diet.

When you have calculated the value of your diet, compare the totals with the recommended allowances for a person of your age. Does your diet add up to the allowances? There is no harm in being a little bit over, but if you are under the allowances, you should look for ways to improve your diet. For the correct calorie intake, your weight is your best guide: if you weigh too much, you are consuming too many calories; if you weigh too little, you are not eating enough to keep your weight at the desirable level.

### FOUR FOOD GROUPS

If you have calculated the nutritive value of a diet for one day, you would agree that this is somewhat time consuming. Fortunately, some short cuts have been developed. The Four Food Groups is one reliable and easily used guide. (See Fig. 4–1.) Each of the Four Food Groups contains a variety of foods that are important in obtaining an adequate diet each day. The milk group is excellent for calcium, riboflavin, and protein. The fruit-vegetable group is not especially outstanding for riboflavin and calcium, and gives very little protein; but this food group is excellent for iron and ascorbic acid, neither of which is provided in appreciable amounts by milk. By use of this simple guide, you can be reasonably certain of obtaining an adequate diet. As you progress in your study of nutrition, you will become thoroughly familiar with the nutritive contributions of foods in each group.

The food groups are:

*Milk group*
> 2 cups for adults
> 2 to 3 cups for children under 9 years
> 3 to 4 cups for children 9 to 12 years
> 3 to 4 cups for teenagers
> 3 cups or more for pregnant women
> 4 cups or more for lactating women

*Meat group*
> 2 or more servings. Count as one serving:
>> 2 to 3 ounces lean, cooked beef, veal, pork, lamb, poultry, fish—without bone
>> 2 eggs
>> 1 cup cooked dry beans, dry peas, lentils
>> 4 tablespoons peanut butter

*Vegetable-fruit group*
> 4 or more servings per day, including:
>> 1 serving of citrus fruit, or other fruit or vegetable as a good source of vitamin C, or 2 servings of a fair source

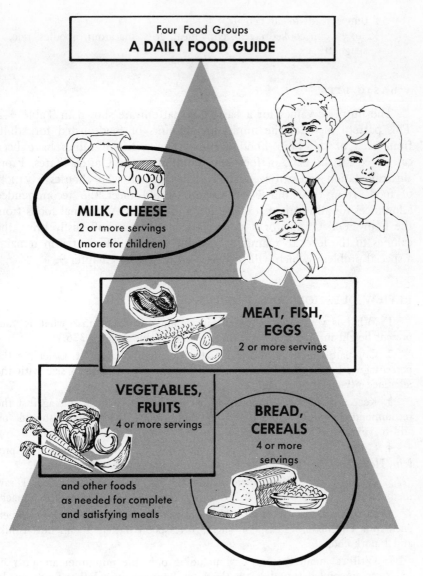

FIGURE 4-1 The Four Food Groups—a daily food guide.

1 serving, at least every other day, of a dark-green or deep-yellow vegetable for vitamin A

2 or more servings of other vegetables and fruits, including potatoes

*Bread-cereals group*

4 or more servings daily (whole grain, enriched, or restored). Count as one serving:

1 slice bread

1 ounce ready-to-eat cereal
½ to ¾ cup cooked cereal, corn meal, grits, macaroni, noodles, rice, or spaghetti

## A BASIC DIET

The nutritive values for a basic diet pattern are shown in Table 4–2. This pattern includes the minimum amounts of foods listed for adults from each of the Four Food Groups. The nutritive values have been calculated on the basis of food consumption in the United States. From this calculation you can see that a young woman who chooses a variety of foods from the Four Food Groups would meet the recommended allowances for all nutrients except iron and calories. Additional foods from the Four Food Groups or desserts, fats, and sweets will easily bring the calories to the level to maintain desirable weight. Sufficient iron remains a special problem, which will be discussed further in Chapter 9.

## REVIEW QUESTIONS AND PROBLEMS

1. What is your present weight in pounds? in kilograms? what is your present height in inches? in centimeters? (See Table A–5, p. 336.)

2. Compare your present weight wth your desirable weight. Calculate the percentage overweight or underweight. How do you compare in size with the reference person of your age?

3. Keep a record of the foods you eat for one day. Check this against the recommended amounts from the Four Food Groups. Which foods should you add to your diet? Why?

4. Using Table A–1 (p. 306), list six foods that are specially rich in protein. How much of these foods would you be likely to eat in one meal?

5. Compare the ascorbic acid values for ½ cup grapefruit juice, 1 raw medium peach, 1 raw plum, 1 baked sweet potato, and ½ cup cooked spinach.

6. List the calorie values for 1 slice enriched bread, 1 tomato, 1 oz. sweetened milk chocolate, 1 teaspoon sugar, 1 teaspoon butter, 1 cup buttermilk, and 1 pork chop.

7. Write a menu for one day including only the minimum amounts of foods recommended for adults in the Four Food Groups. What foods would you ordinarily add to this menu pattern?

8. From Table A–1 determine whether these statements are correct.
   a. A 4-oz. glass of apricot nectar is not a good substitute for 4 oz. of orange juice.
   b. Green peas and broccoli are about equal in value for vitamin A and ascorbic acid.

TABLE 4-2   NUTRITIVE VALUE OF A BASIC DIET PATTERN FOR THE ADULT IN HEALTH *

| Food | Measure | Weight gm | Energy kcal | Protein gm | Fat gm | Carbohydrate gm | Minerals | | Vitamins | | | | | |
|---|---|---|---|---|---|---|---|---|---|---|---|---|---|---|
| | | | | | | | Ca mg | Fe mg | A I.U. | Thiamine mg | Riboflavin mg | Niacin mg | Ascorbic Acid mg |
| Milk | 2 cups | 488 | 320 | 18 | 18 | 24 | 576 | 0.2 | 700 | 0.14 | 0.82 | 0.4 | 4 |
| *Meat Group* | | | | | | | | | | | | | |
| Egg | 1 | 50 | 80 | 6 | 6 | tr | 27 | 1.1 | 590 | 0.05 | 0.15 | tr | 0 |
| Meat, fish, poultry (lean cooked) † | 4 ounces | 120 | 240 | 33 | 10 | 0 | 17 | 3.6 | 35 | 0.32 | 0.26 | 7.4 | 0 |
| *Vegetable-Fruit Group* | | | | | | | | | | | | | |
| Leafy green or deep yellow | ¼ to ⅓ cup ‡ | 50 | 15 | 1 | tr | 3 | 14 | 0.5 | 3700 | 0.03 | 0.04 | 0.3 | 14 |
| Other vegetable | ¼ to ⅓ cup § | 50 | 15 | 1 | tr | 3 | 10 | 0.4 | 240 | 0.03 | 0.03 | 0.3 | 7 |
| Potato | 1 medium | 122 | 80 | 2 | tr | 18 | 7 | 0.6 | tr | 0.11 | 0.04 | 1.4 | 20 |
| Citrus fruit ‖ | 1 serving | 100 | 40 | 1 | tr | 10 | 10 | 0.2 | 160 | 0.07 | 0.02 | 0.3 | 40 |
| Other fruit # | 1 serving | 100 | 60 | 1 | tr | 16 | 12 | 0.5 | 600 | 0.04 | 0.04 | 0.4 | 9 |
| *Bread-Cereal Group* | | | | | | | | | | | | | |
| Cereal, enriched or whole grain ** | ¾ cup | 30 (dry) | 105 | 3 | tr | 22 | 10 | 0.8 | 0 | 0.12 | 0.04 | 0.8 | 0 |
| Bread, enriched or whole grain | 3 slices | 75 | 210 | 6 | 3 | 39 | 63 | 1.8 | tr | 0.18 | 0.15 | 1.8 | tr |
| | | | 1165 | 72 | 37 | 135 | 746 | 9.7 | 6025 | 1.09 | 1.59 | 13.1 †† | 94 |
| *Recommended Dietary Allowances* | | | | | | | | | | | | | |
| Woman (over 23 years) | | | 2000 | 46 | | | 800 | 18 | 4000 | 1.0 | 1.2 | 13 | 45 |
| Man (over 23 years) | | | 2700 | 56 | | | 800 | 10 | 5000 | 1.4 | 1.6 | 18 | 45 |

* Values for foods in the meat, vegetable-fruit, and bread-cereal groups are weighted on the basis of the approximate consumption in the United States.
† Calculations based upon an average weekly intake for meat of 11 ounces beef, 7½ ounces pork, 6½ ounces poultry, 1½ ounces lamb and veal, and 1½ ounces fish.
‡ Dark-green leafy and deep-yellow vegetables include carrots, green peppers, broccoli, spinach, endive, escarole, and kale. It is assumed that an average serving of ½ cup is eaten at least every other day.
§ Other vegetables include tomatoes, lettuce, cabbage, snap beans, Lima beans, celery, peas, onions, corn, cucumbers, beets, and cauliflower. It is assumed that an average serving of ½ cup is eaten at least every other day.
‖ Citrus fruit includes fresh, canned, and frozen oranges, orange juice, grapefruit, and grapefruit juice.
# Other fruit includes apples, peaches, pears, apricots, grapes, plums, prunes, berries, and bananas.
** Cereals include corn flakes, wheat flakes, macaroni, oatmeal, shredded wheat, and enriched rice.
†† The protein in this diet contains about 720 mg trytophan, equivalent to 12 mg niacin; thus, the niacin equivalent of this diet is 25 mg.

37

UNIT **II**

# THE NUTRIENTS

**5**

NATURE AND PROPERTIES | QUALITY OF FOOD PROTEINS | SOURCES |
FUNCTIONS | PROTEIN ALLOWANCES | PROTEIN DEFICIENCY |
SOME FALLACIES AND FACTS

# PROTEINS AND AMINO ACIDS

Proteins are essential components of all living things—plants, animals, and even microorganisms. In fact, every tissue and fluid in the body, except bile and urine, contains proteins.

Most American diets provide an abundance of proteins, but certain groups of people even in this country may not get enough each day. Throughout the world, the shortage of protein is second to the shortage of calories.

## NATURE AND PROPERTIES

Like carbohydrates and fats, proteins contain carbon, hydrogen, and oxygen. In addition, proteins contain about 16 per cent nitrogen. Sulfur, phosphorus, iron, and sometimes other elements such as iodine are found in small amounts. Proteins are built from 20 or so simpler building stones called *amino acids*. Just as the 26 letters of the alphabet can be combined in an amazing number of words, so the different amino acids can be joined to give an almost infinite variety of proteins. For example, the proteins found in bones, or teeth, or fingernails are quite different from those in hair, or muscle, or liver. The proteins in egg are different from those in milk, or wheat, or rice, and so on.

The amount of protein present in a food or in a tissue can be determined in the laboratory by an analysis for the nitrogen content. Each gram of nitrogen found in a food sample is equal to 6.25 gm protein.

Proteins coagulate when they are exposed to heat or to acid. Thus egg

41

white and meat coagulate when they are cooked; if too high heat is used, or if the food is cooked too long, the protein becomes dried out and tough. Perhaps at some time you have added a little vinegar to milk when you did not have the sour milk called for in a recipe. The milk thickens or curdles with the addition of the acid; in other words, the milk protein has been *coagulated*.

## QUALITY OF FOOD PROTEINS

The body can manufacture some of the amino acids required by the tissues, but it is unable to make others. Those amino acids that cannot be manufactured by the body must be present in the protein of the diet, and are called *essential amino acids*. It is a good idea to be able to recognize the names of these essential amino acids when you see them. They are:

| | |
|---|---|
| histidine (infants and children) | phenylalanine |
| isoleucine | threonine |
| leucine | tryptophan |
| lysine | valine |
| methionine | |

Not all food proteins are of the same quality. When a food contains the amino acids in the proportions and the amounts needed by the body for tissue replacement and growth, it is said to provide *complete* protein, or a protein of *high biologic value*. Eggs, milk, cheese, meat, fish, and poultry are examples of complete protein foods.

Some foods lack one or more of the essential amino acids in adequate amounts. Such foods would not meet the growth needs of the tissues, and so these food proteins are said to be *incomplete* or of *poor biologic value*. Generally speaking, plant foods—cereals, vegetables, and fruits—are in this group.

Fortunately, the same amino acids are not missing from all plant foods. When one food provides the amino acids that are missing in another, it is said to *supplement* the second food. Neither corn nor dry beans, when eaten at separate times, provide all the amino acids needed by the tissues. But if they are eaten at the same meal, as Mexicans often do, the two foods will supply all the amino acid needs of adults.

## SOURCES

Most people immediately think of meat, fish, and poultry as good sources of protein. In the daily diet they do provide most protein per serving portion, but it is a mistake to assume that these are the only good sources of protein. The complete protein foods—meat, fish, poultry, eggs, milk, cheese—provide just over three fifths of all the protein in the average diet in the United States.

Legumes (navy beans, pinto beans, chick peas, soybeans, split peas) are rich in protein, as are also nuts of many kinds. Presently, the legumes do not form an important part of the American diet, but their potential uses are great; they are widely used in some parts of the world.

Food technologists have developed procedures to extract the protein from plant foods such as soybeans, cottonseed, wheat, and others. The extracted protein is spun into fibers which are almost pure protein. The fibers can be formulated into products that simulate chicken, beef, ham, bacon, sausage, tuna, and others in terms of appearance, texture, and flavor. These products are sometimes referred to as *textured vegetable proteins*. Because these products are intended as a replacement of meat, it is important that they provide the same variety and quantity of nutrients as contained in meat. Presently, these products are used to supplement expensive animal protein foods in school food service programs and replace meat in the diets of vegetarians.

Breads and cereals contain relatively small amounts of protein per serving. However, the amount of bread and cereal eaten may be sufficiently great to provide an important proportion of the total protein. For example, a boy of 16 who eats eight slices of bread in a day is thus obtaining 16 to 20 gm protein from this source alone.

Although the proteins in breads, cereals, and legumes do not provide enough of all the essential amino acids, we have seen that a proper supplementation of one with the other can "stretch" the supply of complete protein foods. Thus cereal and milk, baked beans and milk, bread and meat, as in a sandwich, are combinations that provide as good quality as that from larger servings of expensive meats and other animal protein foods alone.

The average serving of vegetable contributes 1 to 3 gm protein, and fruits are even lower in protein content. This food group accounts for only a small part of the protein in typical American diets.

The protein value for specific foods is listed in Table A–1, Appendix A. The approximate amount of protein contributed by typical foods of the Four Food Groups is shown in Table 5–1 and Figure 5–1.

## FUNCTIONS

Proteins are digested to amino acids (see Chap. 3) and are absorbed through the walls of the small intestines into the portal blood circulation for delivery to the liver and the tissues of the body. The tissues and organs remove the kinds and amounts of amino acids required for a given function. The need for protein continues throughout life since there is a constant need for new cells to replace those that have broken down. For

TABLE 5–1   AVERAGE PROTEIN COMPOSITION OF SOME FOODS

| Food | Serving | Protein gm | Protein Quality |
|---|---|---|---|
| *Milk group* | | | |
| Milk, whole, skim, buttermilk | 1 cup | 9 | Complete |
| Cheese, American, process | 1 oz | 7 | Complete |
| Cheese, cottage | ¼ cup | 8 | Complete |
| Cheese, cream | 2 tablespoons | 2 | Complete |
| Ice cream | ⅛ qt | 3 | Complete |
| *Meat group* | | | |
| Meat, fish, poultry | 3 oz, fatty | 15–20 | Complete |
| | 3 oz, lean | 20–25 | Complete |
| Egg | 1 whole | 6 | Complete |
| Dried beans or peas | ½ cup cooked | 7–8 | Incomplete |
| Peanut butter | 1 tablespoon | 4 | Incomplete |
| *Vegetable-fruit group* | | | |
| Fruit juice | ½ cup | Trace | |
| Fruits | 1 serving | Trace–1 | Incomplete |
| Vegetables | ½ cup | 1–3 | Incomplete |
| *Bread-cereal group* | | | |
| Breakfast cereals | ½ cup cooked | 2–3 | Incomplete |
| | ¾ cup dry | 2–3 | Incomplete |
| Bread | 1 slice | 2 | Incomplete |
| Macaroni, noodles, rice, spaghetti | ½ cup cooked | 2 | Incomplete |

example, red blood cells have a life-span of 60 to 120 days. When they are broken down, there are equal numbers of new ones to take their places. So it is with every body tissue.

Throughout the period of pregnancy, and in infancy, childhood, and adolescence, protein is continuously required for the building of the marvelous variety of new tissues as well as for the replacement to take care of wear and tear.

Most of the regulatory materials of the body, including enzymes and hormones, are protein in nature. For example, thyroxine, which regulates energy metabolism, and insulin, which regulates the blood sugar level, contain specific kinds and amounts of certain amino acids. The red coloring matter of the blood, *hemoglobin*, is a protein that carries oxygen to the tissues so that the energy materials may be "burned" to supply energy. Other proteins in the blood are necessary to regulate osmotic pressure

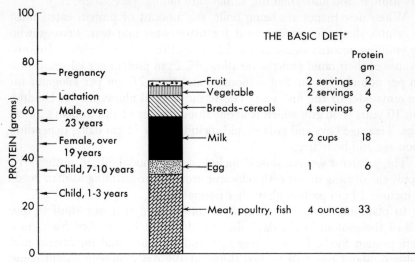

FIGURE 5–1 The Four Food Groups of the Basic Diet meet the recommended allowances for protein for all categories except the pregnant woman. See Table 4–2 (p. 37) for complete calculation.

and to maintain water balance. The digestion of food requires certain enzymes that are constructed from amino acids. The body's defense against disease is brought about by antibodies that are composed of proteins.

Proteins also furnish 4 kilocalories per gram. If the diet contains more protein than is needed, the nitrogen will be removed from the excess amino acids by the liver. The nitrogen is excreted in the form of urea by the kidney. The remainder of the amino acid molecule is then used as an immediate source of energy, or it may be stored in the form of fat. On the other hand, if the diet does not contain sufficient calories from fat and carbohydrate, the protein will be used for energy rather than for building or replacing tissues.

## PROTEIN ALLOWANCES

The protein need of the adult is based on body size. The recommended allowance is 0.8 gm per kilogram body weight. This amounts to 56 gm for the 70-kg man and 46 gm for the 58-kg woman. (See Table 4–1, p. 32.) Hard work and exercise do not increase the protein requirement. On the other hand, advancing age does not decrease the requirement.

Under certain conditions the adult can maintain nitrogen balance with a protein intake as low as 25 to 40 gm. The quality of the protein in these circumstances must be excellent, and sufficient calories must be provided by carbohydrate and fat so that protein is not used for energy. Such reduction of protein intake becomes imperative when the food supply is very limited, and also when the kidneys are failing. (See Chap. 26.)

When new tissues are being built, the amount of protein eaten must be greater than the amount used for tissue wear and tear. Persons who are building new tissues are said to be in *positive nitrogen balance*. Infants, because of their rapid growth, are allowed 2.2 gm protein per kilogram (1.0 gm per pound) for the first 6 months, and then 2.0 gm per kilogram for the remainder of the first year. The recommended allowance for children 7 to 10 years is 36 gm, which is about three fourths of the woman's allowance. Teen-age boys and girls should include 44 to 54 gm daily, depending upon age and body size.

The pregnant woman should include an additional 30 gm protein. To supply the nursing infant with sufficient protein, the lactating woman needs to include 20 gm protein above her normal needs.

In planning diets, it is generally recommended that one third to one half of the protein in the day's diet for the adult be supplied from complete protein foods. During pregnancy and lactation, and for infants and children, about one half to two thirds of the day's protein should come from complete protein foods.

It is also important to provide some complete protein foods at each meal. Tissue building and repair do not take place if all the amino acids are not present in the blood circulation at the same time; this is sometimes referred to as the "all or none law."

### PROTEIN DEFICIENCY

Most people in America have an abundant intake of protein. An individual, however, might be in *negative nitrogen balance*. This means that his body is breaking down protein tissues faster than they are being replaced. Thus the excretions will contain more nitrogen than is being supplied by the diet. Just as overdrawing a bank account is not a good thing, so the excess removal of nitrogen from the tissue is also harmful. When negative nitrogen balance exists, the individual is less able to resist infections, he may withstand the stress of injury or surgery very poorly, and his general health will deteriorate.

Negative nitrogen balance exists when an individual does not eat enough protein or eats protein foods of poor quality. Some persons use crash diets for reducing weight and thus have a very low protein intake. Many elderly persons are unable to chew food well, and they may eat large quantities of bread and no meat, eggs, or milk; although the amount of protein may be sufficient, the quality is inadequate. Negative nitrogen balance occurs in many disease conditions and can be corrected only with a high-protein diet. (See Chap. 26.)

Infantile protein malnutrition, also called kwashiorkor, is rarely seen in the United States, but it is a major world health problem, most especially in Africa, Central and Latin America, and parts of the Orient. (See Fig. 5–2.) The condition usually appears shortly after the infant is weaned from the mother's breast and the food used is chiefly of a carbohydrate nature. The infants fail to grow, the muscles are poorly developed, the appetite is poor, the skin and hair change in texture and color, diarrhea

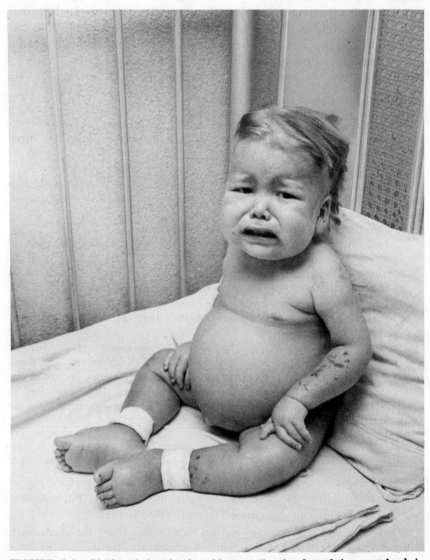

FIGURE 5–2  Child with kwashiorkor. Note swollen hands and feet, patchy hair, mottled skin, uncomfortable appearance. (*Courtesy, UNICEF. Photo by Nagata.*)

follows, the tissues hold water (edema), and death finally results. Those children who do survive sometimes suffer mental retardation because the brain has not had an opportunity to develop during the critical early years of life.

Kwashiorkor can be prevented or treated with inexpensive sources of protein-rich foods. Dry nonfat milk supplied through UNICEF to many infants and children has been highly effective. Many countries are now developing protein-rich foods by combining locally available plant foods. *Incaparina,* the best known of these, is a food powder that can be mixed with water for child feeding. It is made of corn, cottonseed, sorghum, and mineral-vitamin supplements. Fish protein concentrate, soybean protein, peanut protein, and others have been used in various mixtures.

### SOME FALLACIES AND FACTS

1. *Fallacy.* Athletes need more protein than nonathletes.

*Fact.* The protein requirement of the adult depends on the body size and not on the amount of exercise.

2. *Fallacy.* Older people need less protein than young adults.

*Fact.* The need for replacing the protein of tissues continues through out life. Older people need the same amount of protein as the young adult of the same body size.

3. *Fallacy.* Gelatin is an excellent source of protein.

*Fact.* Although gelatin is useful in providing a variety of dishes in the diet, its protein contribution is not important. Dry gelatin is about 90 per cent protein, but the average gelatin dessert would furnish about 2 gm protein. Gelatin lacks some of the essential amino acids; as a sole source of protein it cannot maintain life or support growth.

4. *Fallacy.* Protein foods should not be eaten in the same meal as starches.

*Fact.* There is no reason to separate protein foods and starches. In fact, many common foods contain both protein and carbohydrate. The digestive tract efficiently digests protein, carbohydrate, and fat components of the diet at the same time. Each meal should contain one fourth to one third of the day's protein so that the amino acids will be most efficiently used for tissue synthesis.

### REVIEW QUESTIONS AND PROBLEMS

1. Define amino acid, essential amino acid, complete protein, supplementary protein, biologic value, nitrogen balance, antibody, phenylalanine.

2. How do proteins differ from fats and carbohydrates?

3. Keep a record of the food you eat for one day. Using the approximate values on page 44, estimate the amount of protein in your diet. What foods provided you with complete protein?

4. Why should you include some complete protein at each meal?

5. What happens if you eat more protein than your tissues need for maintenance?

6. How does the protein need of a ten-year-old boy compare with your need?

7. How could you improve these meals for protein?

| I | II |
|---|---|
| Large fruit salad | Baked beans |
| Roll with butter | Brown bread with butter |
| Cucumber–water cress sandwich | Sliced tomato salad |
| Iced tea | Jello with whipped cream |

8. Name three substances in the body that are of a protein nature and that regulate body functions. Tell what each does.

9. What is kwashiorkor? How may it be prevented?

10. A 75-year-old woman refuses to drink milk or to eat meat because she thinks these foods are not good for her. How would you respond to this situation?

## REFERENCES

Breeling, J. L.: "Marketing Protein for the World's Poor," *Today's Health,* 47:42, February 1969.

Cooley, D. G.: "What's So Important About Proteins?" *Today's Health,* 43:46, October 1965.

Robinson, C. H.: *Normal and Therapeutic Nutrition,* 14th ed. New York: Macmillan Publishing Co., Inc., 1972, Chap. 4.

Scrimshaw, N. S.: "Nature of Protein Requirements: Ways They Can Be Met in Tomorrow's World," *J. Am. Diet. Assoc.,* 54:94–102, 1969.

# FATS

"The fat of the land." The word "fat" brings to mind such ideas as wealth, prosperity, and well-being; likewise, the word makes one think of such rich foods as pastries, cookies, cakes, ice cream, butter, cream, and oil. But fat is also associated with overweight, and more recently with heart disease. *Lipid* is another term for fats and fatlike substances.

## NATURE AND PROPERTIES

Fats are composed of three chemical elements: carbon, hydrogen, and oxygen. Fats contain much smaller proportions of oxygen than do carbohydrates.

Most fats are *triglycerides*; that is, they are formed from three molecules of *fatty acids* attached to one molecule of *glycerol*. About 20 fatty acids are commonly found in foods. Each fatty acid consists of a short or long chain of carbon atoms attached to an acid group. *Short-chain* fatty acids contain 4 to 6 carbon atoms; *medium-chain* fatty acids contain 8 to 10 carbon atoms; and *long-chain* fatty acids contain 12 to 20 or more carbon atoms.

Long-chain fatty acids may be saturated, monounsaturated, or polyunsaturated. *Saturated* fatty acids are those having single bonds between the carbon atoms (see Fig. 6–1). They cannot take up any hydrogen. Myristic, palmitic, and stearic acids are three examples of such fatty acids; they are abundant in animal fats, including beef and mutton fat, butter, and others. Coconut oil, although liquid, consists mostly of lauric acid, a saturated fatty acid.

50

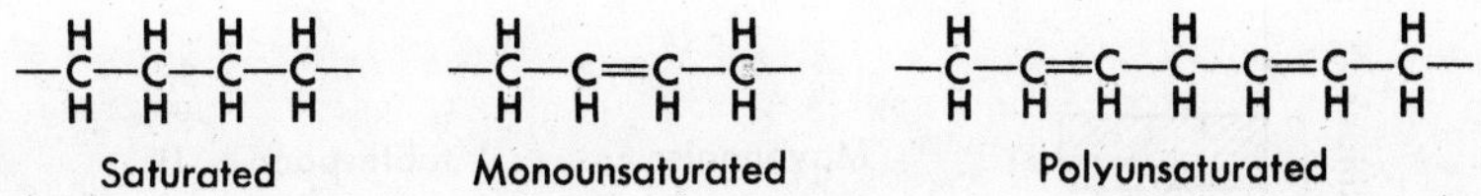

H H H H         H        H        H        H        H
—C—C—C—C—    —C—C=C—C—    —C—C=C—C—C=C—C—
H H H H         H H H H        H H H H H H H
  Saturated       Monounsaturated      Polyunsaturated

**FIGURE 6–1** Fatty acids with one bond between all carbon atoms are saturated; those with a double bond between two or more carbon atoms are unsaturated.

A *monounsaturated* fatty acid is one in which two of the carbon atoms are joined by a double bond. This means that a hydrogen atom could be added to each of the carbon atoms at the double bond. Oleic acid is the most abundant monounsaturated fatty acid. Olive oil is especially high in oleic acid, but most fats contain generous amounts of this fatty acid.

A *polyunsaturated* fatty acid is one in which two or more double bonds are present. Thus, each of four or more carbon atoms could take up a hydrogen atom. *Linoleic* acid has two double bonds and is the most common of the polyunsaturated acids; it is abundant in most vegetable oils.

*Hydrogenation* is the addition of hydrogen to the carbon atoms in unsaturated fats to produce a solid fat. Regular margarines and many cooking fats are prepared from vegetable oils by this process. As might be expected, the addition of hydrogen increases the proportion of saturated fatty acids and decreases the proportion of unsaturated fatty acids.

The flavor and hardness of a food fat depend upon the kinds and amounts of the fatty acids that are present. Food fats are a mixture of saturated and unsaturated fatty acids. For convenience a food fat is called *saturated* if it contains more saturated than polyunsaturated fatty acids; such fats are solid. If polyunsaturated fatty acids exceed the saturated fatty acids, the food fat is said to be *polyunsaturated*; such fats are liquid, such as oils, or very soft, such as some special type margarines.

Fats become rancid if they are exposed to air and light. The change is more rapid at high temperatures. Many manufacturers add antioxidants to fats to lengthen the time that they may be kept.

**FOOD SOURCES**

Some fats are "visible," as in butter, shortenings, and oils, whereas others are "invisible," as in milk, egg yolk, and food mixtures. The milk group and the meat group furnish about half of the fat in our diets. Visible fats and oils are the next important source of fats. The vegetable-fruit group (except olives and avocados) and the bread-cereal group are very low in fat. The fat content of the basic diet is shown in Figure 6–2.

The important way by which fats contribute to the calories of the diet is shown in Table 6–1.

The following classification of fat-rich foods indicates whether saturated fatty acids or polyunsaturated fatty acids predominate.

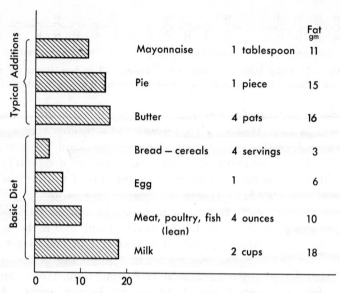

**FIGURE 6–2** The fat content of a diet is rapidly increased with the addition of butter or margarine, salad dressings, and most desserts. See Table 4–2 (p. 37) for calculations of the Basic Diet.

TABLE 6–1   COMPARISON OF FAT CONTENT AND CALORIES

| | Total Fat | |
| --- | --- | --- |
| | *gm* | *kcal* |
| Skim milk, 1 cup | Trace | 90 |
| Whole milk, 1 cup | 9 | 160 |
| Half milk and half cream, 1 cup | 28 | 325 |
| Tossed salad | Trace | 20 |
| Tossed salad with 2 tablespoons blue cheese dressing | 16 | 170 |
| Bread, 1 thin slice | 1 | 65 |
| Bread, 1 slice with 1 pat butter | 5 | 100 |
| Baked potato, one | Trace | 90 |
| Baked potato with 2 tablespoons sour cream | 4 | 140 |
| Lamb chop, lean, one | 6 | 140 |
| Lamb chop, lean with fat, one | 33 | 400 |

*High in saturated fatty acids*

Whole milk, cream, ice cream, cheeses made from whole milk, egg yolk
Medium fat or fatty meats: beef, lamb, pork, ham
Bacon, beef tallow, butter, coconut oil, lamb fat, lard, regular margarine, salt pork, hydrogenated shortenings
Chocolate, chocolate candy, cakes, cookies, pies, rich puddings

*High in polyunsaturated fatty acids*
    Vegetable oils: safflower, corn, cottonseed, soybean, sesame, sunflower
    Salad dressings made from the above oils: mayonnaise, French, and others
    Special margarines: liquid oil listed first on label
    Fatty fish: salmon, tuna, herring

## FUNCTIONS

Normally, about 95 per cent of the fat in food is digested and absorbed. (See Chap. 3.) Fats, as we all know, are important sources of calories; each gram contributes 9 kcal. It is quite normal for the body to have deposits of fat (adipose tissue) that serve as a continuing supply of energy each and every hour. In fact, if we had no reserves of fat in the body whatsoever, we would need to eat much more frequently in order to provide a continuous supply of energy. Fat is said to be *protein-sparing* because its availability reduces the need to burn protein for energy. Carbohydrates and proteins in excess of body needs are also changed into fatty tissue, just as fat in the diet contributes to these stores.

In addition to providing energy, fats are essential (1) to maintain the constant body temperature by providing effective insulation underneath the skin; (2) to cushion the vital organs, such as the kidney, against injury; (3) to facilitate the absorption of the fat-soluble vitamins A, D, E, and K; (4) to provide satiety and to delay the onset of hunger; and (5) to contribute flavor and palatability to the diet.

*Essential fatty acids.* Arachidonic acid, a long-chain polyunsaturated fatty acid, is essential for normal growth and skin health. This fatty acid occurs in only limited amounts in the food supply. However, linoleic acid occurs abundantly in foods that are high in polyunsaturated fatty acids and can be readily converted by the body to arachidonic acid. Linoleic acid is therefore considered to be a dietary essential.

*Phospholipids* are complex fats that also contain phosphorus and nitrogen. The diet supplies small amounts of these, and the body can make them. They are important in brain and nervous tissue. They also assist in the absorption of fat from the small intestine and in the transportation of fat in the blood.

## DAILY ALLOWANCES

No recommendation for the level of fat intake is listed in the table of Recommended Dietary Allowances. The requirement for linoleic acid is met even on very low fat intakes.

Fats account for about 40 per cent of the calories available in the United States, but actual intakes vary widely. Some people eat many fried foods, pastries, rich desserts, cream, salad dressings, and butter or margarine, whereas others consume very little of such high-fat foods. Some people throughout the world, for example, Asians and Africans, consume diets providing as little as 10 per cent of the calories from fat, whereas other people, such as Eskimos, eat large quantities of fat. Based upon American food habits, a palatable diet can be planned with 35 per cent of calories coming from fat.

Many people today are concerned about the relationship of the amount and kind of fat in the diet to heart disease. Research indicates that most Americans would benefit by (1) reducing their daily fat intake to no more than 35 percent of calories, and (2) increasing the proportion of fats consumed from the foods high in polyunsaturated fatty acids. These relationships will be discussed further in Chapter 24.

## CHOLESTEROL

Cholesterol is a white, waxy substance related to fats, but very different in chemical structure. It is abundant in certain foods such as egg yolk, liver, kidney, and brains. Cholesterol is distributed evenly through lean and fatty tissue of meat, poultry, and fish. Other animal fats, including butter, cream, whole milk, whole-milk cheeses, and ice cream, contain smaller amounts of cholesterol. Plant foods do not contain cholesterol.

Cholesterol is a normal constituent of tissues, but it is especially important in brain and nervous tissue and in the liver. It serves as a precursor of vitamin D; that is, cholesterol in the skin can be changed into active vitamin D by exposure to the ultraviolet rays in sunlight. Cholesterol is closely related to the sex hormones and to the hormones of the adrenal gland. Excess cholesterol in the body is removed in the bile.

Each day the body manufactures cholesterol to meet its needs from fats, carbohydrates, and even amino acids. In addition the diet supplies 500 to 800 mg cholesterol, but this intake may be well over 1000 mg for the individual who eats at least two eggs a day and generous amounts of cholesterol-rich foods. Cholesterol sometimes accumulates in the gallbladder to form gallstones. High intakes of cholesterol also increase the level in the blood, one of several risk factors in diseases of the heart. See Chapter 24.

## SOME FALLACIES AND FACTS

1. *Fallacy.* Fried foods are hard to digest.

*Fact.* Digestion of fried foods is as complete as that of other foods. However, because fat coats the food particles, the digestion of fried foods takes somewhat longer.

2. *Fallacy.* Mineral oil is a good substitute for regular oil in low-calorie salad dressings.

*Fact.* Mineral oil is not absorbed through the intestinal wall and thus provides no calories. However, it interferes seriously with the absorption of fat-soluble vitamins A, D, E, and K. Therefore, it should never be used in food preparation.

3. *Fallacy.* Vegetable oils without additives are more nutritious than those preserved with an antioxidant.

*Fact.* The unsaturated fatty acids in vegetable oils are rapidly oxidized in the absence of antioxidants; this results in rancidity of the oil. Tocopherols (vitamin E) are among the most effective antioxidants, and any excess in the oils enters into the normal metabolism of vitamin E.

4. *Fallacy.* Vegetable oils are less fattening than solid fats.

*Fact.* Oils and solid fats are equally high in calories; that is, each gram of fat from either source furnishes 9 kcal.

5. *Fallacy.* Sour cream is lower in calories than sweet cream.

*Fact.* Sour cream has the same number of calories as the sweet cream from which it is made. Usually sour cream is made from light cream.

## REVIEW QUESTIONS AND PROBLEMS

1. What is meant by lipid, saturated fat, polyunsaturated fat, linoleic acid, hydrogenated fat, cholesterol?

2. What chemical elements are present in fats?

3. If a diet contains 90 gm fat, how many kilocalories are provided?

4. List six functions of fats.

5. List the sources of fat that you had in your diet yesterday. Which of these sources furnished linoleic acid? What foods did you eat that contained cholesterol?

6. A person complains that a meal that included fried chicken, French fried potatoes, and apple pie was "heavy." What does he probably mean by this? How do you explain this feeling?

7. A person tells you that he is not going to eat any more eggs, milk, or butter because they are high in cholesterol. How would you respond to this?

8. Examine the labels on several brands of margarine. Which of these brands is the best source of polyunsaturated fatty acids?

## REFERENCES

Grollman, A.: "A Common Sense Guide to Cholesterol," *Today's Health,* **44**:3, August 1966.

Holt, P. A.: "Fats and Bile Salts: Physiologic Considerations," *J. Am. Diet. Assoc.,* **60**:491–95, 1972.

Robinson, C. H.: *Normal and Therapeutic Nutrition,* 14th ed. New York: Macmillan Publishing Co., Inc., 1972, Chap. 6.

# CARBOHYDRATES

## UNIVERSAL ROLE

All peoples of the world depend upon the carbohydrate-rich foods as the principal source of calories. In the United States carbohydrates furnish about half of the calories, whereas in some countries of the world as much as four fifths of the calories is obtained from carbohydrate. The carbohydrate-rich plants are easily grown, give a large yield of food per acre, keep rather well, and are less expensive than foods of animal origin. The foods are highly acceptable in a great variety of ways and are easily digested and used in the body.

Cereal grains, legumes, roots, and sugars are the principal sources of carbohydrate. Rice is the leading staple food of the world, being especially prominent in Oriental diets. Wheat ranks second and is the staple cereal in parts of India, the Near East, Russia, Western Europe, and America. Rye, oats, and millet are important cereals in some dietaries of the world. Corn and legumes such as beans are favored in Central and Latin America. Potatoes, sweet potatoes, taro, plantain, and cassava do not approach the cereal grains in importance; yet they furnish significant amounts of carbohydrate and calories to the diets of some peoples. Although sugars are universally liked, the highest consumption is found in the most highly developed and affluent countries.

In the United States the trend has been toward a steady decline in the use of cereal grains and potatoes, a gradual increase in the use of sugars, and a relatively limited use of legumes.

56

**NATURE AND CLASSIFICATION**

By a complex process known as photosynthesis all green plants use energy from the sun, water from the soil, and carbon dioxide from the air to make carbohydrate. All carbohydrates contain the chemical elements carbon, hydrogen, and oxygen. The hydrogen and oxygen are present in the same proportions as found in water. Carbohydrates may be classed as shown in Table 7–1.

TABLE 7–1   CLASSIFICATION OF CARBOHYDRATES

| Class | Examples | Some Food Sources |
|---|---|---|
| Single sugars (monosaccharides) | Glucose (dextrose, grape sugar, corn sugar, blood sugar) | Fruits, honey, vegetables, corn syrup |
|  | Fructose (fruit sugar, levulose) | Fruits, vegetables, honey, corn syrup |
|  | Galactose | Occurs only from the digestion of lactose |
| Double sugars (disaccharides) | Sucrose $= G + F$ | Cane, beet, maple sugar; small amounts in fruits, some vegetables |
|  | Maltose $= G + G$ | Malting of cereal grains; acid hydrolysis of starch |
|  | Lactose $= Galactose + glucose$ | Milk only |
| Complex carbohydrates (polysaccharides) | Starch | Grains and grain foods, legumes, potatoes and other root vegetables, green bananas |
|  | Glycogen ("animal starch") | Liver and muscle of freshly killed animals; freshly opened oysters |
|  | Dextrin | Partial breakdown of starch by heat or in digestion |
|  | Cellulose | Bran of cereal grains, skins and fibers of fruits and vegetables |
|  | Pectins | Ripe fruits |

**PROPERTIES**

Carbohydrates may be ranked in decreasing order of sweetness: fructose, sucrose, glucose, lactose, dextrin, and starch. Regardless of their sweetness, all carbohydrates furnish 4 kcal per gram. Only a small amount of honey, which is rich in fructose, can be eaten at one time. If one needs to increase the caloric value of a glass of lemonade, for example, he could use about twice as much glucose as sucrose. Lactose is only about one seventh as sweet as sucrose.

Sugars vary greatly in their solubility. Glucose is less soluble than sucrose; when making up a beverage it should be stirred well so that the sugar will not settle to the bottom. Lactose is now seldom used in beverages because of its poor solubility, its higher cost, and its tendency to irritate the intestinal tract when taken in large amounts.

Starches are bland in flavor and not sweet. A green banana is high in starch; as it ripens, the starch is changed to glucose and the sweetness is thereby increased. When corn ripens, it becomes less sweet as the sugars are converted to starch.

The thickening property of starch is well known, as in the making of cornstarch pudding or the cooking of a breakfast cereal such as oatmeal. When mixed with water and cooked, the starch absorbs water, and the mixture thickens.

### SOURCES

When you are planning diets, you should consider the amount of carbohydrate in the food and also the contributions of other nutrients made by a given food. Of the Four Food Groups breads and cereals are the outstanding sources of carbohydrate. This group is important because the amounts of these foods eaten daily may be considerable, and because enriched or whole-grain breads and cereals provide substantial quantities of iron, B-complex vitamins, and some protein.

The whole grain is rich in iron, thiamine, niacin, and other nutrients. In the manufacture of white flour and refined cereals the germ and outer layers of the grain are removed. (See Fig. 7–1.) This refinement results in significant losses of iron and B-complex vitamins. Early in World War II a program of enrichment was initiated to replace the lost nutrients to cereal foods.

*Enrichment* is a legal term used by the Food and Drug Administration to apply specifically to the addition of thiamine, riboflavin, niacin, and iron. When foods are labeled as enriched, they must contain the four nutrients within the ranges specified by the law. Enrichment of bread and flour is required in the majority of states and is voluntary in others. Some states in the South also require the enrichment of corn and rice. About 80 per cent of the white flour and bread in this country are now enriched, and also a substantial proportion of the macaroni, noodles, and spaghetti.

Sweet potatoes and white potatoes are important contributors from the vegetable-fruit group to the carbohydrate intake, because they are daily

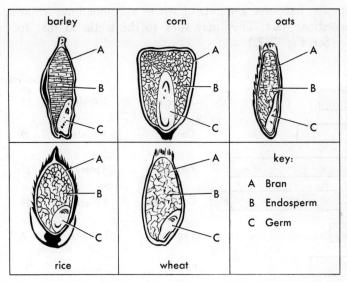

FIGURE 7–1  Structure of cereal grains. *(Courtesy, Cereal Institute, Inc., Chicago.)*

items in many diets. Some fruits, such as bananas and dried fruits, and some vegetables, such as corn and Lima beans, are also relatively high in carbohydrate content. They are not usually daily items in the diet, and therefore the amount of carbohydrate realized from these foods is considerably less than that from potatoes.

Milk is unique in that it is the only dietary source of lactose. Each cup contains 12 gm; thus the daily intake from this source would be 24 to 48 gm lactose, depending upon the amount of milk consumed. Cheese contains only traces of lactose.

Meat, poultry, and fish contain no carbohydrate. The small amount of glycogen present in fresh liver and oysters has usually disappeared before the food reaches the consumer. Legumes and peanuts contain fair amounts of carbohydrate.

Cakes, cookies, pastries, sugars, and sweets are higher in carbohydrate content than breads and cereals. When they are prepared with enriched flour, cakes, cookies, and pastries will contribute B-complex vitamins and iron. Any eggs and milk used in the preparation further increase the nutritive value. Cane and beet sugars are inexpensive, whereas honey, maple syrup, jellies and jams, and candies are moderately high in cost. Sugars and sweets are concentrated so that relatively small amounts will rapidly increase the carbohydrate and calorie intake. On the other hand, they do not contain important amounts of other nutrients; they are often referred to as "empty-calorie" foods. If too many sweets are included, they are likely to take the place of foods that supply other nutrients, because they often destroy the appetite. Excessive amounts of sweets are sometimes irritating to the gastrointestinal tract. They may stick to the teeth, so that tooth decay results. (See Fig. 7–2.)

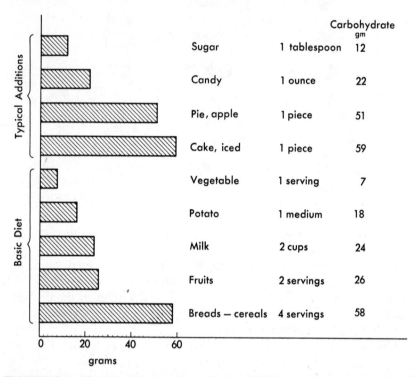

FIGURE 7–2 Desserts and sweets are typical additions to the Basic Diet for additional calories. Some additions provide few nutrients other than carbohydrate. See Basic Diet, Table 4–2 (p. 37), for calculations.

Cellulose, being the fibrous part of the plant, is supplied by the whole grains, raw fruits, and raw vegetables. During cookery some of the fibers disintegrate whereas others are softened.

### FACTS ABOUT CARBOHYDRATE-RICH FOODS

1. Are honey, crude sugar, and brown sugar nutritionally better than cane or beet sugar?

Honey and brown sugar bring flavor variety to the diet. Like cane or beet sugar they are good sources of energy, but the amounts of minerals and vitamins are too small to make a worthwhile addition to the day's diet.

2. Are whole-grain breads more nutritious than white bread?

Cereal foods, whether whole grain or highly milled, are important and inexpensive sources of energy. They also furnish some protein. White breads that have been enriched are just as nutritious as whole-grain breads. Whole-grain breads contain appreciably more fiber than white breads and the percentage of digestibility is, therefore, slightly lower. Unenriched white breads supply much lower amounts of iron and B-complex vitamins.

3. Are rice, macaroni, noodles, and spaghetti good substitutes for potatoes?

It depends upon the choices made. All these foods are high in starch and an average serving of each is similar in calorie and protein value. If the cereal foods are enriched, they would furnish about the same amounts of minerals and B vitamins as potatoes. Fresh potatoes contain some ascorbic acid not provided by cereal foods.

4. Is blackstrap molasses good for anemia?

Blackstrap molasses is relatively rich in iron but it does not have any special virtue over many foods that provide iron. Blackstrap molasses is widely used in livestock feeding. The treatment of anemia depends upon the type of anemia present and should be directed by a physician.

## FUNCTIONS

Glucose, fructose, and galactose are the end products of carbohydrate digestion (see Chap. 3). These single sugars are absorbed from the small intestine into the portal circulation and are carried to the liver.

The form of sugar in the blood is glucose. The blood glucose is rapidly withdrawn by the cells of all body tissues, and is constantly replaced by the liver. The hormone insulin is the primary regulator of the level of sugar in the blood. As soon as the blood sugar rises, the pancreas is stimulated to produce insulin. Three important functions are performed by insulin: (1) the utilization of glucose for energy by the tissues; (2) the conversion of glucose to glycogen in the liver; and (3) the conversion of glucose to fat, as a reserve store of energy.

The amount of carbohydrate in the body at any given moment is about 300 gm (¾ lb) or less. Some of this is present in the blood, and the greater amount is stored in the liver and muscles as glycogen. Any carbohydrate in excess of immediate body needs is converted into fat. Carbohydrate has many functions in the body, such as these:

1. The chief function of carbohydrate is to provide energy to carry on the work of the body and heat to maintain the body's temperature. Glucose is the only form of energy used by the central nervous system, but other tissues also use fats for energy. Glucose and oxygen are carried by the blood to the tissues. In a complex manner involving many enzymes and intermediate reactions, glucose is oxidized to yield the following results:

$$\text{glucose} + \text{oxygen} = \text{energy} + \text{carbon dioxide} + \text{water}.$$

When tissues require much energy for their work, oxidation of glucose will proceed at a rapid rate. If you run, for example, you begin to breathe rapidly. You are then providing additional oxygen to combine with the extra glucose to meet this energy need. The carbon dioxide produced in this reaction is a waste product that is removed through the lungs. The water that results may be reused by the body in a number of ways or may be eliminated by the kidneys, skin, and lungs.

2. Carbohydrate spares protein. This means that the body need not burn protein from the diet or from body stores to meet energy needs when carbohydrate is available. Carbohydrates also furnish chemical elements that can be combined with nitrogen to manufacture nonessential amino acids.

3. The complete oxidation of fats requires some carbohydrate. When too little carbohydrate is available, some fatty acids known as ketones accumulate. This condition is seen in poorly regulated diabetic patients, and is known as *diabetic acidosis* or *coma*. (See Chap. 22.)

4. Nervous tissues and cartilage require small amounts of carbohydrate for their synthesis.

5. Lactose in milk favors the growth of certain intestinal bacteria that synthesize some of the B-complex vitamins. Lactose also increases the absorption of calcium and phosphorus.

6. Cellulose is desirable because it contributes bulk to the diet. It can absorb and hold water so that normal elimination occurs from the bowel.

7. The values of starches and sugars in providing variety and flavor to the diet should not be minimized. Jam on bread, strawberries on cereal, freshly baked dinner rolls, cake with frosting—all of these are taste-appealing and encourage food intake. To be sure, carbohydrates if eaten too liberally contribute to excessive caloric intake and thus to overweight.

### DAILY NEEDS

A recommended allowance for carbohydrate has not been established. Typical American diets furnish 45 to 50 per cent of the calories from carbohydrate, or about 200 to 350 gm carbohydrate. Some people of the world maintain vigorous health with high intakes of carbohydrate, and others are just as healthy on low-carbohydrate diets. Generally, the daily diet should contain not less than 100 gm carbohydrate; this is more than sufficient for efficient oxidation of fats. Note that the Basic Diet furnishes somewhat more than this. (See Table 4–2.)

### REVIEW QUESTIONS AND PROBLEMS

1. Define these terms: photosynthesis, galactose, cellulose, dextrin, maltose, enrichment, legume, monosaccharide, carbohydrate, starch, glycogen.

2. List the foods you ate yesterday. Which of these are important sources of carbohydrate? Which are important sources of fiber? Which are "empty-calorie" foods?

3. Outline the steps in the digestion of a carbohydrate meal, including the names of the enzymes, the site of their activity, and the digestion products that result. (Review Chap. 3.)

4. You sometimes find that a glass of fruit juice quickly makes you feel better. How can you explain this?

5. List four functions of carbohydrates in the body.

6. How many kilocalories would be provided by 250 gm carbohydrate?

7. Why is cellulose important? What foods would you increase in the diet for more cellulose?

8. Look up in Table A-1 the carbohydrate value of 1 piece of layer cake, 1 fresh peach, ½ cup cooked rice, 1 piece of apple pie, 1 sweet potato, 1 teaspoon sugar, 1 sweet roll, ½ cup spinach, 1 candy bar, 1 cup blueberries.

## REFERENCES

Bauer, W. W.: "Why Today's Bread Is Better," *Today's Health*, **44**:60, December 1966.

Council on Foods and Nutrition: "Fortification of Flour and Bread with Iron," *JAMA*, **223**:322, 1973.

Joseph, L.: "Foods and Drinks That Will Cause You the Fewest Calories," *Today's Health*, **51**:41, October 1973.

Robinson, C. H.: *Normal and Therapeutic Nutrition*, 14th ed. New York: Macmillan Publishing Co., Inc., 1972, Chap. 5.

## 8

Fuel and Energy | CALORIE, A UNIT OF HEAT • Energy Needs
of the Body | MEASURING ENERGY NEEDS | BASAL METABOLISM |
VOLUNTARY ACTIVITY | INFLUENCE OF FOOD | CALORIE
ALLOWANCES • Meeting Calorie Needs | CALORIE VALUE OF
FOODS | CALORIE FALLACIES AND FACTS | CALORIE VALUE OF THE
BASIC DIET | CALORIE BALANCE AND BODY WEIGHT

# ENERGY METABOLISM

## Fuel and Energy

Probably no aspect of nutrition is more discussed than that of calories. People say they "eat" too many calories or not enough calories. They associate calories with their weight. We need to know what we mean by calories, how many calories we need each day, and which foods are good and poor sources of calories.

Every engine requires fuel. The automobile runs only so long as it has a supply of gasoline. The furnace heats the house only when oil, gas, or coal is fed into it. The human body, sometimes likened to an engine, requires fuel to carry on all of its activities and to keep it warm. Every moment of our lives some energy is being used by the body—for every breath we draw, every beat of the heart, the blinking of the eyelid, the lifting of the heavy weight, or any activity whatsoever. The carbohydrate, fat, and protein in the foods we eat are the potential sources of energy for all body activities.

### CALORIE, A UNIT OF HEAT

Strictly speaking, we don't "eat" calories. When carbohydrates, fats, and proteins are oxidized in the body, heat is a by-product. Just as we can measure length in centimeters or inches and weight in kilograms or pounds, so we can measure the energy value of a food, or the heat production of the body, in heat units called *calories*. By definition, one large or kilocalorie is the amount of heat required to raise the temperature of 1000 gm of water by 1° C. The large calorie is the unit always used in nutrition, whether it is written with a small "c" *calorie*, or a capital "C" *Calorie*, or as a *kilocalorie* (kcal). It is 1000 times as great as the unit used in chemistry and physics.

The energy value of a food is measured in the laboratory with an instrument called a *bomb calorimeter*. The caloric values for foods obtained with this instrument must be corrected to allow for some losses that occur in the feces and urine. In the body, these are the corrected values for pure carbohydrate, fat, and protein:

| | |
|---|---|
| Carbohydrate | 4 kilocalories per gram |
| Fat | 9 kilocalories per gram |
| Protein | 4 kilocalories per gram |

Thus 5 gm of sugar (1 teaspoon) would yield 20 kilocalories, but 5 gm of fat would yield 45 kilocalories.

If we know the carbohydrate, fat, and protein values for a food, we can easily calculate the calorie value of that food. For example, the calorie value of one cup of milk would be calculated thus:

| | | |
|---|---|---|
| 12 gm carbohydrate | × 4 kcal = | 48 |
| 10 gm fat | × 9 kcal = | 90 |
| 8 gm protein | × 4 kcal = | 32 |
| | Total kcal | 170 |

You will see that this calculation, using figures for milk that have been rounded off, is quite close to the actual value listed in Table A–1, Appendix A. Ordinarily, we don't need to make such calculations, because tables of calorie values are readily available.

## Energy Needs of the Body

### MEASURING ENERGY NEEDS

An individual uses oxygen to burn (oxidize) the simple sugars, fatty acids, and amino acids in his body; the higher the rate of burning (oxidation) in his body, the more oxygen he will need. Therefore, the amount of oxygen used by an individual under certain conditions of rest or activity is measured to calculate the energy expended.

The total daily calorie requirement depends upon the basal metabolism, the amount of voluntary activity, the influence of food, the climate, and needs for growth.

## BASAL METABOLISM

Basal metabolism, sometimes called "the cost of living," accounts for more than half of the calorie requirements of most people. It includes the involuntary activities of the body (activities over which we have no control) while resting but awake. The breathing, the beating of the heart, the circulation of the blood, the metabolic activities within the cells, the keeping of the muscles in good tone, and the maintenance of the body temperature require energy.

The basal metabolism may be measured in a number of ways. One of these consists in measuring the amount of pure oxygen a person breathes in for a given length of time under these conditions: (1) the individual is awake but lying quietly in a comfortable room; (2) he is in the *postabsorptive* state; that is, he has had no food for 12 to 16 hours; (3) his body temperature is normal; and (4) he is not tense or emotionally upset. When the test is performed the nose is clamped so that the person breathes through his mouth from a tank of oxygen. The amount of oxygen he uses is measured, and from that the number of calories is calculated.

For his basal metabolism the adult requires about one kilocalorie per kilogram per hour. Thus, a woman weighing 55 kg (121 lb) would have a basal metabolism of approximately 1320 kcal ($1 \times 55 \times 24$). A man weighing 70 kg (154 lb) would have a basal metabolism of 1680 kcal ($1 \times 70 \times 24$).

Several factors affect the rate of basal metabolism. The first of these is *body size*. The larger a person is, the greater is the amount of lean muscle tissue and the greater is the skin surface area. Thus a tall, well-built man has a greater skin surface and will have a higher basal metabolism than a short, fat man of the same weight.

The amount of *muscle tissue* has an effect on the basal metabolism. An athlete with firm muscles has a higher rate than a nonathlete with poorly developed, flabby muscles. Usually men have a higher rate than women, because men, as a rule, have more muscle tissue, and women have more deposits of fat.

Rapid *growth* increases the basal metabolism greatly. Infants in proportion to body size have a very high rate of metabolism. The metabolism is also high during the rapid growth period of adolescence and the last trimester of pregnancy when the fetus is greatly increasing in size.

After the *age* of 25 years the metabolism declines gradually; thus the calories are reduced somewhat for later years. Many men and women become overweight during middle age because they fail to reduce their calories as their metabolism goes down.

The *thyroid* gland produces thyroxine, an iodine-containing hormone that regulates the rate of energy metabolism. If too much thyroxine is produced, the metabolism will increase; if too little thyroid hormone is manufactured, the metabolism will be correspondingly lower. The level of protein-bound iodine (PBI) in the blood is now widely used by physicians in place of the basal metabolism test to determine the activity of the thyroid.

## VOLUNTARY ACTIVITY

Our daily work may well vary from sitting at a desk to bedside nursing, active housework, or hard manual labor. In our leisure time we might choose to watch television, take a leisurely walk, or go swimming or dancing. The kind of physical activity in which we engage, and the amounts of time spent in each activity, determine the amount of energy the body uses. It is difficult to assign exact values to any activity because individuals vary widely in the efficiency with which they use their bodies. Common activities have been placed in five groups in Table 8–1. The lower level of calories for each group is typical for the average woman, whereas the upper level of calories would more nearly apply to the average man. The figures include the calories for basal metabolism. One can readily see why a typist, classed as sedentary, requires fewer calories than the moderately active homemaker who might also do some gardening in addition to her housework.

Mental effort requires so few calories that it is hardly worth considering. If you are studying and nibbling foods all the while, it is certain that the calories you are consuming are far greater than are needed for your mental effort. Of course, if you are tense or squirm about quite a bit while you study, this would have some effect on increasing your calorie need.

## INFLUENCE OF FOOD

The digestion, absorption, and metabolism of food increase the total calorie requirement slightly. It amounts to about 6 per cent of the total calories. This increase is sometimes referred to as *specific dynamic action*.

## CALORIE ALLOWANCES

The recommended daily allowances for kilocalories are shown in Table 8–2. At best, these recommendations can be only approximate because of

TABLE 8–1 CALORIE EXPENDITURE FOR VARIOUS TYPES OF ACTIVITIES *

| Type of Activity | Kcal per Hour |
|---|---|
| Sedentary activities, such as: Reading; writing; eating; watching television or movies; listening to the radio; sewing; playing cards; and typing, miscellaneous office work, and other activities done with sitting that requires little or no arm movement | 80 to 100 |
| Light activities, such as: Preparing and cooking food; doing dishes; dusting; handwashing small articles of clothing; ironing; walking slowly; personal care; miscellaneous office work and other activities done while standing that require some arm movement; and rapid typing and other activities done while sitting that are more strenuous | 110 to 160 |
| Moderate activities, such as: Making beds; mopping and scrubbing; sweeping; light polishing and waxing; laundering by machine; light gardening and carpentry work; walking moderately fast; other activities done while standing that require moderate arm movement; and activities done while sitting that require more vigorous arm movement | 170 to 240 |
| Vigorous activities, such as: Heavy scrubbing and waxing; handwashing large articles of clothing; hanging out clothes; stripping beds; other heavy work; walking fast; bowling; golfing; and gardening | 250 to 350 |
| Strenuous activities, such as: Swimming; playing tennis; running; bicycling; dancing; skiing; and playing football | 350 and more |

* Page, L., and Fincher, L. J., *Food and Your Weight*. Washington, D.C.: Home and Garden Bulletin No. 74, U.S. Department of Agriculture, 1964, p. 4.

individual variations. For persons who are lighter or heavier than the reference individual, the allowances would be decreased or increased. Women who have average physical activity require about 35 kcal per kilogram (16 kcal per pound), and men with average physical activity require about 38 kcal per kilogram (17 kcal per pound). The allowances for persons who are sedentary would be decreased, while those for persons engaged in hard physical labor would be much more.

The allowances for infants and for children are very high in proportion to their body size so that there is ample energy for growth as well as the high level of physical activity. Note, for example, that the 30-kg child between 7 and 10 years requires about 2400 kcal—a level that is more than his mother needs and only 300 kcal less than his father needs. (See Figure 8–1.)

TABLE 8–2 RECOMMENDED DAILY ALLOWANCES FOR ENERGY

| Age Years | Weight kg | lb | Energy kcal | Age Years | Weight kg | lb | Energy kcal |
|---|---|---|---|---|---|---|---|
| Infants | | | | Females | | | |
| 0.0–0.5 | 6 | 14 | kg × 117 | 11–14 | 44 | 97 | 2400 |
| 0.5–1.0 | 9 | 20 | kg × 108 | 15–18 | 54 | 119 | 2100 |
| | | | | 19–22 | 58 | 128 | 2100 |
| Children | | | | 23–50 | 58 | 128 | 2000 |
| 1–3 | 13 | 28 | 1300 | 51+ | 58 | 128 | 1800 |
| 4–6 | 20 | 44 | 1800 | | | | |
| 7–10 | 30 | 66 | 2400 | | | | |
| | | | | Pregnancy | | | +300 |
| Males | | | | Lactation | | | +500 |
| 11–14 | 44 | 97 | 2800 | | | | |
| 15–18 | 61 | 134 | 3000 | | | | |
| 19–22 | 67 | 147 | 3000 | | | | |
| 23–50 | 70 | 154 | 2700 | | | | |
| 51+ | 70 | 154 | 2400 | | | | |

Ordinarily, no calorie adjustments need to be made for climate. Most Americans live in well-heated buildings in winter and wear warm clothing. Many people now also work in air-conditioned buildings in the summer.

## Meeting Calorie Needs

### CALORIE VALUE OF FOODS

In the United States about 45 to 55 per cent of the total calories in the diet come from carbohydrate; 35 to 45 per cent of the calories come from fat; and about 15 per cent of the calories come from protein.

The caloric value of many foods is given in Table A–1, Appendix A. If you will examine this table you will find that you could draw some general conclusions about the caloric value of food groups. Some foods contain much water and some fiber and are low in calories. Vegetables and fruits, as a class, are in this group. The variation in calories between a tomato, for example, and a sweet potato lies in the much greater carbohydrate content of the sweet potato. Fresh fruits are much lower in calories than canned or frozen fruits, which have been packed in syrup.

Many foods contain little water but appreciable amounts of carbohydrate: flour, cereal foods, bread, sugar, candy, jellies, and others. Weight for weight these foods rank much higher in calories than vegetables and fruits.

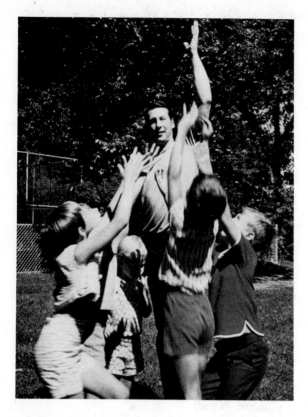

FIGURE 8–1 Vigorous physical activity increases the energy requirement. Throughout life physical activity should be encouraged as one way to maintain normal weight. (*Courtesy, National Dairy Council, Chicago.*)

The highest concentration of calories occurs in foods that contain much fat. Lean meat, poultry, and fish are moderate in calorie content, but fatty meats and fish are high in calories. Oils, butter, margarine, cooking fats, and cream are concentrated sources of calories because of their high fat content.

Many cooked foods are higher in calories because of the ingredients used and the method of preparation. Cakes, cookies, pies, and pastries contain much flour, sugar, shortening, eggs, and milk, and are, of course, high in calories. A piece of lean meat may be only moderately high in calories if it is broiled, but if it is dipped in egg, crumbs, and then fried, the calorie value could be twice as high. Deep-fat fried foods are, generally speaking, high in calories.

## CALORIE FALLACIES AND FACTS

1. *Fallacy.* Potatoes, bread, meat, and milk are fattening. Grapefruit is not fattening.

*Facts.* No single food can be called fattening or nonfattening. A calorie from one food is the same as a calorie from another food. Some foods provide more calories than others. One becomes fat only if the total calorie intake is greater than the calorie expenditure of the body.

2. *Fallacy.* Boiled potatoes are more fattening than baked potatoes.

*Facts.* Potatoes of the same weight will have the same number of calories whether boiled or baked. The "hidden" calories in the form of butter or cream would rapidly increase the number of calories.

3. *Fallacy.* Margarine has fewer calories than butter.

*Facts.* One tablespoon of margarine or of butter contains 100 kilocalories and equal amounts of fat and vitamin A. One tablespoon of whipped margarine will have somewhat less calories because air has been beaten in and the volume is greater; but gram for gram, or pound for pound, whipped margarine would be equal to regular margarine or butter in calories.

4. *Fallacy.* Toast has fewer calories than bread.

*Facts.* A slice of bread loses some weight when it is toasted because it dries out. The calorie content of that slice of bread does not change with toasting.

## CALORIE VALUE OF THE BASIC DIET

The minimum number of servings of the Four Food Groups supplies almost 60 per cent of the calorie needs of the average woman. Note in Figure 8–2 that the milk and meat groups are roughly equal in their

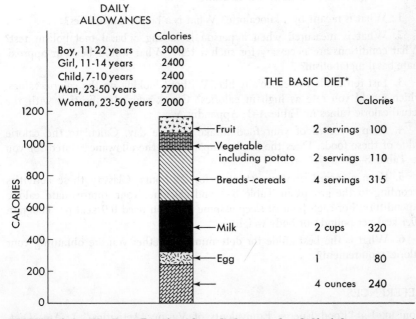

DAILY ALLOWANCES

| | Calories |
| --- | --- |
| Boy, 11-22 years | 3000 |
| Girl, 11-14 years | 2400 |
| Child, 7-10 years | 2400 |
| Man, 23-50 years | 2700 |
| Woman, 23-50 years | 2000 |

THE BASIC DIET*

| | | Calories |
| --- | --- | --- |
| Fruit | 2 servings | 100 |
| Vegetable including potato | 2 servings | 110 |
| Breads-cereals | 4 servings | 315 |
| Milk | 2 cups | 320 |
| Egg | 1 | 80 |
| | 4 ounces | 240 |

**FIGURE 8–2** The Basic Diet furnishes a little more than half of the energy requirements for girls and women. The full energy requirement is met by eating additional foods from the Four Food Groups and by including fats, sugars, and desserts. See Table 4–2 (p. 37) for complete calculation.

calorie contribution; likewise, the vegetable-fruit group and the bread-cereal group are about equal in their contribution.

## CALORIE BALANCE AND BODY WEIGHT

For the adult the best guide to the calorie requirement is the body weight. If the amount of energy needed by the body is less than the amount of energy supplied by the diet, the extra energy will be stored as fat, and the individual will gain weight. This is the problem that many men and women face. On the other hand, insufficient energy in the diet to meet body needs means that the adipose tissue will be used up, and thus weight is lost.

The adult in good health and who has a desirable body weight should aim to keep his weight constant. If people will weigh themselves regularly and will learn to avoid many hidden calories, to refuse second servings, to select low-calorie snacks, and to engage in a regular program of exercise, the maintenance of weight is not difficult. If a pound is gained, the effort should be made to lose it promptly so that there is no accumulation from month to month and year to year. (See also Chap. 21.)

## REVIEW QUESTIONS AND PROBLEMS

1. What is meant by a kilocalorie? What is a bomb calorimeter?

2. What is measured when a person is having a basal metabolism test? What conditions are necessary for such a test? What would be your approximate basal metabolism?

3. List ten foods you especially like. Without looking up the calorie values, which would you rate as high in calories? Check your classification with the actual calorie values in Table A–1, Appendix A.

4. Keep a record of your food intake for one day. Calculate the calorie value of these foods. Does the total compare with the allowance stated for you in Table 8–2?

5. Keep a record of your activities for 24 hours. Classify these activities according to the groups in Table 8–1 and calculate your approximate calorie expenditure. For each hour of sleep assume that you need 0.9 kcal per kilogram (0.4 kcal per pound) of body weight.

6. What is the best guide for determining whether you are obtaining your calorie requirement?

## REFERENCES

Konishi, F.: "Food Energy Equivalents of Various Activities," *J. Am. Diet. Assoc.*, 46:186–88, 1965

Leverton, R. M.: *Food Becomes You*, 3rd ed. Ames: Iowa State University Press, 1965, Chaps. 4 and 5.

Page, L., and Fincher, L. J.: *Food and Your Weight*. Home and Garden Bulletin No. 74. Washington, D.C.: U.S. Department of Agriculture, 1964.

Robinson, C. H.: *Normal and Therapeutic Nutrition*, 14th ed. New York: Macmillan Publishing Co., Inc., 1972, Chap. 7.

## 9

# MINERAL ELEMENTS

### NATURE AND DISTRIBUTION

Mineral elements are inorganic substances as contrasted to such organic compounds as proteins, fats, and carbohydrates. The mineral elements do not exist as such in foods, but are combined in salts; for example, sodium chloride. They may also be combined with organic compounds; for example, iron in hemoglobin and sulfur in almost all proteins. Unlike carbohydrates, fats, and proteins, mineral elements cannot be used for energy. They are found in all body tissues and fluids.

It is often said that valuable things come in small packages. About 15 to 20 mineral elements account for only 4 per cent of the body weight; that is, 2 to 3 kg (5 to 6 lb) in the average adult. They vary in amount from 1000 to 1500 gm calcium, which alone accounts for one half of all mineral matter in the body, to 20 to 25 mg iodine, to cobalt which is present in such minute traces that measurement is difficult. Yet the absence of any one of these elements can cause serious problems. An excess of some of them can be toxic.

A summary of the kinds and average amounts of mineral elements in the body is presented in Table 9–1. *Macronutrients* are those major elements that occur in the largest amounts, whereas *micronutrients* or *trace* elements are found in very small amounts indeed.

TABLE 9–1 MINERAL ELEMENTS IN THE ADULT BODY *

| | Per Cent of Body Weight | Man gm | Principal Locations in Body |
|---|---|---|---|
| **Macronutrients** | | | |
| Calcium (Ca) | 1.5–2.2 | 1050–1540 | 99% in bones and teeth |
| Phosphorus (P) | 0.8–1.2 | 560– 840 | 80–90% in bones, teeth |
| Potassium (K) | 0.35 | 245 | Fluid inside cells |
| Sulfur (S) | 0.25 | 175 | Associated with protein |
| Chlorine (Cl) | 0.15 | 105 | Fluid outside cells |
| Sodium (Na) | 0.15 | 105 | Fluid outside cells |
| Magnesium (Mg) | 0.05 | 35 | 60% in bones and teeth |
| **Micronutrients** | | | |
| Iron (Fe) | 0.004 | 2.8 | Chiefly in hemoglobin; stores in liver and other organs |
| Manganese (Mn) | 0.0003 | 0.21 | |
| Copper (Cu) | 0.00015 | 0.11 | |
| Iodine (I) | 0.00004 | 0.02 | Thyroid gland |
| Fluorine (F) | | | Bones and teeth |
| Zinc (Zn) | | | |
| Molybdenum (Mo) | | | |
| Selenium (Se) | | | |
| Cobalt (Co) | | | Part of vitamin $B_{12}$ molecule |
| Chromium (Cr) | | | |

Present but not known to be essential: aluminum, arsenic, barium, boron, bromine, lead, nickel, silicon, strontium

* Calculations based on elementary composition of the body as stated by H. C. Sherman, *Chemistry of Food and Nutrition*, 8th ed. (New York: Macmillan Publishing Co., Inc., 1952), p. 227.

## FOOD CHOICES FOR MINERAL ELEMENTS

If one burns a sample of food, the mineral matter or ash remains. The ash can be analyzed for the kinds and amounts of each mineral element present. Tables of food composition show the values for various elements found in foods.

Daily allowances for six mineral elements—calcium, phosphorus, iron, iodine, magnesium, and zinc—have been listed by the Food and Nutrition Board. (See Table 4–1, p. 32.) In your study of the mineral elements you should become thoroughly familiar with the food sources of calcium and iron. Recommended amounts of foods from the Four Food Groups furnish sufficient amounts of all the mineral elements needed by humans except possibly iron, iodine, and fluorine. Sources of these elements will be discussed further in this chapter. Usually, calculations for the normal diet need include only calcium and iron. For certain therapeutic diets calculations for sodium and/or potassium are required.

## GENERAL FUNCTIONS

For convenience mineral elements are often discussed separately. However, within the body they function together in building body tissues and in the regulation of body metabolism. Some of the important ways in which mineral elements function together are discussed below. Specific functions will also be listed under the headings for each element.

*Bone formation.* Bone consists of a soft, pliable, but tough protein material into which minerals are deposited. Most of the calcium, phosphorus, and magnesium, and smaller amounts of other mineral elements, are deposited in the bones and teeth. During the last two months of pregnancy most of the ossification of the bones of the fetus occurs. The infant at birth has a well-formed skeleton, but the bones are still quite soft. Throughout childhood, adolescence, and into the early twenties the bones continue to harden as well as to grow in length and in diameter. The individual who has ample calcium, phosphorus, and protein in his diet during the growing years will be taller than the one who is poorly nourished.

As well as providing the framework for the body, bones serve as a storehouse for the mineral elements they contain. They are never fixed for life. The blood can withdraw mineral elements from the bone according to the daily soft-tissue and fluid needs of the body. These withdrawals are ordinarily replaced from the diet. However, an individual who has a poor diet for a long time may have very weak, thin bones because of the day-to-day withdrawals. As much as 10 to 40 per cent of the calcium can be removed from the bones before it will show up on x-ray.

*Tooth formation.* Teeth, like bones, contain a ground substance of protein. The tooth enamel and dentine are hard substances containing appreciable amounts of calcium and phosphorus. The first teeth form in the fetus at the fourth to sixth week of pregnancy and begin to calcify by the twentieth week. The permanent teeth calcify soon after birth up to about three years of age. Wisdom teeth may calcify as late as eight to ten years of age. The teeth are fully mineralized before they erupt. The enamel and dentine are not supplied with blood vessels. Therefore, a decayed tooth cannot repair itself, so that proper care of the teeth once they have erupted is vital.

*Soft tissues* contain many mineral elements in their structure, including potassium, sulfur, phosphorus, iron, and others. In fact, every cell in the body contains iron and phosphorus as part of its structure.

*Enzymes and hormones.* Tiny amounts of mineral elements are constituents of specific enzymes or hormones, or they are the agents that initiate (activate) and speed up (catalyze) the activity of enzymes. These are a few examples: copper is required for the incorporation of iron into the hemoglobin molecule; zinc is necessary for the formation of insulin by the pancreas; cobalt is a constituent of vitamin $B_{12}$; sulfur is part of the thiamine molecule; and magnesium activates the enzymes involved in the use of carbohydrates, fats, and proteins.

*Nerve irritability and muscle contraction.* Body fluids contain exact amounts of sodium, potassium, calcium, and magnesium. These elements control the passage of materials into and out of the cell. They regulate the transmission of the nerve impulses and the contraction of muscles. If, for example, the amount of calcium is lowered, the individual might have twitching and cramping of the muscles and convulsions, and the rhythm of the heart might be affected. This condition is known as tetany. Potassium in too small or great concentration will also affect the contraction of the muscles and the work of the heart.

*Water balance.* The balance of fluid between the inside and the outside of each cell depends upon the correct concentrations of sodium and potassium. Sodium occurs primarily in the extracellular fluid, and potassium is found chiefly in the intracellular fluid. These balances are upset in edema or dehydration. (See Chap. 10.)

*Acid-base balance.* The body fluids are maintained at a constant pH at all times. The pH is a measure of the acidity or alkalinity. The mechanisms for maintaining acid-base balance are complex, but compounds containing sodium and phosphorus are important contributors to this function. (See Chap. 10 for further discussion.)

## Macronutrients

### CALCIUM

*Functions.* About 99 per cent of the body calcium is found in the bones and teeth where it is combined with phosphorus and other elements to give rigidity to the skeleton. The bones also serve as the storehouse for calcium needed for a number of cellular functions. Calcium is required for the complex process of blood coagulation. Together with other elements it regulates the passage of materials into and out of cells; controls the transmission of nerve messages; and brings about the normal contraction of muscles, including the heart.

*Utilization.* Calcium absorption from the gastorintestinal tract is regulated according to the body needs for maintenance and growth. A child who is growing rapidly would therefore absorb a greater proportion of the calcium in his diet than the adult who simply needs to maintain the proper levels of calcium in the bones and soft tissues. The daily absorption ranges from 10 to 40 per cent.

Since calcium salts are more soluble in acid solution, most of the absorption takes place from the upper small intestine. Vitamin D is essential for efficient absorption. Lactose from milk also improves the uptake of calcium.

The parathyroid hormone governs the correct amount of calcium in the blood. When the blood level of calcium is low, calcium is removed from the bones. When the blood level goes up, calcium is deposited in the bones or is excreted in the urine. Vitamin D is also essential for the normal deposit of calcium and phosphorus in the bones and teeth.

Calcium is excreted in the feces and the urine. Much of the calcium in the feces comes from the insoluble salts that could not be absorbed.

*Daily allowances.* The calcium allowance for schoolchildren and adults throughout life is 800 mg. During periods of rapid growth in teenagers and during pregnancy and lactation the calcium allowance is 1200 mg. (See Table 4–1, p. 32.)

*Food sources.* Any kind of milk—fresh whole, skim, evaporated, dry, or buttermilk—is an equally good source of calcium. Hard cheeses such as American and Swiss are excellent. You would need to eat 1½ cups of ice cream or cottage cheese to get the same amount of calcium as that in one cup of milk. Cream cheese and butter, although dairy products, are not sources of calcium. (See Fig. 9–1.)

Kale, turnip greens, mustard greens, and collards are good sources of calcium. Broccoli, cabbage, and cauliflower rate as fair sources. Such other greens as spinach, chard, and beet greens contain oxalic acid, which combines with calcium in the intestines to form an insoluble salt. This insoluble compound cannot be absorbed into the blood. Therefore, these greens should not be counted on for calcium, but they do not affect the utilization of calcium from other foods.

Among the fruits, oranges contribute some calcium, although oranges cannot take the place of milk. Canned salmon is a fairly good source of calcium if the tiny bones are eaten. Clams, oysters, lobster, dried beans, and peas are moderate sources, but these foods are not eaten often enough to make an appreciable contribution. Meats and cereal foods are poor sources. (See Fig. 9–2.)

*Deficiency.* Calcium deficiency becomes evident only after years of inadequate intake. Therefore, an adequate diet becomes a kind of insurance against future problems. Osteoporosis is a frequent bone disease observed principally in older women. The posture is poor, the bone mass

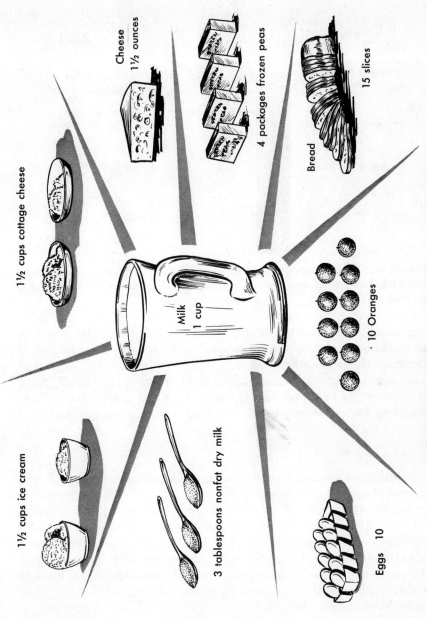

1½ cups cottage cheese

Cheese
1½ ounces

4 packages frozen peas

Bread
15 slices

Milk
1 cup

10 Oranges

1½ cups ice cream

3 tablespoons nonfat dry milk

Eggs 10

FIGURE 9–1  Calcium equivalents for 1 cup of milk.

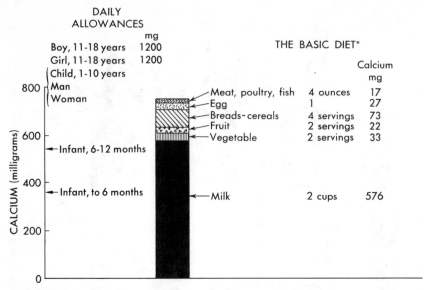

**FIGURE 9-2** Milk furnishes about three fourths of the calcium allowance for adults. The addition of 1 to 2 cups for boys and girls supplies their greater needs during growth. See Table 4-2 (p. 37) for complete calculation.

is reduced, the bones break readily, and healing is slow. The causes of the condition are complex, but nonmilk drinkers are more frequently susceptible than those who drink milk throughout life.

Rickets, infrequently seen in infants and toddlers in the United States, is a deficiency related to vitamin D, calcium, and phosphorus metabolism. (See Chap. 11.)

PHOSPHORUS

Probably no mineral element has more functions than phosphorus. It is essential for (1) building bones and teeth, (2) phospholipids that regulate the absorption and transport of fats, (3) DNA (deoxyribonucleic acid) and RNA (ribonucleic acid), which are nucleic acids essential for protein synthesis and genetic coding, (4) ATP (adenosine triphosphate) and ADP (adenosine diphosphate), which are necessary for storing and releasing energy according to the body needs, (5) enzymes that are required to utilize carbohydrates, fats, and proteins, and (6) buffer salts in the regulation of acid-base balance.

The phosphorus allowances for individuals of various ages are the same as those for calcium. (See Table 4-1, p. 32.) If the diet supplies enough calcium and protein, it will furnish enough phosphorus. Milk, meat, poultry, fish, egg yolk, legumes, and nuts are rich sources.

## MAGNESIUM

About 60 per cent of the body magnesium is found in the bones and teeth. Together with other mineral elements, magnesium regulates nervous irritability and muscle contraction. Magnesium activates many enzymes including those involved in energy metabolism. Like calcium, the salts of magnesium are rather insoluble, and much of the dietary magnesium is not absorbed. Most absorption occurs from the upper gastrointestinal tract.

The adult allowance for magnesium is 300 to 350 mg per day. Magnesium is a constituent of the chlorophyll of plants; so one would expect green leaves to be rich in this mineral element. Nuts, cereal grains, and seafoods are especially rich in magnesium. Recommended amounts of the Four Food Groups will furnish the daily needs.

Dietary deficiency of magnesium is not likely. However, some disease states give rise to symptoms of deficiency. Patients with diabetic acidosis, chronic alcoholism, kwashiorkor, and severe malabsorption diseases sometimes show the characteristic symptoms of tremor and nervous irritability.

## Micronutrients

### IRON

*Functions.* The total content of iron in the adult body is only 3 to 5 gm. Most of this iron is present in *hemoglobin*, a protein that consists of an iron-containing compound, *heme*, attached to a protein, *globin*. Hemoglobin is carried in the circulation in the red blood cells. It picks up oxygen in the lungs and transports the oxygen to the tissues so that oxidation reactions can take place in the cells. From the cells the hemoglobin carries carbon dioxide to the lungs to be exhaled.

*Myoglobin* is an iron-containing protein similar to hemoglobin and is present in muscle tissue. Iron is also a constituent of many enzymes that are required for the use of glucose and fatty acids for energy.

*Utilization.* Iron salts are relatively insoluble, and the proportion absorbed from the gastrointestinal tract is small and varies widely. The amount absorbed depends upon the body's need for iron. The well-nourished adult absorbs only 5 to 10 per cent of the iron in his diet, but somewhat larger percentages are absorbed by children during periods of rapid growth, by pregnant women, and by people who have anemia.

Iron salts are more soluble in acid, so most of the absorption takes place from the upper part of the small intestine. Vitamin C improves the absorption of iron, as do also the organic acids present in some fruits. The iron in plant foods is somewhat less absorbed than that in animal foods. Antacid medications interfere with the absorption of iron.

Iron is used very economically by the body. When the red blood cells are destroyed after their normal life-span of about 120 days, the hemoglobin is broken down. The iron that is released is used over and over again. Small daily losses amounting to about 1.0 mg do occur in the urine and from the skin. On the average, the menstrual losses account for 15 to 30 mg per month or 0.5 to 1.0 mg per day.

*Daily allowances.* The well-nourished woman should receive 18 mg iron per day, whereas the healthy man needs 10 mg. Infants and children need liberal amounts of iron to take care of the expanding blood circulation as they grow. More than 18 mg iron are required by the pregnant woman; an iron supplement is essential. (See Table 4–1, p. 32.)

*Food sources.* Foods in the meat group are good sources of iron, any kind of liver or organ meat being especially rich. (See Fig. 9–3.) Oysters and clams are rich in iron, but other seafoods are somewhat lower than meat. Egg yolk is an excellent source of iron, but egg white contains only traces. Legumes and nuts are fairly rich in iron. When dry beans are baked with molasses, the iron contribution is good.

Dark-green leafy vegetables of all kinds are especially rich in iron. Fruits are fair contributors. Dried prunes, apricots, peaches, and raisins

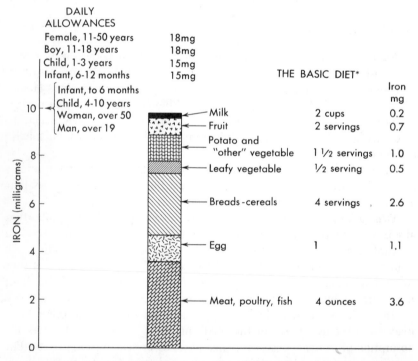

FIGURE 9–3 The Basic Diet supplies sufficient iron for the adult male. It is difficult to meet the recommended allowances for women and children unless fortified foods or dietary supplements of iron are used. See Table 4–2 (p. 37) for complete calculation.

are rich in iron, but their infrequent use means that the daily intake is not importantly affected.

The enrichment program for flours, breads, and cereals has had a significant effect on the iron intake during the last 25 years (see p. 58). Of the foods not included in the Four Food Groups, dark molasses is the only good source of iron, although it is used infrequently. Molasses in gingerbread or in baked beans, or the addition of one tablespoon molasses to milk (some children like this for variety), can make an important contribution to the iron intake.

From Figure 9–3 it becomes evident that the Basic Diet including recommended amounts of the Four Food Groups does not furnish enough iron for the girl or woman. In fact, typical American diets that are adequate in all other nutrients furnish about 6 mg iron per 1000 calories. The Food and Nutrition Board has stated that fortification of the food supply with iron is desirable.

**Deficiency.**  Iron-deficiency anemia is widespread in the United States, most especially in infants and in young women. Such anemia principally results from diets that have long been deficient in iron. Anemia can also result from hemorrhage following an accident or surgery or from chronic blood loss as from a bleeding ulcer.

In anemia the blood is unable to supply the full oxygen needs of the tissues. With even a little physical effort the person becomes very tired, looks pale, and may have a poor resistance to infection. When anemia is suspected, the diagnosis should be made by a physician because there are many kinds of anemia and likewise a variety of causes. Iron-deficiency anemia is most effectively treated with iron salts and an adequate diet. High-iron diets are impractical, since it is very difficult to obtain dietary intakes of more than 15 to 20 mg. Such levels are too low for effective treatment of anemia.

## IODINE

Iodine is stored chiefly in the thyroid gland, but it is also present in trace amounts in all cells. It is an essential constituent of two hormones, thyroxine and triiodothyronine, that regulate energy metabolism.

The adult allowance for iodine ranges from 80 to 140 mcg (see Table 4–1, p. 32). The iodide content of the soil in many geographic areas, for example the Midwest, is low, so that foods grown on these soils supply too little iodine to meet daily needs. On the other hand, foods grown along the seacoast, saltwater fish, and shellfish are good sources. Since people cannot be certain where the foods they consume are produced, the most reliable way to ensure adequate intake is through the use of iodized salt.

Too little iodine results in decreased production of thyroxine and a lowered rate of energy metabolism. In an attempt to produce more hormone the thyroid gland enlarges. This condition is called *simple* or *endemic goiter*. With a mild deficiency the only symptom may be slight enlargement of the thyroid gland, visible at the neckline. However, if the condition persists, the woman who has a simple goiter and who fails to get sufficient iodine during pregnancy will be unable to supply the fetus; thus, the baby is more severely affected than she was. When the deficiency is severe, growth is retarded and mentality is dulled.

More people in the United States today have simple goiter than was true some years ago because of less emphasis on the use of iodized salt. Endemic goiter is still a major problem in some Central and South American countries, Asia, and Africa. The most severe form of deficiency, *cretinism*, is seldom seen in the United States; in this condition the individual is stunted in growth and does not progress in mentality beyond the preschool years.

### ZINC

Allowances for zinc are listed for the first time in the table of recommended allowances. (See Table 4–1, p. 32.) The allowance for adults is 15 mg; for pregnancy, 20 mg; and for lactation, 25 mg. Zinc is widely distributed in plant and animal foods that are good sources of protein, and there is little likelihood of zinc deficiency when people consume a varied diet.

Zinc has a number of important functions: (1) it is part of the enzyme that transfers carbon dioxide from the tissues to the lungs; (2) it is essential for the production of insulin by the pancreas; and (3) it is related in some way to a normal sense of taste.

### FLUORIDE

Fluorine exists in the body in compounds called fluorides. Minute traces of fluoride are decidedly beneficial in protecting the teeth from decay. They may also be useful in maintaining the bone structure. To be of most value, fluorides must be supplied to the young child before the permanent teeth have erupted. In communities where fluoridation of the water supply has been used for some years, tooth decay has decreased up to 60 per cent.

Fluoride is best provided in the water supply. In a few communities the natural content in water is sufficient to protect the teeth. Many major cities and hundreds of smaller communities now add 1 part fluoride to 1 million parts water (about 1 mg per quart). This inexpensive, safe, and effective public health measure for protection of the teeth deserves the fullest public support.

In some parts of the world natural supplies of drinking water contain excessive amounts of fluoride (over 1.5 parts per million of water). People who live in these areas have *mottled* teeth; that is, their teeth have a chalky white appearance, and later become discolored. Such teeth are resistant to decay, and no signs of other health changes have been found in these people.

## OTHER TRACE ELEMENTS

A number of trace elements function primarily as parts of enzyme or vitamin molecules, or as catalysts for chemical reactions. They include:

*Chromium:* involved in carbohydrate metabolism
*Cobalt:* a constituent of vitamin $B_{12}$
*Copper:* a catalyst for hemoglobin formation
*Manganese:* enzyme systems; normal bone structure; blood formation
*Molybdenum:* enzyme systems
*Selenium:* related to activity of vitamin E

The amounts of these elements required by the body are not known, but at any rate they are very small. The mixed diet supplying adequate amounts of other nutrients will furnish sufficient amounts of these elements.

## SOME FALLACIES AND FACTS

1. *Fallacy.* A diet low in calcium leads to nervousness.
   *Fact.* When the diet is inadequate, calcium is readily withdrawn from the bones to supply the minute amounts needed to regulate the response of the nerves. There is no evidence that a low-calcium intake leads to nervousness.
2. *Fallacy.* Fluoridated waters are poisonous.
   *Fact.* Fluoride in water (1 part per million) reduces tooth decay in children by about 60 per cent. There is less osteoporosis in older people who have lived in areas with fluoridated water. If the water contains fluoride in excess of 1.5 parts per million, some staining (mottling) of the teeth occurs, but this is not harmful to health or to the soundness of the teeth.
3. *Fallacy.* Cocoa and chocolate interfere with the absorption of calcium.
   *Fact.* The amounts of cocoa and chocolate normally eaten do not interfere with the absorption of calcium. Although they contain some oxalic acid, one would need to eat abnormally large amounts of chocolate and cocoa to have any noticeable effect. Hot cocoa, chocolate pudding, and chocolate milk are quite appropriate in the menus of children as well as adults. However, the child should not be given these foods so often that he refuses to take regular milk.
4. *Fallacy.* Foods purchased in American markets are likely to be lacking in important trace elements.

*Fact.* The wide variety of foods used in the diet supplies ample amounts of all trace elements known to be needed except iodine and fluorine. See discussion on pages 83 and 84. Farmers use chemical and organic fertilizers in order to realize high yields of foods that are excellent in nutritive quality. Present-day techniques of food processing retain most of the nutritive values.

A summary of the mineral elements and review questions appear at the end of Chapter 10.

## REFERENCES

Cohen, N. L., and Briggs, G. M.: "Trace Minerals in Nutrition," *Am. J. Nurs.,* 68:807–11, 1968.

Council on Foods and Nutrition: "Iron Deficiency in the United States," *JAMA,* 203:407–14, 1968.

Council on Foods and Nutrition: "Iron in Enriched Wheat Flour, Farina, Bread, Buns, and Rolls," *JAMA,* 220:855–59, 1972.

Finch, C. A.: "Iron Metabolism," *Nutr. Today,* 4:2–7, Summer 1969.

Goulding, P. C.: "Why Doctors Vote Yes to Fluoridation," *Today's Health,* 43:8, October 1965.

Knutson, J. W.: "Fluoridation," *Am. J. Nurs.,* 60:196, 1960.

Robinson, C. H.: *Normal and Therapeutic Nutrition,* 14th ed. New York: Macmillan Publishing Co., Inc., 1972, Chaps. 8 and 9.

Staff Report: "Iodized Salt," *Nutr. Today,* 4:22–25, Spring 1969.

# FLUID AND ELECTROLYTE BALANCE

Two of the important functions of mineral elements mentioned in Chapter 9 are the maintenance of water balance and acid-base balance. These functions will be further described in this chapter together with a discussion of sodium and potassium, which are especially concerned in the maintenance of these balances.

## Water

Next to oxygen, water is most important for life. We can survive, at best, for only a few days without water; persons who have been lost in the desert have sometimes perished within 24 hours.

### DISTRIBUTION

About 50 to 60 per cent of the total body weight is made up of water. The proportion varies somewhat, with fat persons having less body water than lean persons. Infants and young children have more body water than older persons.

About three fourths of the water in the body is within the cells; this is referred to as *intracellular* fluid. The remaining water is in the blood and lymph circulation and in the fluids around the cells and tissues. This is called *extracellular* fluid.

## FUNCTIONS

Every cell in the body contains water. Muscle tissue contains as much as 80 per cent, fat tissue about 20 per cent, and bone about 25 per cent water.

Water is the solvent for materials within the body. The foods we eat are digested by enzymes in an abundance of digestive juices; the nutrients are carried in solution across the intestinal wall; the blood transports nutrients to all body tissues; materials dissolved in water are transported across the cell membranes; chemical reactions take place in the presence of water; and body wastes are carried by the blood for elimination by the kidneys, lungs, skin, and bowel.

Water is also a lubricant, for it avoids friction between moving body parts. Water regulates the body temperature through its evaporation from the skin, thus giving a cooling effect. On very humid days we feel uncomfortable because water does not evaporate very readily.

## NORMAL WATER LOSSES

Water is lost from the body through the kidneys, skin, lungs, and bowel. Usually, most of the water is lost in the urine. The amount of urine is related to the daily intake of water and other fluids, and varies from about 500 to 2000 ml. Because the nitrogenous and other materials must be kept in solution, about 500 ml urine is the minimum excretion.

An appreciable amount of water is lost through the skin by *insensible* and *visible* perspiration. Insensible perspiration is so called because one is not aware of it; it evaporates as rapidly as it is formed. On the other hand, with vigorous activity, especially in warm weather, we lose much additional water through visible perspiration. A baseball player, for example, might lose 3 to 5 liters of fluid through perspiration. Appreciable amounts of urea, salts, and traces of other mineral elements are also lost in the visible perspiration. When we perspire a great deal, the urine volume is reduced.

The adult loses about 350 ml water in the air exhaled through the lungs. The amount of water lost in the feces is small, averaging about 100 to 150 ml daily.

## WATER REQUIREMENT

The daily water requirement is about 1 ml per kcal; a requirement of 2000 kcal necessitates a water intake of 2000 ml. Infants have proportionately greater water losses, and should be allowed about 150 ml (5 oz) water for each 100 kcal. Thirst is a good guide for adequate fluid intake, except for sick persons and for infants.

## SOURCES OF WATER

The fluids we drink account for the chief intake of water. There is no harm in drinking water with meals provided it is not used to wash foods down without chewing them.

Foods contribute a fair amount of water, as may be seen from Table 10-1.

TABLE 10-1  WATER CONTENT OF FOODS

| | Water Per Cent | | Water Per Cent |
|---|---|---|---|
| Milk | 87 | Fruits and vegetables | 70–95 |
| Egg | 74 | Bread | 35 |
| Cooked meat, poultry, fish | | Dry cereals, crackers | 3–7 |
|     Well done | 40–50 | Cooked cereals | 60–85 |
|     Medium to rare | 50–70 | Nuts, fats, sweets | 0–10 |
| Cheese, hard | 35–40 | | |

Water also results from the oxidation of glucose, fatty acids, and amino acids. The amount of water produced in the body from metabolism is about 300 to 450 ml daily.

## WATER BALANCE

Ordinarily the water sources to the body and the water losses from the body are in balance, as the following example shows:

| Sources of Water | | Losses of Water | |
|---|---|---|---|
| Water, tea, coffee | 1100 | Urine | 1200 |
| Milk (2 cups) | 420 | Feces | 100 |
| "Solid" foods | 480 | Skin and lungs | 1000 |
| Metabolic water | 300 | | |
| | 2300 | | 2300 |

*Dehydration* results when the intake is less than the body needs. This can occur when, for some reason, there is no food or fluid intake, or when the losses from the body are abnormally high: excessive perspiration because of marked activity in hot weather; severe diarrhea; vomiting; fever with increased losses through the skin; hemorrhage; severe burns with the accompanying water losses from the skin; uncontrolled diabetes with frequent urination. Dehydration is a serious medical problem requiring prompt attention. Fluids are given by mouth when possible; intravenous fluids are given when the patient is unable to take sufficient fluid by mouth. In dehydration there has often been loss of electrolytes as well so that these will require replacement with the water.

*Edema* is the accumulation water in the body. It occurs when the body is unable to excrete sodium in sufficient amounts. This is not unusual in diseases of the heart when the circulation is impaired, or when the kidneys are unable to excrete wastes normally. Edema also occurs following prolonged protein deficiency, because the tissues are no longer able to maintain normal water balance.

## Electrolytes

### DISTRIBUTION

Electrolytes are chemical compounds that can break up into their ions when dissolved in water. They are called electrolytes because they carry electrical charges. *Cations* carry positive electrical charges; *anions* carry negative electrical charges. The total cations are exactly equal to the total anions.

The electrolytes in body fluids are measured in units called milliequivalents (mEq). The normal electrolyte composition of blood plasma and interstitial fluid is shown in Table 10–2. Note that the principal cation in blood plasma and interstitial fluid is sodium, and the principal anion is chloride. Within the cells, however, the principal cation is potassium, and the chief anion is phosphate.

TABLE 10–2  ELECTROLYTE COMPOSITION OF BLOOD PLASMA

| Cations | mEq per Liter | Anions | mEq per Liter |
|---|---|---|---|
| Sodium ($Na^+$) | 142 | Chloride ($Cl^-$) | 103 |
| Potassium ($K^+$) | 5 | Bicarbonate ($HCO_3^-$) | 27 |
|  |  | Phosphate ($HPO_4^{--}$) | 2 |
| Calcium ($Ca^{++}$) | 5 | Sulfate ($SO_4^{--}$) | 1 |
|  |  | Organic acids$^-$ | 6 |
| Magnesium ($Mg^{++}$) | 3 | Proteinate$^-$ | 16 |
| Total | 155 | Total | 155 |

In health the concentrations of the electrolytes in the extracellular fluid and in the intracellular fluid are maintained within very narrow ranges. Very little sodium enters into the cell, and very little potassium leaves the cell into the interstitial fluid or the blood plasma. Therefore, a change in the level of any of the electrolytes in the blood plasma is of great significance in the treatment of disease conditions.

## SODIUM

Sodium is found principally in the extracellular fluid. It helps to maintain the fluid and acid-base balance of the body.

Sodium in the diet is almost completely absorbed from the gastrointestinal tract. Any excess is rapidly excreted in the urine. A person who is perspiring heavily will also lose much sodium through the skin. The amount of sodium that is excreted is regulated by adrenal hormones that exert their control over the kidneys. When the sodium intake is high, the excretion of the kidneys is increased; but if the body stores of sodium, or the dietary supply, are low, only traces of sodium will be excreted by the kidneys.

No recommendations have been made for the daily sodium requirement. The daily diet provides far more than is needed, chiefly from salt used in cooking and at the table. Other sodium compounds used in food processing and preparation—baking powder and baking soda, for example—are also important sources. Milk, meat, poultry, fish, and eggs are well supplied with sodium.

When the kidney or heart is not functioning normally, sodium may accumulate in the tissues and water will also be held (edema). The need for diets restricted in sodium is fully discussed in Chapter 25. Dietary deficiency of sodium does not occur. However, excessive perspiration, severe vomiting or diarrhea, or diseases of the adrenal gland may lead to depletion of body sodium.

## POTASSIUM

Just as sodium is the principal mineral element in fluids surrounding the cells, so potassium is the principal mineral element within the cell. Potassium is essential for the synthesis of proteins, for enzyme functions within the cells, and for maintenance of the fluid balance. A small amount of potassium is also found in the extracellular fluid, and aids in the regulation of muscle contraction and nervous irritability.

No recommendation has been made for the daily intake of potassium. Most foods supply liberal amounts and dietary deficiency does not occur.

Problems of potassium deficiency are sometimes seen following severe vomiting, diarrhea and diabetic acidosis. Excessive potassium is a problem in renal failure. (See Chap. 26.)

## Acid-Base Balance

### pH

Body fluids are maintained at a pH ranging between 7.35 and 7.45, which is slightly alkaline. The pH is a measure of acidity or alkalinity. A pH of 7.0 is exact neutrality. A pH below 7 indicates acid; the lower the number, the greater the acidity. A pH above 7 indicates alkalinity; the higher the number, the greater the alkalinity.

A pH of 7.0 to 7.2 is abnormally low; it is called *acidosis* in relation to the normal level. It is seen in uncontrolled diabetic patients who are excreting large quantities of ketones (see Chap. 22). It also occurs in severe starvation, and in renal failure.

A pH above 7.5 is labeled as *alkalosis*. It results when there is prolonged, severe vomiting so that there is much loss of stomach acid. Alkalosis also occurs with excessive ingestion of soluble antacids such as sodium bicarbonate because such compounds are rapidly absorbed from the gastrointestinal tract.

#### REACTION OF FOODS

Some foods are potentially *alkali-producing* because they contain important amounts of calcium, sodium, potassium, and magnesium. Other foods are *acid-producing* because they contain greater amounts of sulfur, chlorine, and phosphorus than they do of the alkali-producing elements. Still other foods are low in mineral elements and are considered to be neutral.

*Acid-producing:* meat, poultry, fish, eggs, cheese, legumes, cereal foods, corn, almonds, chestnuts, coconut, prunes, plums, cranberries
*Alkali-producing:* fruits, vegetables, milk, peanuts, walnuts, Brazil nuts
*Neutral:* butter, margarine, oils, cooking fats, sugar, syrup, starch, tapioca

Certain fruits such as lemons, grapefruit, oranges, and peaches contain organic acids that give a sour (acid) taste. These acids are weak and they do not increase the acidity of the stomach. The hydrochloric acid in the stomach is a strong acid that is useful for the digestion of proteins. The organic acids in fruits are oxidized, just as are the carbohydrates, to yield energy, carbon dioxide, and water.

Plums, cranberries, and prunes contain an organic acid that is not metabolized by the body. The excretion of this acid increases the acidity of the urine; therefore, these fruits are sometimes recommended with other acid-producing foods to help counteract the formation of certain types of renal calculi.

## REGULATION OF ACID-BASE BALANCE

A number of acids are normally produced in the metabolism of food-stuffs. The body has several efficient mechanisms for taking care of these acids so that the normal acid-base balance is not disturbed.

A principal acid produced in metabolism is carbonic acid. This is released through the lungs by exhalation of carbon dioxide. When the carbon dioxide content of the blood increases, the individual breathes more rapidly and more deeply to get rid of more carbon dioxide.

Minerals function in *buffer* salts. A buffer is a substance that can react with an acid or an alkali without much change occurring in the pH. The sodium phosphate and carbonate buffer systems are important. Proteins are also good buffers.

The kidneys are the final regulators of acid-base balance. When excess acid is being produced, the kidneys secrete a highly acid urine, so that little change takes place in the pH of the blood. The kidneys also synthesize the ammonium ($NH_4^+$) ion which can combine with acid so that the body loses less of its sodium.

The healthy individual maintains acid-base balance regardless of the composition of his diet. Moreover, there is no evidence that shows the merits of an acid-producing or alkali-producing diet. In certain pathologic conditions such as renal failure or renal calculi these characteristics of the diet may be adjusted.

### REVIEW QUESTIONS AND PROBLEMS

1. Define these terms: insensible perspiration, water balance, ossification, pH, osteoporosis, fluoridation, cretinism.

2. List the ways in which water assists in making the nutrients of food available to the cells of the body.

3. Record your fluid intake for one day. Include water, tea, coffee, soft drinks, milk, fruit juices, and soup.

4. What reasons might account for edema? For dehydration?

5. Which mineral elements are listed in the Recommended Dietary Allowances? What are your daily allowances? How do these compare with those of a 14-year-old girl?

6. What other mineral elements are known to be essential for human nutrition? Why are there no allowances listed in the table of Recommended Dietary Allowances?

7. What is meant by intracellular fluid? By extracellular fluid? What mineral elements would you expect to find in each.

8. What mineral elements are especially important for each of the following: building hemoglobin; construction of bones and teeth; function of the thyroid gland; maintenance of water balance; release of energy from fats, carbohydrates, and proteins.

TABLE 10–3   SUMMARY OF MINERAL ELEMENTS

| Element | Function | Utilization | Daily Allowances Food Sources |
|---------|----------|-------------|-------------------------------|
| Calcium | 99% in bones, teeth<br>Nervous stimulation<br>Muscle contraction<br>Blood clotting<br>Activates enzymes | 10 to 40% absorbed<br>Aided by vitamin D<br>and lactose; hindered<br>by oxalic acid<br>Parathyroid hormone<br>regulates blood levels | RDA, adults: 800 mg<br><br>Milk, cheese, ice cream<br>Mustard and turnip<br>greens<br>Cabbage, broccoli<br>Clams, oysters, salmon |
| Phosphorus | 80–90% in bones,<br>teeth<br>Acid-base balance<br>Transport of fats<br>Enzymes for energy<br>metabolism | Vitamin D favors<br>absorption and use<br>by bones<br>Dietary deficiency<br>unlikely | RDA, adults: 800 mg<br><br>Milk, cheese, ice cream<br>Meat, poultry, fish<br>Whole-grain cereals,<br>nuts, legumes |
| Magnesium | 60% in bones, teeth<br>Transmit nerve<br>impulses<br>Muscle contraction<br>Enzymes for energy<br>metabolism | Salts relatively<br>insoluble<br>Acid favors absorption<br>Dietary deficiency<br>unlikely | RDA, adults: 300–350<br>mg |
| Sodium | Extracellular fluid<br>Water balance<br>Acid-base balance<br>Nervous stimulation<br>Muscle contraction | Almost completely<br>absorbed<br>Body levels regulated<br>by adrenal; excess<br>excreted in urine and<br>by skin | No recommended<br>intake<br>Table salt<br>Baking powder, soda<br>Milk, meat, poultry,<br>fish, eggs |
| Potassium | Intracellular fluid<br>Protein synthesis<br>Water balance<br>Transmit nerve<br>impulse<br>Muscle contraction | Almost completely<br>absorbed<br>Body levels regulated<br>by adrenal; excess<br>excreted in urine | No recommended<br>intake<br>Ample amounts in<br>meat, cereals, fruits,<br>fruit juices, vegetable |
| Iron | Mostly in hemoglobin<br>Muscle myoglobin<br>Oxidizing enzymes | 5–20% absorption<br>Acid and vitamin C<br>aid absorption<br>Daily losses in urine<br>and feces<br>Menstrual losses<br>Anemia is common | RDA, men: 10 mg<br>women: 18 mg<br>Organ meats, meat,<br>fish, poultry, eggs<br>Whole-grain and<br>enriched cereal<br>Green vegetables; dried<br>fruits |
| Iodine | Form thyroxine for<br>energy metabolism | Chiefly in thyroid<br>gland<br>Deficiency leads to<br>endemic goiter | RDA: 100–140 µg<br><br>Iodized salt<br>Shellfish, saltwater fish |
| Fluorine | Prevent tooth decay | | Fluoridated water |
| Zinc | Enzymes for transfer<br>of carbon dioxide<br>Taste | Little likelihood of<br>deficiency or excess | RDA, adults: 15 mg<br>Plant and animal<br>proteins are good<br>sources |

9. A woman patient asks you why it is important to drink milk. What would you tell her?

10. Write a menu for one day, including foods from the Four Food Groups. Do not use liver. Calculate the iron content of your menu. Adjust the menu so that it includes 18 mg iron.

11. What is meant by anemia? What lack in the diet may cause it?

12. Of what importance is fluorine? How is it best supplied?

13. List three acid-producing foods; three alkali-producing foods.

## REFERENCES

Abbey, J. C.: "Nursing Observations of Fluid Imbalance," *Nurs. Clin. North Am.*, 3:77–86, March 1968.

Anthony, C. P.: "Fluid Imbalances, Formidable Foes to Survival," *Am. J. Nurs.*, 63:75–77, 1963.

Burgess, R. E.: "Fluids and Electrolytes," *Am. J. Nurs.*, 65:90–95, October 1965.

Carlisle, N.: "Water, Thirst, and Your Health," *Today's Health*, 40:26, August 1962.

Fenton, M.: "What to Do About Thirst," *Am. J. Nurs.*, 69:1014–17, 1969.

**11**

Introduction to Vitamin Study | DEFINITIONS | CLASSIFICATION
AND PROPERTIES | MEETING DAILY NEEDS | SELECTION OF FOODS ·
Fat-Soluble Vitamins | VITAMIN A (RETINOL) | VITAMIN D |
VITAMIN E (TOCOPHEROLS) | VITAMIN K (MENADIONE,
PHYLLOQUINONE) | SOME FALLACIES AND FACTS · **Summary**
of Fat-Soluble Vitamins.

# VITAMINS: INTRODUCTION AND FAT-SOLUBLE VITAMINS

## Introduction to Vitamin Study

Undoubtedly the discovery of vitamins in the twentieth century will go down in history as one of the major factors in the improvement of health of people throughout the world. The fact that these substances in such small amounts affect the course of health in so many ways has also led to widespread abuse of them. Many people, lacking full understanding of how vitamins function, place emphasis upon vitamin intake from one source or another, while ignoring other equally important nutrients. Other people somehow expect that a vitamin pill will solve many nutritional problems. Let us now look at some of the facts concerning vitamins.

### DEFINITIONS

*Vitamins* are chemical compounds of an organic nature that occur in minute quantities in foods and are necessary for life and growth. They do not provide energy, but they facilitate the use of the energy nutrients. Nor are vitamins important constituents of major body structures; yet as constituents of enzymes they regulate the building of such structures.

*Precursors* or *provitamins* are compounds that can be changed into the active vitamin.

*Avitaminosis* means "without vitamins." It denotes a deficiency or lack of sufficient vitamin to carry out normal body functions. Some defi-

96

ciencies are so mild that a diagnosis can be made only by biochemical tests of the blood and urine. As deficiencies become more severe, clinical signs typical of the specific vitamin lack begin to appear.

*Hypervitaminosis* is an excessive accumulation of a vitamin in the body leading to toxic symptoms. Excessive intakes of vitamins A and D can be toxic.

Vitamin *antagonists* or *antivitamins* are substances that interfere with the functioning of a vitamin.

## CLASSIFICATION AND PROPERTIES

Vitamins are generally classified as fat-soluble and water-soluble. However, within each classification the vitamins differ in their chemical structure, their distribution in foods, and in their functions. Moreover, the deficiencies produced by lack of each vitamin are specific.

Fat-soluble vitamins are absorbed from the intestinal tract with fats and require bile for their absorption. Anything that interferes with fat absorption will also reduce the absorption of the fat-soluble vitamins. These vitamins are stored in the body, especially in the liver. They are stable to ordinary cooking and processing procedures. The level in foods is reduced by wilting, drying, and rancidity.

Water-soluble vitamins are readily absorbed, but the body does not store them to any appreciable extent. Therefore, they must be provided on a daily basis in the diet. Ascorbic acid and thiamine are readily destroyed during food preparation by the action of heat, by alkalies, and by solubility in liquids that are discarded. Riboflavin is sensitive to light, and much of the riboflavin in milk is destroyed if a clear glass bottle remains in sunlight for several hours.

## MEETING DAILY NEEDS

The recommended allowances for all age-sex categories for three fat-soluble and seven water-soluble vitamins are listed in Table 4–1 (p. 32). No recommended allowances have been established for vitamin K, biotin, choline, and pantothenic acid. As you study each of the vitamins, you should refer to the table of allowances so that you become familiar with the range for the various age-sex groupings.

The rapidly growing child needs proportionately more of the vitamins than the mature adult. The recommended allowances in each instance provide a generous margin of safety. The classic deficiency diseases can probably be prevented with half or less of the daily allowances. However, these lower levels would not encourage optimum nutrition.

## SELECTION OF FOODS

Values for five vitamins are given for commonly used foods in Table A–1, Appendix A. Most foods are poor sources of vitamin D and hence no values are published. Analyses have been made for a number of B-complex vitamins not included in Table A–1, but the nurse is rarely required to refer to these data. The diet that supplies sufficient thiamine, riboflavin, and niacin will also furnish enough of the other B factors.

In selecting food sources for vitamins we should keep in mind (1) how much of a given food we would ordinarily eat, (2) how often the food is eaten, and (3) how stable the vitamin may be after processing or cooking. Parsley is an excellent source of vitamin A, but it will make little difference in the average diet, because it is so often left on the plate or, when eaten, is consumed in such small amounts. A raw fruit might be a good source of ascorbic acid but might contain little of the vitamin after drying or canning.

Wheat germ, dried yeast, and fish-liver oils are rich sources of several vitamins but are generally regarded as dietary supplements rather than basic items of the diet. Liver and other organ meats are outstanding sources of vitamin A and B-complex vitamins; yet their contribution to the diet will be important only if these foods are included on a fairly regular basis— for example, once a week.

## Fat-Soluble Vitamins

### VITAMIN A (RETINOL)

*Nomenclature.* Preformed vitamin A is also known as retinol, retinoic acid, and retinal. The precursors of vitamin A are alpha-, beta-, and gamma-carotene and cryptoxanthin.

*Function.* Vitamin A is important (1) for the normal structure of the bones and teeth; (2) for the maintenance of the epithelium or outer layer of the skin, and the mucous membranes that line the nose and respiratory tract, the mouth and gastrointestinal tract, the eyes, the genitourinary tract, and the glands of secretion; and (3) for the formation of *visual purple*, which enables the retina of the eye to adapt to dim light.

Bile is essential for the absorption of carotenes from the intestines. Mineral oil can seriously interfere with the absorption of vitamin A; if it is used as a laxative, it should not be taken near mealtimes. The liver stores vitamin A, and well-nourished individuals usually have a sufficient supply to last for several months.

*Deficiency.* Night blindness (nyctalopia) is a form of vitamin A deficiency sometimes seen in this country. It is experienced when the visual purple is slowly produced in the eye because of lack of vitamin A. The affected person has difficulty in adjusting to the glare of automobile highlights or in trying to find a seat in a darkened theater, for example.

Skin changes and infections caused by lack of vitamin A are rarely seen in the United States, but are fairly prevalent in the Far East. With the lack of the vitamin the skin becomes *keratinized* (dry and scaly). Soft, moist epithelium normally offers protection against bacteria, but when it becomes dry and hard, infections of the respiratory tract, the mouth, the eye, and the genitourinary tract occur easily. Additional vitamin A does not provide further protection against infection to individuals who are well nourished, but it would be indicated for those persons whose vitamin A store has become depleted. *Xerophthalmia* is the severe eye disease caused by changes in the epithelium of the eye and is the cause of some blindness in the Orient.

**Recommended allowances.**   Vitamin A is measured in retinol equivalents (R.E.) and international units (I.U.). The latter designation will no longer be used when food tables have been converted to retinol equivalents.

The allowance for vitamin A from 11 years throughout life is 1000 R.E. (5000 I.U.) for males, and 800 R.E. (4000 I.U.) for females. During pregnancy and lactation the allowances are increased to 1000 R.E. and 1200 R.E., respectively. Intakes ranging from 400 R.E. (2000 I.U.) to 700 R.E. (3300 I.U) are recommended for infants and children.

**Sources.**   The animal stores most of its vitamin A in the liver; hence the liver of any animal—beef, veal, pork, lamb, chicken—is a rich source of the vitamin. Fish-liver oils are excellent sources, but are considered supplements rather than foods. Liver once a week or every ten days will go far toward ensuring the full weekly allowance. Many people do not like liver. However, with many other good sources of vitamin A, there is little excuse for an inadequate intake.

Whole milk, cream, butter, and whole-milk cheeses are good sources of vitamin A. One egg yolk furnishes one tenth of the daily allowance of the adult. Fortified margarine contains the same levels as butter.

Dark-green leafy vegetables and deep-yellow vegetables and fruits are rich in carotene, which can be converted into vitamin A by the intestinal wall. Among the carotene-rich foods are carrots, sweet potatoes, pumpkin, yellow winter squash, cantaloupe, yellow peaches, apricots, spinach, kale, turnip greens, dark salad greens, broccoli, and green asparagus. (See Fig. 11-1.)

**Toxicity.**   Vitamin A given to children in doses of 25,000 to 50,000 I.U. daily for several months has led to loss of appetite, failure to grow, fretfulness, drying and scaling of the skin, thinning of the hair, swelling and tenderness of the long bones, joint pains, and enlargement of the liver and spleen. These symptoms may also occur in adults after a somewhat longer period of excessive intake. The intakes far in excess of needs result when

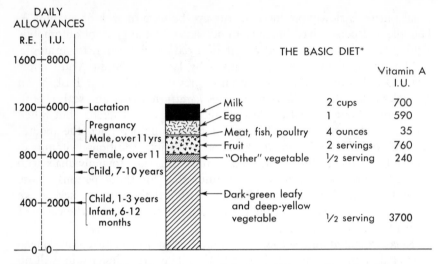

**FIGURE 11–1** The Four Food Groups of the Basic Diet provide a liberal allowance of vitamin A. Note the contributions made by dark-green leafy and deep-yellow vegetables. Breads, cereals, and white potato do not provide vitamin A. See Table 4–2 (p. 37) for complete calculation.

infants are given the wrong dosages of supplements, or when individuals persist in taking vitamin pills of high potency for prolonged periods of time without medical indication for need. The condition is corrected when the individual stops taking the supplement.

### VITAMIN D

**Nomenclature.** There are about ten forms of vitamin D. The two most common forms are known as *ergocalciferol* and *cholecalciferol*. Precursors of vitamin D are ergosterol in plants and 7-dehydrocholesterol in the skin.

**Functions.** Vitamin D is essential for the normal absorption of calcium and phosphorus from the gastorintestinal tract. It is also required for the normal calcification of the bones and teeth.

**Deficiency.** Rickets is the deficiency disease seen in children who fail to get enough vitamin D. Calcium and phosphorus are inadequately deposited in the bones. The soft, pliable bones yield to pressure, the joints enlarge, and there is delayed closing of the skull bones. The child may have an enlarged skull, chest deformities, spinal curvature, and bowed legs. (See Fig. 11–2.)

Rickets is rarely seen in the United States because of the use of vitamin-D milk for infant feeding. Premature infants are more susceptible to rickets than full-term infants. Insufficient calcium and phosphorus intakes may also be responsible for rickets.

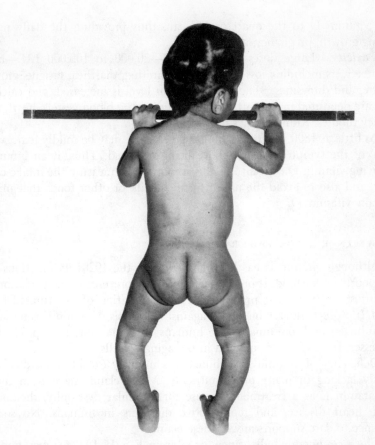

FIGURE 11-2 Early skeletal deformities of rickets often persist throughout life. Bowlegs that curve as shown here indicate that the weakened bones have bent as a result of standing. *(Courtesy, Dr. Rosa Lee Nemir and the Upjohn Company, Kalamazoo.)*

*Osteomalacia* is adult rickets sometimes seen in women of the Orient who have had a grossly inadequate intake of calcium, phosphorus, and vitamin D and have had several pregnancies.

*Meeting daily needs.* An allowance of 400 I.U. vitamin D is recommended for infants, children, adolescents, young men and women to age 22 years, and pregnant or lactating women. Adults probably get enough vitamin D through exposure of the skin to sunlight. However, clothing, soot, fog, and window glass cut off the ultraviolet light and prevent the change of the precursor in the skin to the active vitamin. People who work at night and sleep in the day, invalids who do not get out in the sun, and people who wear religious habits may require a vitamin D supplement.

*Sources.* Foods are not good sources of vitamin D except when they are fortified. Almost all fresh milk or evaporated milk is fortified with 400

I.U. vitamin D to the quart or tall can, thus providing the daily needs during growth, pregnancy, and lactation.

*Toxicity.* Large doses of vitamin D—20,000 to 100,000 I.U.—have severe effects including loss of appetite, vomiting, diarrhea, fatigue, growth failure, and drowsiness. The blood calcium level is increased, and calcium salts are deposited in the soft tissues, including the blood vessels, heart, and kidney tubules. Kidney stones may form.

As little as 1800 I.U. of vitamin D given daily may be mildly toxic, with some of the symptoms listed above being observed. Thus, if an infant is receiving vitamin D concentrate, it is important to measure the intake carefully, and also to avoid the use of fortified milk or other foods that might contain vitamin D.

### VITAMIN E (TOCOPHEROLS)

Although vitamin E has been known since the 1920s its functions are still poorly understood. It protects vitamin A by preventing the oxidation in the intestine. It likewise prevents the rapid oxidation of unsaturated fatty acids. It protects the red blood cell against hemolysis. Vitamin E is required by animals, and presumably by humans, for the normal reproductive processes. It may have a function in the aging of cells.

Deficiency of vitamin E in humans is unlikely except when diets are grossly lacking in many other nutrients. Many claims have been made for vitamin E as a treatment or cure for muscular dystrophy, rheumatic fever, heart disease, and reproductive disorders in humans. No sound evidence to date supports any of these claims.

The recommended allowance for vitamin E is 15 I.U. for men and 12 I.U. for women. The requirement is increased in diets that are high in polyunsaturated fatty acids.

Vitamin E is widely distributed in foods, with vegetable oils, shortening, and margarines furnishing about two thirds of the day's intake. Whole-grain cereals, legumes, nuts, and dark green vegetables are also good sources.

### VITAMIN K (MENADIONE, PHYLLOQUINONE)

Vitamin K is needed for the formation of prothrombin, a substance necessary for blood clotting. Intestinal bacteria normally synthesize a substantial amount of vitamin K. Because vitamin K is fat soluble, absorption is facilitated by the presence of bile. Anything that interferes with the absorption of fat will likewise interfere with the absorption of vitamin K. Only a limited amount of the vitamin is stored in body tissues.

Hemorrhage is the principal finding in vitamin K deficiency. It results from failure to synthesize vitamin K in the intestine or inability to absorb the vitamin. Some newborn infants have a tendency to hemorrhage because their intestinal bacteria are not sufficiently developed for synthesis of the vitamin. The hemorrhagic tendency may also develop in patients who have been treated with oral sulfa drugs or antibiotics, or in whom there is interference with the production or flow of bile.

The requirement for vitamin K is not known. Green leaves are an excellent source of the vitamin; cereals, fruits, and nonleafy vegetables are rather poor sources. Vitamin K preparations are sometimes given to the newborn infant to protect against hemorrhage.

*Dicoumarol* is a vitamin K antagonist. It counteracts the effect of vitamin K in the formation of prothrombin and thus prevents blood clotting. It has been an effective aid in treating heart diseases in which blood clots tend to form and that might endanger the patient's life.

## SOME FALLACIES AND FACTS

1. *Fallacy*. Supplements of vitamins, especially vitamins A and C, will help to prevent colds and other infections.

*Facts*. A normal diet based upon the Four Food Groups will furnish enough of all vitamins to maintain good health. It is true that some of the functions of vitamins include the maintenance of normal mucous membranes, the synthesis of antibodies, and healthy body tissues. But this does not mean that "if a little bit is good, more is better." In fact, if too much vitamin A is taken over several months, toxic effects may result (see p. 99). An excess of vitamin C would be excreted in the urine and would be of no value in building up additional resistance to an already healthy tissue.

2. *Fallacy*. Vitamin concentrates should never be used.

*Facts*. Sometimes vitamin concentrates are prescribed by a physician because of various disease conditions that may be present. Someone who is ill may have a very poor appetite and may be unable to eat the kinds and amounts of foods for an adequate diet. Other persons may have a disease of the gastrointestinal tract that reduces the absorption of the vitamins present in a normally adequate diet. Still other persons may have a deficiency disease because they did not understand what foods are necessary for health, or because they did not have enough money to buy a satisfactory diet. Once a deficiency disease is present, the most rapid way to cure it is to give large doses of vitamins in addition to improving the quality of the diet. Of course, these are all situations requiring a physician's diagnosis and prescription.

3. *Fallacy*. Vitamins from food sources are better than those from pills.

*Facts*. Each vitamin has a definite chemical composition. Thus, 1 mg of vitamin from a food source or from a concentrate may be expected to have the same value. But if the foods you eat for energy, protein, and minerals also furnish the vitamins you need, why spend additional money for vitamin pills that you do not need?

TABLE 11–1  SUMMARY OF FAT-SOLUBLE VITAMINS

| Vitamin | Metabolism and Function | Deficiency or Excess | Meeting Body Needs |
|---|---|---|---|
| Vitamin A precursors: Carotenes | Bile needed for absorption of carotenes<br>Mineral oil prevents absorption<br>Stored in liver<br>Bone and tooth structure<br>Healthy skin and mucous membranes<br>Vision in dim light | Night blindness<br>Lowered resistance to infection<br>*Severe:* drying and scaling of skin; eye infections; blindness<br><br>Overdoses are toxic: skin, hair, and bone changes | Men: 1000 R.E. (5000 I.U.)<br>Women: 800 R.E. (4000 I.U.)<br>Liver, kidney<br>Egg yolk, butter, fortified margarine<br>Whole milk, cream, cheese<br>Dark-green leafy and deep-yellow vegetables<br>Deep-yellow fruits |
| Vitamin D precursors: Ergosterol in plants 7-Dehydro-cholesterol in skin | Some storage in liver<br>Aids absorption of calcium and phosphorus<br>Calcification of bones, teeth | *Rickets*<br>Soft bones<br>Enlarged joints<br>Enlarged skull<br>Deformed chest<br>Spinal curvature<br>Bowed legs<br>*Osteomalacia* in adults (infrequent in U.S.)<br>Even small excess is toxic | Infants, children, adolescents, and pregnant women: 400 I.U.<br><br>Fortified milk<br>Concentrates: calciferol, viosterol<br>Fish-liver oils<br>Exposure to ultraviolet rays of sun |
| Vitamin E tocopherols | Prevents oxidation of vitamin A in intestine<br>Protects red blood cells<br>Limited stores in body<br>Polyunsaturated fats increase need | Deficiency not a problem in humans | Men: 15 I.U.<br>Women: 12 I.U.<br><br>Salad oils, shortenings, margarines<br>Whole grains, legumes, nuts, dark leafy vegetables |
| Vitamin K | Forms prothrombin for normal blood clotting<br>Dicoumarol is an antagonist | Hemorrhage, especially in newborn infants, and biliary tract disease | No recommended allowances<br><br>Synthesis by intestinal bacteria<br>Dark-green leafy vegetables |

## REVIEW QUESTIONS AND PROBLEMS

1. Explain the meaning of each of these terms: antagonist, antivitamin, avitaminosis, calciferol, carotene, ergosterol, keratinization, menadione, precursor, provitamin, rickets, tocopherol, viosterol, xerophthalmia.

2. If an individual is on a very low-fat diet, what effect might this have on the fat-soluble vitamins?

3. State the vitamin most directly concerned with each of the following items and indicate the relationship of the vitamin: visual purple, blood clotting, healthy skin, formation of bones and teeth, normal mucous membranes, carotene, ergosterol.

4. If your intake of vitamins A and D is more than you need, what happens to the excess?

5. Keep a record of your own diet for two days. Which foods provided you with vitamin A? What improvements are needed, if any?

6. Examine the labeling on fresh milk, evaporated milk, nonfat dry milk, and margarines. What information do you find concerning vitamins A and D?

7. What problems may arise if an individual uses vitamin A and D supplements in addition to an adequate diet?

## REFERENCES

Bieri, J. G., and Evarts, R. P.: "Tocopherols and Fatty Acids in American Diets," *J. Am. Diet. Assoc.*, **62**:147–51, 1973.

Cooley, D. G.: "What Is a Vitamin? " *Today's Health*, **41**:20, January 1963.

Hodges, R. E.: "Vitamin E and Coronary Heart Disease," *J. Am. Diet. Assoc.*, **62**:638–42, 1973.

Palmisano, P. A.: "Vitamin D: A Reawakening," *JAMA*, **224**:1526, 1973.

Robinson, C. H.: *Normal and Therapeutic Nutrition*, 14th ed. New York: Macmillan Publishing Co., Inc., 1972, Chap. 10.

# WATER-SOLUBLE VITAMINS

ASCORBIC ACID $\left(\text{VIT C}\right)$

*Functions.* Ascorbic acid (vitamin C) is essential for building *collagen,* the connective tissue protein that "cements" the cells and tissues together. The effect of this material is to provide firm tissues of all kinds: strong blood vessels, teeth firmly held in their sockets, and bones firmly held together. The body tissues maintain a normal saturation of vitamin C, but excessive intakes are excreted in the urine.

Ascorbic acid improves the absorption of iron from the intestines; it is needed to convert folacin to folinic acid (see p. 113); it is required for the formation of hormones such as thyroxine and adrenaline; it participates in the metabolism of amino acids; and it is essential for wound healing. By maintaining normal tissue health, vitamin C helps to protect against infections. However, it has not been established that massive doses will prevent or cure colds; in fact, large excesses of ascorbic acid may be harmful to some persons.

*Deficiency.* Severe deficiency of ascorbic acid leads to *scurvy.* This was the disease that figured so importantly in the sea journeys of explorers in the sixteenth century and accounted for the death of so many sailors. Scurvy is characterized by easy bruising and hemorrhaging of the skin, loosening of the teeth, bleeding of the gums, and disruption of the cartilages that support the skeleton.

Scurvy is occasionally seen in infants who have had a cow's milk formula for several months without vitamin C supplements. One of the out-

106

standing symptoms found in the infant is the extreme tenderness of the skin to touch. (See Fig. 12–1.)

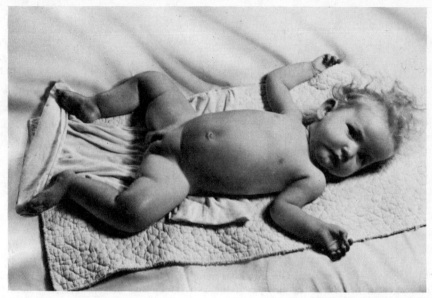

FIGURE 12–1 Infants who have been bottle-fed but who have no supplement of vitamin C will have scurvy. They assume this position because of the pain and tenderness of the skin. (*Courtesy, Dr. Bernard S. Epstein and the Upjohn Company, Kalamazoo.*)

*Meeting daily needs.* A minimum intake of 10 mg ascorbic acid daily will prevent scurvy, but higher intakes are recommended for optimum health. The recommended allowance for adults is 45 mg; for infants, 35 mg; and for children, 40 mg. (See also Table 4–1, p. 32.)

Ascorbic acid is sometimes called the "fresh-food" vitamin. It occurs in the growing parts of the plant, but it is absent from the dormant seed. Only the vegetable-fruit group contributes to the vitamin C intake. (See Fig. 12–2.) Human milk from a healthy mother supplies sufficient amounts for the young infant. Pasteurized milk contains only traces.

Raw fresh fruits and vegetables all contain vitamin C, but some foods are more outstanding than others. Oranges, grapefruits, tangerines, limes, and lemons are especially rich. Cantaloupe, strawberries, guava, and fresh pineapple are good sources. Blueberries, peaches, apples, pears, and banana are lower in vitamin C; if they are eaten in large amounts, they may be important for this vitamin.

The dark-green leafy vegetables so rich in carotene are also important for ascorbic acid. Tossed salad, or freshly prepared cabbage slaw, or fresh

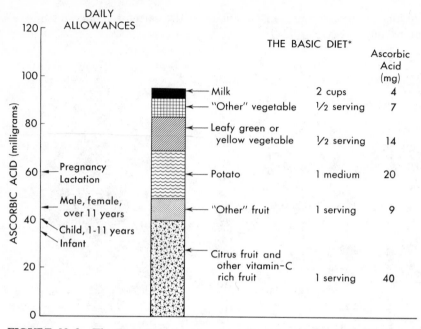

**FIGURE 12-2** The Basic Diet furnishes more than the ascorbic acid allowance for all age categories. Note the absence of the meat group and the bread-cereal group. For complete calculations of the Basic Diet see Table 4-2 (p. 37).

tomatoes are excellent sources. Broccoli is one of the outstanding sources; one serving, even after cooking, is equal in vitamin content to that of an orange.

Potatoes and sweet potatoes contain much less vitamin C, but it is sometimes said that "the lowly potato has prevented more scurvy than the lordly orange." This statement applies, of course, to those people who include appreciable amounts of fresh potato in the daily diet and who exercise care in proper preparation so that the vitamin is retained.

Canned and frozen citrus juices and fruits and tomato juice contain almost as much ascorbic acid as the fresh fruit. Cooked or canned non-acid fruits and vegetables lose more of the ascorbic acid. Frozen vegetables and fruits contain most of the vitamin C of the fresh product. On the other hand, dried foods contain only traces. Some food processors now add ascorbic acid to dehydrated potatoes. Labels should be read for this information.

### THIAMINE

*Functions.* Thiamine (vitamin $B_1$) is a coenzyme in many enzyme systems. These are involved principally in the breakdown of glucose to yield energy. Thiamine also aids in the formation of *ribose*, a sugar that is an essential constituent of DNA and RNA, the carriers of the genetic code. The adequate functioning of thiamine maintains healthy nerves, a good mental outlook, a normal appetite, and good digestion.

*Deficiency.* Thiamine deficiency may account for signs of fatigue, irritability, a feeling of depression and moodiness, poor appetite, a tingling and numbness of the legs, and constipation because of poor tone of the gastrointestinal tract. As you know, many other reasons could also explain such symptoms, and a diagnosis of thiamine deficiency could be made only with laboratory tests. *Beriberi*, sometimes called "rice-eater's disease" because it is often seen in people whose chief diet is refined rice, is the severest form of thiamine deficiency. It is still seen frequently in the Orient. The symptoms include polyneuritis (disease of the nerves, especially of the legs and hands), heart disease, and edema. Severe deficiency is sometimes seen in alcoholics who fail to get enough thiamine over long periods of time.

*Meeting daily needs.* The thiamine allowance is 0.5 mg per 1000 calories. Thus, an adult whose calorie allowance is 2000 would need 1.0 mg thiamine daily. For older adults 1.0 mg is allowed even though the calorie intake may be less than 2000.

Each of the Four Food Groups contributes importantly to the daily thiamine intake. (See Fig. 12–3.) Meats, especially pork and liver, are rich in thiamine and account for about one fourth of the average intake. Dry beans and peas, peanuts, peanut butter, and eggs are good sources.

Enriched and whole-grain breads and cereals supply about one third of the daily thiamine intake. Although individual foods of the fruit-vegetable and milk groups contain lower concentrations of thiamine, the intake of recommended amounts of foods from these groups accounts for about 40 per cent of the daily thiamine need.

### RIBOFLAVIN

*Functions.* Like thiamine, riboflavin (vitamin $B_2$) is concerned with the breakdown of glucose for energy. It is a component of many enzymes that are essential for a healthy skin and for good vision in bright light. If the individual ingests riboflavin in excess of his body needs, the urinary excretion will increase; if the intake is inadequate, the body conserves its supply very carefully and the urinary excretion will be practically stopped.

*Deficiency.* Riboflavin deficiency leads to *cheilosis*, a cracking of the skin at the corners of the lips and scaliness of the skin around the ears and nose. There may be redness and burning as well as itching of the eyes and extreme sensitivity to strong light.

*Meeting daily needs.* The requirement for riboflavin is related to the calorie and protein intake of the individual. The recommended allowance

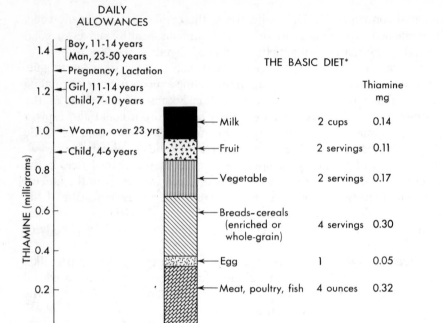

DAILY
ALLOWANCES

THE BASIC DIET*

| | Thiamine mg |
|---|---|
| Milk | 2 cups 0.14 |
| Fruit | 2 servings 0.11 |
| Vegetable | 2 servings 0.17 |
| Breads- cereals (enriched or whole-grain) | 4 servings 0.30 |
| Egg | 1 0.05 |
| Meat, poultry, fish | 4 ounces 0.32 |

1.4 — Boy, 11-14 years / Man, 23-50 years

— Pregnancy, Lactation

1.2 — Girl, 11-14 years / Child, 7-10 years

1.0 — Woman, over 23 yrs.

— Child, 4-6 years

THIAMINE (milligrams)

FIGURE 12–3  The thiamine needs of children and women are met by the Basic Diet. Additional foods from any of the Four Food Groups to satisfy the calorie requirement will also fulfill the thiamine need. See Table 4–2 (p. 37) for complete calculation.

for the reference woman is 1.2 mg and for the reference man is 1.6 mg. The allowances are somewhat higher in proportion to body size for growing children and during pregnancy and lactation.

About half of the intake of riboflavin daily is furnished by milk alone. Cheese is a good source, although some of the vitamin has been lost in the whey. Important but smaller contributions are made by meat, especially organ meats, dark-green leafy vegetables, and enriched cereal foods. (See Fig. 12–4.)

### NIACIN

*Functions.*  Niacin also is required for the stepwise breakdown of glucose in metabolism. Thus, if niacin, or thiamine, or riboflavin is missing in the diet, the metabolism will fail at the point of the missing enzyme. Moreover, each of these vitamins is needed for a specific step and cannot be replaced by any other. Niacin is essential for a healthy skin, normal function of the gastrointestinal tract, and maintenance of the nervous system.

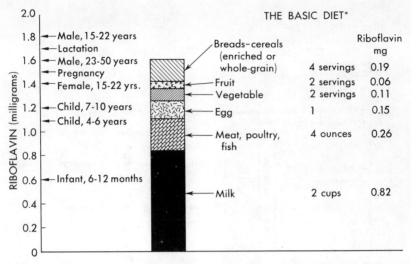

DAILY
ALLOWANCES

THE BASIC DIET*

FIGURE 12-4 The Basic Diet supplies sufficient riboflavin to meet the recommended allowances for all groups except teen-age boys. Note the importance of the milk and meat groups. See Table 4-2 (p. 37) for complete calculation.

*Deficiency.* Pellagra, the deficiency disease resulting from lack of niacin, is seldom seen in the United States. It occurs in areas of extreme poverty in some parts of the world where diets are low in both niacin and protein. Dermatitis, especially of the skin exposed to the sun, soreness of the mouth, swelling of the tongue, diarrhea, and mental changes including depression, confusion, disorientation, and delirium are typical of the advancing stages of the disease, which ends in death if not treated. The disease is sometimes referred to by the "4 D's"—dermatitis, diarrhea, dementia, and death.

*Meeting daily needs.* The recommended niacin allowance is 6.6 mg per 1000 calories. This can be supplied by preformed niacin in the diet and by tryptophan, an essential amino acid that is a precursor of niacin. Each 6 gm protein in the diet supplies about 60 mg tryptophan which is equal to 1 mg niacin.

The Basic Diet (see Fig. 12-5) supplies 13 mg niacin from food. In addition, the protein of the diet furnishes 720 mg tryptophan or 12 mg niacin; thus, the diet is equal to 25 mg niacin—about twice the daily need of the reference woman. Excess niacin in the diet is excreted and not stored.

The meat group, especially organ meats and poultry, is the chief source of preformed niacin. Dark-green leafy vegetables and whole-grain or enriched breads and cereals are fair sources. Milk contains little preformed

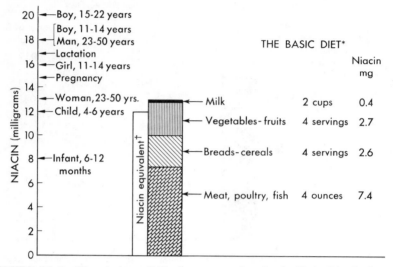

FIGURE 12–5 The niacin available from tryptophan in the Basic Diet is about 12 mg. The preformed niacin from the meat and bread-cereal groups brings the total well above the needs for all age groups. See Table 4–2 (p. 37) for complete calculation.

niacin. All good sources of complete proteins, including milk, cheese, eggs, meat, poultry, and fish, are good sources of the precursor tryptophan. Niacin is more stable to cooking procedures than thiamine or ascorbic acid.

### VITAMIN B₆

*Functions.* Three forms of vitamin $B_6$ exist: pyridoxine, pyridoxal, and pyridoxamine. The functions of vitamin $B_6$ are closely related to protein metabolism: the synthesis and breakdown of amino acids; the conversion of trytophan to niacin; the production of antibodies; the formation of heme in hemoglobin, and others.

*Deficiency.* Vitamin $B_6$ deficiency occurs rarely. The symptoms of deficiency include loss of appetite, nausea, vomiting, dermatitis, soreness of the lips and tongue, nervous irritability, and anemia. Some years ago vitamin $B_6$ deficiency was observed in infants who had received a formula in which vitamin $B_6$ had been inadvertently destroyed by high heat. These infants had a reduced growth rate, nervous irritability, anemia, and convulsions; they recovered promptly when adequate vitamin $B_6$ was provided.

*Meeting daily needs.* More vitamin $B_6$ is required when diets are high in protein than when they are low in protein. The adult allowance is 2.0 mg per day. (See also Table 4–1, p. 32.)

Meats, organ meats, whole-grain cereals, soybeans, peanuts, and wheat germ are rich sources. Milk and green vegetables supply smaller amounts.

### VITAMIN B$_{12}$

*Functions.* Of all vitamins, vitamin B$_{12}$ is the most complex. The trace element cobalt is an essential part of the molecule. Vitamin B$_{12}$ is required for the production of red blood cells in the bone marrow, for the synthesis of proteins, and for the metabolism of nervous tissue. A protein substance, known as *intrinsic factor*, is produced in the stomach, and is essential for the absorption of vitamin B$_{12}$.

*Deficiency.* Pernicious anemia is the disease resulting from vitamin B$_{12}$ deficiency. It is caused by lack of intrinsic factor in the stomach and not by dietary deficiency. Since the vitamin present in the diet cannot be absorbed without intrinsic factor, the normal functions of the vitamin cannot be performed. Patients with pernicious anemia have a macrocytic type of anemia; that is, the red blood cells are large and reduced in number. The patients frequently have a sore mouth, poor appetite, and gastrointestinal disturbances. The nervous system is affected so that the individual shows poor coordination in walking, for example; his mental processes may also be affected. Parenteral injections of vitamin B$_{12}$ effectively control the condition; they must be used throughout the life of the patient. Macrocytic anemia also develops in patients with severe malabsorption as in sprue, or in those whose stomach has been removed.

*Meeting daily needs.* For adults 3 mcg vitamin B$_{12}$ is recommended daily; 0.3 mcg for infants, 1 to 2 mcg for children, and 4 mcg during pregnancy and lactation. Milk, eggs, cheese, and meat supply ample vitamin B$_{12}$ even though the intakes of these animal foods may be relatively low. Plant foods supply practically no vitamin B$_{12}$, and use of an exclusively vegetarian diet for a long period of time will lead to some of the symptoms of deficiency.

### FOLACIN

The formation of red blood cells and the metabolism of protein are important functions of folacin, but it must be remembered that folacin and vitamin B$_{12}$ are both needed; they cannot replace each other. Folacin is converted to its active form, *folinic acid*, by ascorbic acid. Some folacin is synthesized in the small intestine.

Folacin deficiency occurs from (1) its lack in the diet, or (2) failure to absorb the vitamin in diseases such as sprue. It is not uncommon to find folacin deficiency in pregnancy; apparently the fetus has a high requirement for folacin. The principal characteristic of folacin deficiency is a macrocytic anemia. A sore mouth and diarrhea are usually present.

The recommended allowance for folacin is 400 mcg for adults and 50 to

300 mcg for children. The word "folacin" is derived from *folium*, meaning green leaf, and thus indicates that green, leafy vegetables are a good source. Organ meats, meat, fish, and whole-grain cereals are excellent sources.

### OTHER B-COMPLEX VITAMINS

*Biotin* occurs in extremely minute amounts in the body and in foods. It is required for many enzymes that participate in the metabolism of carbohydrates, fats, and amino acids. It is closely related to folacin and pantothenic acid in its activities.

No recommended allowances have been set for biotin. Average diets supply 100 to 300 mcg daily. A protein, *avidin*, found in raw egg white is an antagonist to biotin. The protein combines with biotin in the small intestine and prevents absorption of the vitamin. However, the amount of egg white that needs to be ingested is far in excess of the number of eggs that would be eaten in a day. No deficiency of biotin has been observed on typical diets.

*Pantothenic acid* is an essential constituent of a complex enzyme known as *coenzyme* A. This enzyme is a key, as it were, to the breakdown of carbohydrates and fats to produce energy. It is also involved in the synthesis of cholesterol and of steroid hormones.

No recommended allowance has been set for pantothenic acid. The word "pantothenic" means "from everywhere," and the vitamin is widely distributed in foods. Deficiency of pantothenic acid occurs only when the diet is markedly deficient in other vitamins. Meat, whole-grain cereals, and legumes are rich in the vitamin, and milk, fruits, and vegetables are moderate sources.

### SOME FALLACIES AND FACTS

1. *Fallacy.* Cooked vegetables are poor sources of ascorbic acid and thiamine.

*Facts.* Some losses of vitamins do occur with cookery. Properly cooked vegetables can still be good sources of the water-soluble vitamins if these rules are observed: (1) Do not soak vegetables or peel them a long time before cooking. (2) Cook vegetables until just done—crisp, tender, not soft, mushy. (3) Serve vegetables as soon as they are cooked. (4) Do not use baking soda to keep the green color.

2. *Fallacy.* Vegetarian diets supply all the nutrients needed.

*Facts.* If no animal foods whatsoever are eaten, the diet will not supply sufficient vitamin $B_{12}$. Deficiency of vitamin $B_{12}$ in children results in reduced rate of growth.

3. *Fallacy.* Raw milk should be used instead of pasteurized milk because it is a better source of vitamins.

*Facts.* Some ascorbic acid is lost in pasteurization but milk is normally low in this vitamin. Fruits and vegetables are the foods to depend upon for vitamin C. There is practically no loss of other vitamins by pasteurization. The most important reason for pasteurization of milk is to destroy pathogenic bacteria that might be present.

TABLE 12–1   SUMMARY OF WATER-SOLUBLE VITAMINS

| Vitamins | Metabolism and Function | Deficiency | Meeting Body Needs |
|---|---|---|---|
| Ascorbic acid Vitamin C | Strong blood vessels Teeth firm in gums Hormone synthesis Resistance to infection Improve iron absorption | *Scurvy:* Bruising and hemorrhage Bleeding gums Loose teeth | Adults: 45 mg Citrus fruits Strawberries, cantaloupe Tomatoes, broccoli Raw green vegetables |
| Thiamine Vitamin B₁ | Healthy nerves Good digestion Normal appetite Good mental outlook Breakdown of glucose for energy | Fatigue Poor appetite Constipation Mental depression Neuritis of legs *Beriberi:* Polyneuritis Edema Heart failure | 0.5 mg per 1000 calories Pork, liver, other meats, poultry Dry beans and peas, peanut butter Enriched and whole-grain bread Milk, eggs |
| Riboflavin Vitamin B₂ | Enzymes for protein and glucose metabolism Healthy skin Normal vision in bright light | *Cheilosis:* Cracking lips Scaling skin Burning, itching, sensitive eyes | Men: 1.6 mg Women: 1.2 mg Milk, cheese Meat, poultry, fish Dark-green leafy vegetables Enriched and whole-grain breads |
| Niacin | Enzymes for energy metabolism Normal digestion Healthy nervous system Healthy skin Tryptophan a precursor: 60 mg = 1 mg niacin | *Pellagra:* Dermatitis Sore mouth Diarrhea Mental depression Disorientation Delirium | 6.6 mg per 1000 calories Meat, poultry, fish, Dark-green leafy vegetables Whole-grain or enriched breads, cereals Tryptophan in complete proteins |

TABLE 12–1 (Continued)

| Vitamins | Metabolism and Function | Deficiency | Meeting Body Needs |
|---|---|---|---|
| Vitamin B$_6$ Pyridoxine, pyridoxal, pyridoxamine | Enzymes for protein metabolism Conversion of tryptophan to niacin Formation of heme | Gastrointestinal upsets Weak gait Irritability Nervousness Convulsions | Adults: 2.0 mg Meat, whole-grain cereals, dark-green vegetables, potatoes |
| Vitamin B$_{12}$ Cobalamin | Formation of mature red blood cells Synthesis of DNA, RNA Requires intrinsic factor from stomach for absorption | Pernicious anemia: lack of intrinsic factor, or after gastrectomy Macrocytic anemia; neurologic degeneration | Adults: 3 mcg Animal foods only: milk, eggs, meat, poultry, fish |
| Folacin | Active form is folinic acid Maturation of red blood cells Synthesis of DNA, RNA Not a substitute for vitamin B$_{12}$ | Macrocytic anemia in pregnancy, sprue | Adults: 400 mcg Deep green leafy vegetables, meats, fish, poultry, eggs, whole-grain cereals |

## REVIEW QUESTIONS AND PROBLEMS

1. Define each of the following terms: anti-pernicious anemia factor, beri-beri, biotin, cheilosis, cyanocobalamin, dermatitis, extrinsic factor, folacin, folinic acid, macrocytic, niacin equivalent, pellagra, pyridoxine, scurvy.

2. Which vitamins are most directly concerned with each of the following: scurvy, wound healing, healthy skin, pellagra, normal red blood cells, break-down of glucose for energy, intercellular substance for firm skeletal structure, tryptophan, bleeding gums?

3. If your daily intake of ascorbic acid, thiamine, riboflavin, or niacin is greater than your body needs, what happens to the excess?

4. What vitamins are added to flours and cereal foods through the enrich-ment program? Collect labels of several enriched foods and evaluate them according to your daily need for these vitamins.

5. Suppose a person is allergic to citrus fruits. What foods could you recommend to meet the day's needs for ascorbic acid?

6. Record your own food intake for two days. Which foods in your diet are providing you with riboflavin; niacin; thiamine; ascorbic acid? What changes do you need to make to improve your intake?

7. Normally you do not need to be concerned about the food sources for B-complex vitamins other than thiamine, riboflavin, and niacin. Explain why this is true.

8. Vitamin $B_{12}$ must be given by injection to patients who have pernicious anemia. Explain why this is true.

## REFERENCES

Erhard, D.: "The New Vegetarians," *Nutr. Today*, 8:4–12, November–December 1973.

Robinson, C. H. *Normal and Therapeutic Nutrition*, 14th ed. New York: Macmillan Publishing Co., Inc., 1972, Chaps. 11 and 12.

Sherlock, P., and Rothschild, E. O.: "Scurvy Produced by a Zen Macrobiotic Diet," *JAMA*, 199:794–98, 1967.

Stare, F. J.: "Good Nutrition from Food, Not Pills," *Am. J. Nurs.*, 65:86, February 1965.

Stare, F. J., and McWilliams, M.: *Living Nutrition*. New York: John Wiley & Sons, Inc., 1973, Chap. 16.

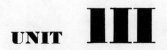

# PRACTICAL PLANNING

# FOR GOOD NUTRITION

**13**   Factors in Meal Planning | FOUR FOOD GROUPS IN MEAL
PLANNING | MEAL PATTERNS | ACHIEVING ATTRACTIVE, PALATABLE
MEALS | SNACKS · Nutrition for Older Persons | NUTRITIONAL
NEEDS | PROBLEMS OF FOOD INTAKE | DIETARY PLANNING |
COMMUNITY PROGRAMS · Pregnancy | NUTRITION BEFORE
PREGNANCY | DEVELOPMENT DURING PREGNANCY | NUTRITIONAL
ALLOWANCES | DIETARY PLANNING | SPECIAL PROBLEMS ·
Lactation | SOME FALLACIES AND FACTS

# MEAL PLANNING FOR ADULTS

A family may sit down, day by day, at the same table and partake of
the same choice of food with apparently different results. A six-year-old
boy seems to grow slowly, the teen-age boy may be a foot taller and 15 lb
heavier in a year's time, one parent may gain weight, and the other maintains constant weight. The six-year-old is often finicky about his food, the
teen-ager never seems to get filled up, and the parent whose weight never
changes appears to have a hearty appetite. If there are toddlers, preschool
children, or grandparents at this table, the homemaker makes particular
adaptations for them and yet tries to keep the meal as uniform as possible.

The ideas expressed above suggest that meal planning and food service
should be individualized within a unified pattern. The purposes of this unit
are to consider the particular emphases on nutritional requirements that
must be made in each phase of the life cycle, to study ways by which food
habits can be improved, and to learn something about meal planning,
food safety, and how to interpret information available to consumers. These
are practical aspects of nutrition that will be of equal value to you either
in your personal and family life or in your professional career.

## Factors in Meal Planning

### FOUR FOOD GROUPS IN MEAL PLANNING

Preceding chapters have emphasized why you need protein, minerals,
and vitamins as well as calories, and have shown how your needs are met

by using the Four Food Groups as a basis for planning. To satisfy the nutritional needs, one should first set up a skeleton plan for the day that includes the stated minimum amounts of foods from each of the four groups. See Table 13–1 for an example of such a plan.

TABLE 13–1  FOUR FOOD GROUPS IN A BASIC MENU PLAN

| Skeleton Menu Plan Based on Four Food Groups | Sample Menu | Typical Additions for Calories |
|---|---|---|
| *Breakfast* | | |
| Citrus fruit | Orange juice | |
| Cereal | * | |
| Egg | Egg, fried | Butter for egg |
| Bread | Whole-wheat toast | Butter for toast |
| | | Jelly for toast |
| Milk | Milk | Sugar, cream for coffee |
| *Luncheon* | | |
| Meat, poultry, fish— small serving | Sandwich 2 slices bread | |
| Bread | 1 ounce bologna | Butter or mayonnaise |
| | 1 ounce cheese | for sandwich |
| Milk | Milk | |
| Fruit | Stewed plums | Sugar for plums |
| | | Cookie |
| *Dinner* | | |
| Meat, poultry, fish— small serving | Baked meat loaf | Gravy |
| Potato | Mashed potato | |
| Dark-green or deep- yellow vegetable | Parslied carrots | Butter on carrots |
| Bread | Hard roll | Butter for roll |
| | | Tossed green salad |
| | | Russian dressing |
| | | Chocolate cake with icing |

* Note that cereal was omitted in the sample menu and used as a slice of bread for the sandwich. Two to four eggs per week are sufficient.

*Additions for the pregnant woman:* 1 cup milk at dinner or at bedtime.

The teen-age mother-to-be should include 5 to 6 cups milk daily.

When you examine the skeleton outline, you realize that not enough food is listed to meet the calorie needs of the man and the calorie and iron allowances of the woman. The man may, therefore, add any foods he desires so that he maintains normal weight: fats, such as butter or margarine for bread and vegetables, or salad dressings; sugar for cereals and fruits, jam, jellies, or marmalade on breads and rolls; desserts of many kinds, some of which add appreciable amounts of protein, minerals, and vitamins. Fruits are low in calories but increase the mineral and vitamin intake; puddings and ice cream add to the level of calcium, and somewhat to the amount of protein, as well as being somewhat higher in calories; cakes, cookies, pies, and pastries are high in calories and contribute in a variable way to protein, minerals, and vitamins, depending upon the specific ingredients used.

The teen-age girl and woman must select foods added to the skeleton menu pattern with care because their caloric requirements are lower than those of the man and their iron requirements are much higher. A serving of liver weekly, enriched or whole-grain breads and cereals, frequent use of dried fruits, molasses, and legumes enhance the intake of iron. Nevertheless, the recommended allowance of 18 mg iron is not likely to be met without the use of an iron supplement.

## MEAL PATTERNS

*Breakfast.* Far too many people skip breakfast, giving such excuses as not being hungry, wishing to lose weight, or not having enough time. Appetite for breakfast is largely a matter of habit; for many people breakfast is the most enjoyable meal of the day. It breaks the night's fast, helps to ensure energy for the morning's work, and reduces irritability. A light breakfast will provide one fourth of the day's calories even if one is reducing. (See Fig. 13–1.) As a matter of fact, people who do not eat breakfast often eat more frequently during the rest of the day, choosing high-calorie snacks, such as pretzels, soft drinks, candy, and so on. Each meal of the day should include some protein food for satiety value and for optimum use of amino acids. Breakfast is a good time to include fruit that is rich in vitamin C, whereas other fruits may be included at lunch and dinner. A good breakfast need take little time to prepare. Two examples of quickly prepared breakfasts are:

| | |
|---|---|
| Orange juice (frozen) | Stewed prunes |
| Wheat flakes *with* | Scrambled eggs |
| Whole or skim milk and sugar | Enriched toast |
| Toasted English muffin *with* | Butter or margarine |
| Butter and orange marmalade | Coffee |
| Coffee, if desired | Milk for children |
| Milk for children | |

*Luncheons.* Good lunches need not be elaborate. The following examples could be adapted to a carried lunch, one purchased in a cafeteria, or one prepared at home.

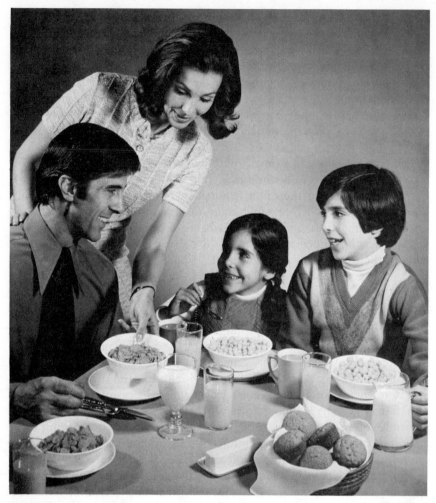

**FIGURE 13-1** Schoolchildren and parents start the day right by eating a breakfast that provides one fourth to one third of the Recommended Dietary Allowances. Breakfasts are more enjoyable when the family eats together. (*Courtesy, Cereal Institute, Inc., Chicago.*)

Fresh fruit salad with cottage cheese
Crisp roll with butter or margarine
Baked custard with caramel sauce
Milk

Split-pea soup (canned)
Sandwich
    Rye bread—2 slices
    Baked ham
    Lettuce
    Mustard, mayonnaise
Sliced tomato and cucumber on
    lettuce
Fresh peach
Milk

*Dinner.* The dinner meal customarily includes meat, poultry, or fish, with cheese, eggs, or legume dishes occasionally substituted. White or sweet potato, rice or pasta, plus vegetable, rolls or bread, butter, dessert, and beverage complete the meal. The vegetable should be deep-yellow or dark-green leafy at least every other day. If a salad is not served at luncheon, one should be included in the evening meal. The dessert should be light and simple with a heavy meal.

### ACHIEVING ATTRACTIVE, PALATABLE MEALS

In addition to planning meals for good nutrition, the following should also be kept in mind:

1. Select appealing color combinations. A dinner of baked fish with mushroom sauce, mashed potato, and creamed cabbage is lacking in color. Adding a touch of minced parsley and pimento to the fish, and the substitution of broccoli for the cabbage, would improve the appearance of this meal.

2. Include some soft and chewy foods. The tossed salad and hard roll add crispness to the sample meal shown in Table 13–1.

3. Vary the shapes of food portions. Several round mounds of food on the same plate are monotonous to the eye.

4. Provide satiety but avoid meals that are so heavy as to give one a feeling of fullness and discomfort. A meal with a hearty soup, meat, potatoes, and vegetables may end with fruit for dessert, for example.

5. Consider the flavor and odor of foods. Rubbing a salad bowl with garlic lends some interest to a salad, but a heavy hand with onion, garlic, pepper, and other seasonings is objectionable. Cabbage and onions in the same meal are poor choices, because they are both strongly flavored vegetables. To vary the flavors: combine some bland and spicy; include some sweet and some tart foods.

6. Adapt meal patterns to the family pattern of living. It makes little difference whether dinner is served at noon or night or whether breakfast is light or substantial in size. When the members of the family are engaged in much activity, the caloric needs are much greater, and the meals will be correspondingly heavier.

7. Prepare foods in a variety of ways. Any good cookbook will give numerous ways to cook meats, eggs, fruits, vegetables, cereal foods. Ground meat, for example, may appear in meat loaf, in chili con carne, in spaghetti sauce, in a macaroni casserole, as well as in hamburgers.

8. Good meals need not require a great deal of preparation time. Today's homemaker makes use of canned soups, frozen and canned fruits and vegetables, mixes, and many other convenience foods to save time. With careful selection, such foods do not cost much more than home-prepared products and may save much time. (See Fig. 13–2.)

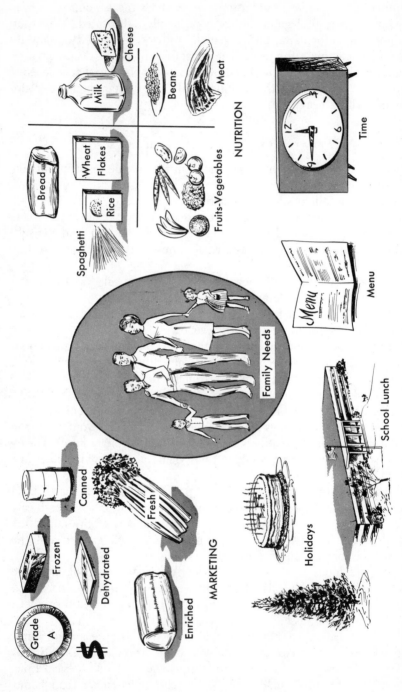

FIGURE 13–2 Good meal management includes consideration of nutrition, family needs, economics, time, attractive meals served in pleasant surroundings.

SNACKS

The coffee break and eating between meals are a well-established custom. Snacks should be planned as part of the daily meals. They should not replace breakfast or lunch. Some people eat snacks to gain weight; others find it easier to lose weight if they have five or six small meals a day rather than three larger meals; still others realize only too late that snacks can be the undoing of effective weight control. Soft drinks, doughnuts, cakes, sweet rolls, pretzels, potato chips, and the like are often a liability, because the additional calories are appreciable although the nutrient contribution is small. More nutritious snacks in increasing order of caloric value are:

Raw vegetables—celery and carrot sticks; tomato juice
Fresh fruits and fruit juices
Milk, skim or whole
Milk beverages
Ice cream, plain or with sauce
Hamburger on bun, pizza

## Nutrition for Older Persons

Aging is a process that covers the entire life-span. The metabolic changes that characterize aging are poorly understood. *Gerontology* is the study of the aging process. *Geriatrics* is the branch of medicine concerned with the prevention and treatment of diseases in older persons.

There is, of course, no specific age that characterizes a person as "old"; some people are "old" at 50 years, and others are "young" at 70 years. About 20 million people in the United States today are over 65 years old. Most of these people are productive, live in their own homes, and enjoy good health. Good nutrition, heredity, and environment play dominant roles in the maintenance of health.

NUTRITIONAL NEEDS

As you well know, it is altogether too common for people to gain weight as they become older. This weight gain is explained in part by a progressively lower basal metabolism after 25 years of age. In addition, older men and women are usually less active than they were in their youth.

The recommended energy allowance at 51 years and thereafter for men is 2400 kcal and for women is 1800 kcal. The allowances for thiamine, riboflavin, and niacin are slightly lower to correspond to these lower calorie requirements. The allowances for protein and most minerals and vitamins are the same as for younger adults. (See Table 4–1, p. 32.) Provided that she does not have an anemia, the woman who reaches 51 years can meet her iron needs with a daily intake of 10 mg.

### PROBLEMS OF FOOD INTAKE

People over 65 years of age are no more like one another than teenagers are like one another. The nurse is likely to encounter a great variety of problems concerned with adequate nutrition of older persons. She needs to be alert to these problems and to use ingenuity, patience, and kindness in solving them.

1. Inability to chew is a frequent source of difficulty because of poorly fitting dentures or absence of teeth.

2. Appetite usually declines in later years because the senses of smell and taste are less acute, the secretion of gastric juices may be reduced, and the satisfactions of sociability with family and friends may be lacking. Chronic disease and medications often interfere with the appetite.

3. Complaints of heartburn, belching, indigestion, and flatulence are frequent. Specific foods are often blamed for these effects, but no firm rules can be given that apply to all persons. Thus, one individual experiences discomfort every time he eats onions, and another enjoys onions and tolerates them well. Concern for the individual would omit onion for the former and include them for the latter.

4. Constipation is a common problem of the older individual and is related to the reduction of muscle tone of the gastrointestinal tract and to lessened activity. It is aggravated by eating too many soft, low-fiber foods and failing to drink sufficient fluid.

5. Chronic diseases of the heart, kidney, circulatory system, gastrointestinal tract, and joints impose needs for modified diets (see Unit IV) or interfere with tolerance for foods and ability to manage one's own diet.

6. A lifetime of poor dietary habits contributes to signs of nutritional deficiency including fatigue, anemia, fragility of bones, poor wound healing, and reduced resistance to infection.

7. Living alone, physical handicaps, inability to shop, poor cooking facilities, low income, frustration, boredom, and fear of the future all reduce the desire to eat or the capacity to prepare adequate meals.

8. Faddism and misinformation are responsible for much poor nutrition. Older people are especially likely to fall prey to the food quack who makes promises of good health, vigor, and even cure of disease.

### DIETARY PLANNING

The lifetime pattern of eating is not easily changed, and the older woman who has always liked rich desserts or the man accustomed to eating hearty rich foods will find it difficult to adjust to the lower calorie require-ments. The Four Food Groups still furnish the basis for meal planning because they provide all the nutrients needed by the older man and woman. (See Table 13–1.) Since the Basic Diet provides 1165 kcal (see Table 4–2, p. 37), the woman of 51 years or older will need to restrict her intake of calorie-rich foods lest she rapidly gain weight. Some useful points to keep in mind when planning meals for older persons are noted below.

1. Consider the food likes and dislikes of the individual. Learn to use essential foods in dishes acceptable to the person. For example, milk may be disliked as a beverage but well accepted in puddings, custards, cream soups, and cream sauces, on cereals, and so on.

2. Use fried foods, rich desserts, highly seasoned foods, and strongly flavored vegetables with discretion and according to the patient's tolerance.

3. If chewing is difficult, adjust the meals to include finely minced or chopped meats, soft breads, fruits, and vegetables.

4. Serve four or five small meals when the appetite is poor.

5. Breakfast is the meal most enjoyed by many older persons, and every effort should be made to provide pleasing variety.

6. Dinner at noon rather than in the evening is preferred by some.

7. If coffee and tea produce insomnia, they should be restricted to meals early in the day.

8. Encourage a liberal fluid intake daily. Adjust the fiber content of the diet if constipation is a problem.

### COMMUNITY PROGRAMS

*Home-delivered meals,* widely known as "Meals on Wheels," is a pro-gram that provides a hot noon meal, and a cold evening meal for elderly persons who are unable to prepare their own meals. The program is sponsored by community agencies, for example, hospitals and churches. *Congregate feeding programs* are federally funded to provide one meal a day for at least five days a week to elderly persons who come to a central site for the meals. Nutrition education, socialization, periodic health checks, and recreational activities are important components of this program.

## Pregnancy

The orderly sequence of fetal development and growth, the mechanisms for nourishment of the fetus, the storage of nutrients in anticipation of labor and delivery, and the development of the mammary glands represent a level of anabolism unequaled in any other time of life. All these needs can be met only through a diet planned to meet these increased requirements.

## NUTRITION BEFORE PREGNANCY

The young woman who is in good health prior to conception and who maintains good nutrition has the best chance of a pregnancy without complications, a healthy baby, and the ability to nurse. During early pregnancy, often before the woman is even aware that she is pregnant, critical development of the fetus takes place.

Two of every five first babies are born to young women under 20 years of age. These young women must still meet the growth needs of their own maturing bodies as well as the nutritional demands of the fetus. Yet, girls in their teens have, far too often, had diets that were inadequate in calcium, iron, and protein. Pregnant girls under 17 years are in an especially high risk category. They have more frequent complications of toxemia, anemia, and long difficult labor. Babies born to them are more often of low birth weight and have a higher rate of neonatal mortality.

## DEVELOPMENT DURING PREGNANCY

During the first two weeks after conception the embryo is fixed in its position in the uterus. The placenta, which is the organ that transfers nutrients from the maternal circulation to the fetus, is well developed early in pregnancy. During the second to eighth weeks there is a rapid development of the skeleton and the organs so that the tiny fetus is a clearly distinguishable human being. By the twelfth week the fetus still weighs only about 30 gm.

The total weight gain during pregnancy should average about 11 kg (24 lb). The weight gain throughout pregnancy should be gradual and steady. During the first trimester a total gain of 0.65 to 1.4 kg (1.4 to 3.0 lb) is normal; for the second and third trimesters a weekly gain of 350 gm (0.8 lb) should be expected. (See Fig. 13–3.)

The weight gain is accounted for in part as follows: fetus, 3300 gm (7½ lb); uterus, 900 gm (2 lb); placenta and membranes, 1450 gm (3 lb); breast tissue, 900 gm; increase in blood volume, 1500 gm. In addition there are considerable stores of protein, fat, calcium, and phosphorus in preparation for delivery and lactation.

## NUTRITIONAL ALLOWANCES

The recommended allowances for some of the nutrients for girls and women prior to and during pregnancy and lactation are shown in Table 13–2. (See also Table 4–1 [p. 32] for other nutrients required.) If one compares these allowances with the value of the basic diet (Table 4–2, p. 37), it is apparent that calcium, iron, and vitamin D are nutrients that require particular emphasis.

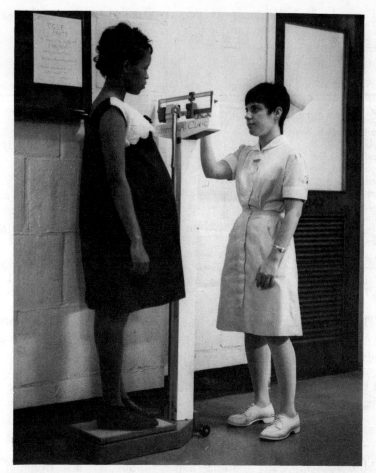

FIGURE 13-3  A steady rate of weight gain should be maintained throughout preg-nancy. A total gain of 10 to 12 kg (22 to 26 lb) is normal. *(Courtesy, School of Nursing, Thomas Jefferson University, Philadelphia.)*

## DIETARY PLANNING

The addition of 1½ cups milk to the basic diet pattern (see Table 13-1) meets additional calcium required by the woman, and supplies vitamin A and B-complex vitamins. The teen-age girl needs to consume 5 to 5½ cups milk daily to meet her calcium requirements.

If plain milk is disliked, it may be flavored with chocolate, coffee, molasses, or fruit purées such as strawberry or apricot. Milk may also be used on cereals and in soups and puddings. One ounce of American or Swiss cheese supplies about the same amount of protein and calcium as one cup of milk. Skim milk fortified with vitamins A and D may be substituted for part or all of the whole milk.

**TABLE 13–2** RECOMMENDED DIETARY ALLOWANCES FOR GIRLS AND WOMEN BEFORE AND DURING PREGNANCY AND LACTATION

| Nutrient | Girl 15–18 Years | Woman 19 Years and Over | Pregnancy | Lactation |
|---|---|---|---|---|
| Energy, kcal | 2100 | 2100–2000 * | +300 | +500 |
| Protein, gm | 48 | 46 | + 30 | + 20 |
| Vitamin A, R.E. (I.U.) | 800 (4000) | 800 (4000) | 1000 (5000) | 1200 (6000) |
| Vitamin D. I.U. | 400 | — | 400 | 400 |
| Ascorbic acid, mg | 45 | 45 | 60 | 80 |
| Folacin, mcg | 400 | 400 | 800 | 600 |
| Niacin, mg | 14 | 14–13 * | + 2 | + 4 |
| Riboflavin, mg | 1.4 | 1.4–1.2 * | + 0.3 | + 0.5 |
| Thiamine, mg | 1.1 | 1.1–1.0 * | + 0.3 | + 0.3 |
| Calcium, mg | 1200 | 800 | 1200–1600 † | 1200–1600 † |
| Iodine, mcg | 115 | 100 | 125–140 † | 150–165 † |
| Iron, mg | 18 | 18 | 18+ | 18 |

\* The second figure in the range applies to women 23 years and over.
† The second figure in this range applies to the teen-age girl.

The iron allowance cannot be met from foods alone. Ferrous salts to provide 30 to 60 mg iron are usually prescribed by the physician. A supplement of 200 to 400 mcg of folacin is also recommended. Ordinarily it is not necessary to use other mineral or vitamin supplements, providing that the milk used is fortified with vitamin D. Iodized salt should be used instead of plain salt.

SPECIAL PROBLEMS

*Mild nausea.* Early morning nausea during the first trimester can usually be overcome by eating some high-carbohydrate food, such as dry toast, crackers, or hard candy before arising. Fatty and fried foods should be restricted. Several small meals a day, rather than three large meals, may be more desirable. Fluids should be taken between meals and not at meal time.

*Food cravings.* Women often experience cravings for certain foods during pregnancy. When these foods are a part of a nutritious diet or don't displace essential foods, these cravings can be satisfied. *Pica,* or craving for abnormal substances such as laundry starch, clay, chalk, or coal, is found among some women, especially in low-income groups. Consuming large amounts of these substances seriously interferes with the intake of nutritious foods, and should be corrected by education and by assuring the means to obtain an adequate diet.

*Anemia.* Iron-deficiency anemia during pregnancy increases the likelihood of premature birth. The baby at birth is less well supplied with hemoglobin and thus is likely to become anemic during the first year of life. Macrocytic anemia caused by insufficient folacin sometimes occurs in pregnancy. These anemias are prevented or treated by supplements of iron and folacin, respectively.

*Constipation* is rather common during the latter part of pregnancy. It can usually be avoided by placing more emphasis upon raw fruits and vegetables, some whole-grain breads and cereals, a liberal intake of liquids, and a regular program of exercise.

*Toxemia of pregnancy.* This condition is characterized by increased blood pressure, swelling of the hands, face, and ankles, and proteinuria. A sudden gain in weight after the 20th week of pregnancy indicates water retention. The causes of toxemia are little understood, but lack of prenatal care and poverty are associated with the condition. Restriction of calories, protein, and/or sodium have often been tried in the past. These dietary restrictions are no longer considered to be useful, and are potentially dangerous.

## Lactation

The lactating woman will produce 550 to 850 ml (20 to 30 oz) of milk each day, representing 20 to 30 gm protein and 400 to 600 kcal. In order to produce this milk, her nutritive allowances are increased as shown in Table 13–2. The calorie needs are best met by choosing more foods from the four food groups. She should continue to consume the amounts of milk recommended for pregnancy.

### SOME FALLACIES AND FACTS

1. *Fallacy.* People over 50 years of age have much lower needs for protein, minerals, and vitamins than do younger adults.

*Fact.* The requirements for most nutrients are the same for adults of any age. Older people need fewer calories and so they must select foods with care to ensure adequate intake of protein, minerals, and vitamins.

2. *Fallacy.* Milk and cheese are constipating, and therefore should be omitted by some older persons.

*Fact.* Milk and cheese are almost completely digested and leave little residue. Constipation is corrected by including sufficient amounts of raw fruits and vegetables, whole-grain breads and cereals, and liquids, and not by the omission of milk and cheese.

3. *Fallacy.* As long as the mother receives plenty of vitamins the fetus will receive all of its nutritional needs regardless of the mother's nutritional status.

*Fact.* Vitamin supplements cannot make up for inadequate intakes of protein, calcium, iron, and other minerals. If the mother is poorly nourished, both mother and baby will be adversely affected.

4. *Fallacy.* The obese pregnant woman should use a low calorie diet so that the baby will be small and delivery will be less difficult.

*Fact.* Calorie restriction and weight loss are not recommended during pregnancy. Small babies are at greater risk during the early months of life. Weight loss should be planned after the birth of the baby.

5. *Fallacy.* Pregnant women should restrict their salt intake.

*Fact.* Pregnant women probably have higher requirements for sodium, and salt restriction can be dangerous. The pregnant woman should be allowed to salt her food to taste.

## REVIEW QUESTIONS AND PROBLEMS

1. Write a menu for one day that is satisfactory for a healthy young man or woman. How would you change this menu for a 25-year-old pregnant woman? What further changes are necessary for the teen-age mother-to-be?

2. Why is good nutrition so important prior to pregnancy?

3. Compare the nutritional needs of a woman of 25 years and of 65 years. How would you adapt the menu you wrote (question 1) for the older woman.

4. As a nurse, what problems might you find in feeding the elderly patient? What measures can you take to meet them?

5. Why is anemia such a serious problem in pregnancy?

6. Describe the normal pattern of weight gain during pregnancy. Why is a low-calorie diet undesirable?

7. What is meant by pica?

8. List five ways to increase milk intake by a person who does not like to drink milk.

## REFERENCES

Anderson, E. H., and Lesser, A. J.: "Maternity Care in the United States: Gains and Gaps," *Am. J. Nurs.*, 66:1539–44, 1966.

Beck, J.: "Guarding the Unborn," *Today's Health*, 46:38, January 1968.

Breeling, J. L.: "Are We Snacking Our Way to Malnutrition," *Today's Health*, 48:48, January 1970.

*Food Guide for Older Folks*, Home and Garden Bulletin No. 17. Washington, D.C.: U.S. Department of Agriculture, 1972.

Foster, H. A.: "Understanding the Senior Citizen," *Nurs. Care*, 6:27–31, June 1973.

Irwin, T.: "How to Handle the Problems of Aging," *Today's Health*, 47:28, July 1969.

Jacobson, H. N.: "Maternal Nutrition," *Modern Med.*, 39:102–105, October 18, 1971.

Pelcovits, J.: "Nutrition Education in Group Meals Programs for the Aged," *J. Nutr. Educ.*, 5:118–20, April 1973.

*Prenatal Care.* Washington, D.C.: Children's Bureau, U.S. Department of Health, Education, and Welfare, 1967.

Schmitt, M. H.: "Superiority of Breast Feeding. Fact or Fancy?" *Am. J. Nurs.*, 70:1488–93, 1970.

Stone, V.: "Give the Older Person Time," *Am. J. Nurs.*, 69:2124–27, 1969.

*Your Retirement Food Guide*. Long-Beach, Calif.: American Association for Retired Persons, 1971.

Infant Feeding | GROWTH AND DEVELOPMENT | BREAST FEEDING |
BOTTLE FEEDING | SUPPLEMENTARY FEEDINGS | FOOD HABITS •
**Preschool and School Children** | NUTRITIONAL NEEDS | FOOD
SELECTION AND HABITS | SCHOOL FOOD SERVICES • **Preadolescent
and Adolescent Youth** | NUTRITIONAL NEEDS | FOOD SELECTION
AND HABITS

# NUTRITION FOR GROWTH AND DEVELOPMENT

## Infant Feeding

### GROWTH AND DEVELOPMENT

Infants vary widely in their growth patterns, and it is not wise to compare one infant with another; yet, there is some value in being familiar with typical patterns of development and growth. On the average, infants gain 140 to 225 gm (5 to 8 oz) per week during the first five months, and double their birth weight in this time. For the remainder of the year the weight increase is about 110 to 140 gm (4 to 5 oz) per week; the birth weight is tripled by the age of 10 to 12 months. The initial height of 50 to 55 cm (20 to 22 in.) has increased to 75 cm (30 in.) or more by the end of the first year.

The body content of water at birth is high and that of fat is low. The relative lack of subcutaneous fat and the proportionately high surface area explain why additional precautions must be taken to keep infants warm. The bones are comparatively soft in the newborn baby, but they continue to add mineral substance throughout childhood and adolescence. Teeth begin to erupt at five to six months. By the end of the year the infant will have five to ten teeth.

The baby is born with a large head and short arms and legs. In the first years of life the nervous system continues to develop rapidly so that the brain will have reached 90 per cent of adult size at the age of four years. Severe malnutrition during the first months of life leads to inadequate development of the central nervous system, and the poorly nourished infant and child may never reach his full mental potential.

The newborn infant's stomach has a capacity of about 30 gm, and at one year can hold about 240 gm. The ability to digest protein, simple sugars, and emulsified fats is present at birth in the full-term infant. During the early months of life the production of digestive enzymes increases so that starchy foods and fats may be gradually included.

### BREAST FEEDING

No one would deny that breast feeding, whenever possible, is best for the infant. Human milk provides benefits of easy digestion, desirable rates of growth and development, and protection against infections. Most women can nurse their babies if they desire to do so and if they eat the foods necessary to build up the stores of nutrients for milk production.

About 15 to 45 ml of a thick, yellowish fluid called *colostrum* is produced during the first few days after delivery. Although this small amount of milk does not provide much nutrient intake, it provides the infant greater protection against infection. Placing the infant at the breast early also helps to stimulate the milk flow.

Self-demand feeding permits the baby to nurse when he is hungry, rather than according to an arbitrary time schedule. The mother soon learns to recognize when the baby is hungry and not crying for relief of some other discomfort. Infants nurse as often as every two hours during the first few weeks, but soon regulate to an approximate three- or four-hour schedule. About the second month the baby begins to sleep through the 2 or 3 A.M. feeding. By five months he usually does not awaken for a feeding at 10 to 11 P.M.

Breast-fed babies should be weaned about the fifth month or later. A bottle or cup feeding is substituted at a convenient feeding time. When the baby has become accustomed to this—after about a week or two— a second bottle or cup is offered. As much as two or three months are needed for full weaning. Breast-fed babies, like bottle-fed babies, require the addition of foods from time to time as discussed later in this chapter.

### BOTTLE FEEDING

*Nutritional needs.* The calorie, protein, mineral, and vitamin needs of the infant are very high in proportion to his body size. See Recommended Dietary Allowances, Table 4–1. The infant under 6 months requires 117 kcal per kg (50 to 55 kcal per lb) and for the remainder of the first year 108 kcal per kg (50 kcal per lb). At these caloric levels the relatively high protein and calcium needs are met by the formula.

To take care of the rapid rate of growth and the expanding blood circulation the infant's iron allowance is 10 mg up to 6 months of age, and 15 mg for the second half of the first year. Particular attention is also called to the need for 35 mg ascorbic acid since this is not supplied by the formula.

*Cow's milk.* Most infants are given cow's milk formulas. Cow's milk contains almost three times as much protein and more than three times as much calcium as human milk. It contains about the same amount of fat and somewhat less lactose. (See Table 14-1.) Ounce for ounce, cow's milk and human milk contain about 20 calories.

TABLE 14-1   COMPOSITION OF HUMAN AND COW'S MILK *
(PER 100 GM OF MILK)

| Nutrient | Human Milk | Cow's Milk | Nutrient | Human Milk | Cow's Milk |
|---|---|---|---|---|---|
| Calories | 77 | 66 | Iron, mg | 0.1 | trace |
| Protein, gm | 1.1 | 3.5 | Vitamin A, I.U. | 240 | 150 |
| Fat, gm | 4.0 | 3.7 | Thiamine, mg | 0.01 | 0.03 |
| Carbohydrate, gm | 9.5 | 4.9 | Riboflavin, mg | 0.04 | 0.17 |
| Calcium, mg | 33 | 117 | Niacin, mg | 0.2 | 0.1 |
| Phosphorus, mg | 14 | 92 | Ascorbic acid, mg | 5 | 1 |

* Watt, B. K., and Merrill, A. L.: *Composition of Foods—Raw, Processed, Prepared*, Handbook No. 8. Washington, D.C.: U.S. Department of Agriculture, 1964, p. 39.

*Proprietary premodified milk formulas* comprise about 90 per cent of all formulas used in infant feeding. These formulas have been developed to resemble the composition of human milk. Cow's milk is the usual base for these formulas, but it has been modified in some or all of the following ways: to lower the protein and calcium concentration; to increase the lactose content; to substitute vegetable oil for butterfat, thus furnishing a higher intake of linoleic acid and minimizing the spitting up associated with the butyric acid of butterfat; to adjust the mineral and vitamin levels to meet recommended allowances; and to heat denature the protein so that a soft, flocculent curd results.

Premodified formulas are available (1) as single strength, ready to feed, in quart cans or in 4 oz or 8 oz disposable nursing bottles, (2) as concentrated liquid which is measured into sterilized bottles and diluted with boiled water, and (3) as powdered formula, now seldom used.

Special formulas are also available for therapeutic purposes. For infants who are allergic to milk, nutritionally adequate formulas of soybean or meat base are substituted. Enzyme deficiency such as galactosemia or lactose intolerance requires meat base or amino acid formulas. A low-phenylalanine formula (Lofenalac *) is used for phenylketonuria, an inborn error of metabolism.

*Home-prepared formulas* are made with fresh whole milk or evaporated milk. To make such formulas comparable to human milk, these changes are required; (1) the milk is diluted with water; (2) cane sugar, corn syrup, or dextrimaltose is added to increase the carbohydrate level; and (3) the formulas are heated to reduce the size of the protein curd and to assure safety from bacterial contamination. Each formula must be calculated to meet the individual infant's needs. Although these formulas may be slightly less expensive than proprietary formulas, their preparation entails precautions in sanitation that may not be adequately observed by mothers who lack education.

### SUPPLEMENTARY FEEDINGS

Neither human nor cow's milk will meet the full nutritive needs of the infant during the first year of life. Several factors require consideration when planning for supplementary feedings.

*Iron-deficiency anemia* is perhaps the most common nutritional problem in the first year of life. Although supplementary foods furnish some iron the amount is usually not enough to meet the needs of the rapidly growing infant. Therefore, many pediatricians recommend that iron-fortified formulas be continued when the infant substitutes cup feedings for the bottle. Commercial infant cereals fortified with iron are preferable to family-type cereals that are not as highly enriched.

*Salt*: Babies, like adults, require some sodium and they respond to the taste of salt. During the early months the formula supplies most of the sodium intake. Thereafter, supplementary foods provide increasing amounts of sodium, often far in excess of needs. Nutritionists have criticized the excessive use of salt for two reasons: (1) the infant becomes accustomed to ingesting higher levels that are continued throughout life, a practice that may have some influence on the incidence of hypertension; (2) the intake of excessive salt increases the excretory load on the kidneys. The sodium level of many proprietary infant foods now comes within the levels recommended by a committee of pediatricians and nutritionists.

*Overnutrition* is a relatively common problem during the first year, and sometimes sets the pattern for later obesity. It can be prevented by allowing the infant to take what he wants from his bottle feeding rather than urging him to finish it, and by using some moderation in the amounts of supplementary feedings that are given.

Skim milk formulas are not desirable for infants. Although they reduce the caloric intake and thereby decrease the fat deposits in the body, they

* Mead Johnson and Company, Evansville, Indiana.

also are likely to reduce the rate of growth of other tissues. Skim milk formulas that are planned to meet caloric requirements for normal growth supply excessively high ratios of protein and carbohydrate and very low levels of fat. A high protein intake increases the load upon the kidneys for excretion of nitrogenous products, and a high intake of lactose could contribute to diarrhea.

*Baby foods.* Processed baby foods possess several advantages over home-prepared foods before the baby is ready for table foods: convenience; variety; uniform consistency and composition; high retention of nutritive values; and safety from bacteriologic contamination.

*Sequence of feeding.* Practices vary widely on the sequence with which foods are added and on the age of introducing these foods. Some babies need supplements earlier than others; some are ready for changes in texture sooner than others. A typical sequence and suggested daily schedule are shown in Tables 14–2 and 14–3. (See Fig. 14–1.)

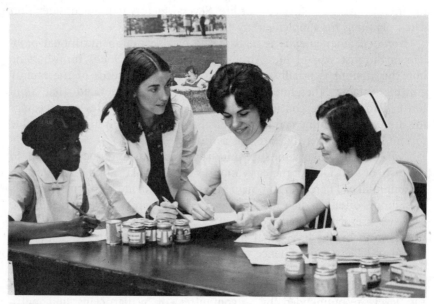

FIGURE 14–1 Nutritionist, student, and staff discuss uses of supplemental foods for infant feeding. (*Courtesy, Handicapped Children's Unit, St. Christopher's Hospital for Children, Philadelphia.*)

### FOOD HABITS

Good food habits in infancy and childhood will lead in later life to a liking for a wide variety of foods and the willingness to accept change. Parents have a wonderful opportunity as well as a tremendous responsibility for the development of good food habits in the young infant.

TABLE 14–2  SEQUENCE FOR FOOD ADDITIONS TO INFANT'S DIET

| Age | Food Addition and Its Nutritive Contribution |
|---|---|
| 2–4 weeks | 400 I.U. vitamin D from the formula. Avoid larger amounts |
| 2–4 weeks | Orange or grapefruit juice or other source of vitamin C; twice as much tomato juice needed; start with 1 teaspoon diluted with boiled water; increase gradually to 3 oz full strength |
| 2–3 months | Cereal for iron, thiamine, calories; mix precooked cereal with formula; give thin consistency at first; increase to 2 to 5 tablespoons by 7 to 8 months |
| 3–4 months | Mashed ripe banana, applesauce, strained pears, apricots, prunes, or peaches; start with 1 teaspoon and increase to 3–4 tablespoons by one year |
| 3–5 months | Strained asparagus, green beans, carrots, peas, spinach, squash, or tomatoes; start with 1 teaspoon, increasing to 3–4 tablespoons by end of the year |
| 4–6 months | Egg yolk for iron, vitamin A, thiamine, protein; mash hard-cooked egg with a little formula; use ¼ teaspoon at first; avoid egg white since it often gives allergic reaction |
| 5–7 months | Strained meats for protein, iron, B complex; sometimes prescribed as early as 6 weeks of age |
| 5–8 months | Crisp toast, zwieback, arrowroot cookies, teething biscuits |
| 7–8 months | Baked or mashed potato or enriched pasta for calories and some additional iron and B complex; small amounts |
| 9 months | Peeled raw apple |
| 8–10 months | Chopped vegetables and fruits |
| 10 months | Whole egg; plain puddings, such as custard, Junket |

1. Hold the young baby while he receives his formula to provide the feelings of satisfaction, security, and warmth. (See Fig. 14–2.)

2. Regulate the feeding schedule to the baby, not to the clock.

3. Introduce only one new food at a time.

4. Give new foods at the beginning of the meal when the baby is hungry.

5. Serve only small portions of a new food; a taste is enough.

6. Don't show your dislike of a food by the expression on your face or by refusing to eat the food yourself.

7. Babies, like adults, are more hungry at some times than others. Don't expect them to finish every bottle or everything at every meal.

TABLE 14–3   TYPICAL SCHEDULES FOR FIVE-MONTH AND YEAR-OLD INFANTS

| Five-Month Infant | Year-Old Infant |
|---|---|
| 6 A.M. Formula, 6–7 oz | 6:00 A.M. Orange juice, 3 oz<br>Zwiebach |
| 8 A.M. Orange juice, 3 oz | 7:30 A.M. Cereal, 2–5 tablespoons<br>Milk, 8 oz *<br>Chopped fruit, 1–2 table-<br>spoons |
| 10 A.M. Formula, 6–7 oz<br>Cereal, 2–3 tablespoons | 11:30 A.M. Chopped meat, ½–1 oz<br>or |
| 2 P.M. Formula, 6–7 oz<br>Egg yolk, ½–1<br>Vegetable, ¼ to 2 table-<br>spoons | Egg, 1<br>Potato, 2–4 tablespoons<br>Chopped vegetable, 2–4<br>tablespoons<br>Milk, 8 oz * |
| 6 P.M. Formula, 6–7 oz<br>Cereal, 2–3 tablespoons | 5:30 P.M. Cereal or potato, 2–5<br>tablespoons<br>Milk, 8 oz * |
| 10 P.M. Formula, 6–7 oz | Chopped fruit, 1–2 table-<br>spoons<br>Toast or zwieback |

* Iron-fortified formula is recommended throughout the first year.

8. Expect that the baby will feel his food and be messy. Don't scold him for spilling accidents. (See Fig. 14–3.)

9. Use a cup that does not tip easily, a deep bowl with rounded edges, and a spoon that can be managed by the baby. Provide safe and comfortable seating.

## Preschool and School Children

### NUTRITIONAL NEEDS

Any table of allowances must be interpreted according to the growth pattern of the individual child, the activity, the appetite, and the amount of musculature or body fatness. The growth patterns of children vary widely. Some children, by heredity, are destined to be short and stocky; others, tall and thin. Some children will have their rapid growth spurts at an earlier age than others. If a child does not have a satisfactory nutrient intake he will not reach the full growth of his hereditary pattern. The amount of physical activity varies widely and influences the calorie requirements.

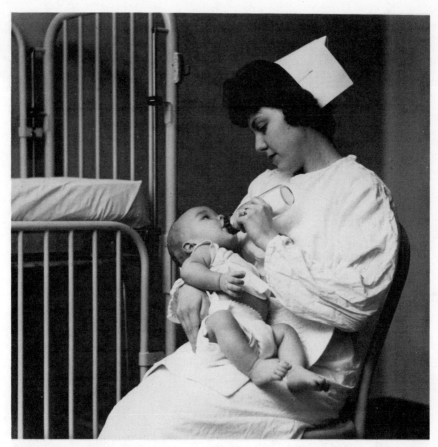

FIGURE 14-2 The baby should always be held while he is being fed. (*Courtesy, Ross Laboratories, Columbus, Ohio.*)

During the second year the baby gains 3.5 to 4.5 kg (8 to 10 lb). Following the second birthday and to the ninth year, the increase in height and weight is at a much slower rate; the annual gain in weight is about 2 to 3 kg (4 to 7 lb). The muscles increase in size, the baby fat is lost, the legs become longer, and the bones become harder. There is a great development in motor coordination, in changing body proportions, and in mental development.

The daily allowances for children of one to ten years are relatively high for all nutrients, when the size of the child is taken into account. See Table 4-1 for a complete list of recommended allowances. Seven- to ten-year-old children have calorie needs higher than those of their mothers. Because of the possibility of anemia, additional iron is recommended in the preschool years.

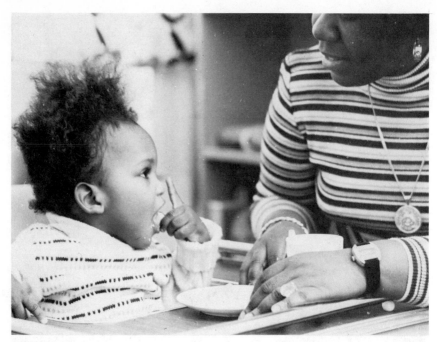

FIGURE 14-3 A toddler enjoys feeding himself. Touching food is important at this stage. (*Courtesy, Handicapped Children's Unit, St. Christopher's Hospital for Children, Philadelphia.*)

## FOOD SELECTION AND HABITS

The Four Food Groups provide the basis for planning the diet for young children. The following list indicates the range in the amounts that are ordinarily eaten.

| | |
|---|---|
| 2 to 3 cups | vitamin D milk |
| 3 to 4 per week | eggs |
| 1 to 4 tablespoons | chopped meat, poultry, fish; some cottage cheese or peanut butter may be substituted |
| ⅓ to ⅔ cup | citrus fruit juice; or whole orange; or twice as much tomato juice |
| ¼ to ½ cup | fruits such as applesauce, peeled apple, apricots, banana, pears, peaches, prunes, etc. |
| 1 serving | raw vegetables: carrots, cabbage, tomatoes, lettuce, rutabagas |
| 2 to 4 tablespoons | white or sweet potatoes |
| ⅓ to ⅔ cup | enriched or whole-grain cereal |
| 1 to 3 slices | enriched or whole-grain bread |
| | butter or margarine for bread and for seasoning vegetables |

Few foods need to be omitted entirely from the diet of children, but some discretion in food selection is necessary. The appetite is ordinarily a good guide, but parents have a responsibility to provide a choice of foods within the framework of the Four Food Groups. When the child is permitted to eat freely from sweets and other empty-calorie foods, he will not obtain sufficient nutrients.

Young children prefer plain, blandly flavored foods that are only lightly seasoned. Mixtures, as in casseroles, are well accepted only as the child becomes older. Some foods that require chewing are essential, but meats that are not chopped or ground may be tough for the preschool child. Lukewarm, rather than hot, foods are preferred. Vegetables are least well liked of all food groups. Strongly flavored vegetables may not be accepted until late school years; some children never learn to like them.

Children sometimes go on food jags; that is, they will eat only certain foods—for example, peanut-butter-and-jelly sandwiches. Usually these diversions of appetite do not last too long if the parents make no particular point of them. If milk is refused as a beverage, it can be given in puddings, or will be accepted if it is occasionally flavored or even colored with vegetable color! American cheese is a good substitute.

Children require snacks to provide for their relatively high energy needs and to avoid excessive hunger at mealtimes. The snacks should be selected largely from the Four Food Groups: fruits and fruit juices; milk; occasionally ice cream; crackers and peanut butter; molasses or peanut butter cookies; small sandwiches.

By the time a child is ready for school his food likes have increased, but he faces other problems relative to maintaining good nutrition. Mornings in many homes are too often rushed, so that breakfast is a hurried meal or may be skipped entirely. A child who is ill at ease at school may eat poorly at lunch. A short lunch period may be upsetting to the slow eater. Children of this age who are extremely active may become unduly tired before meals.

Observation of the following points will encourage good food habits.

1. Serve meals in a pleasant place and a calm unhurried atmosphere.

2. Provide meals that are colorful, varied in texture and flavor, and attractively served.

3. Don't serve the same food over and over again even if it is a favorite. Even well-liked foods can become tiresome.

4. Provide eating utensils and dishes that are easy for the child to hold and to use. Many vegetables, fruits, meats, and bread may be served as finger foods.

5. Allow sufficient time for meals; breakfast need not be hurried if children are awakened early enough.

6. Don't let the child become too tired before meals. Plan for adequate rest and early bedtime.

7. Plan for snacks as carefully as the meal. Snacks can provide good nutrition. They should not be eaten so close to meals that the appetite is spoiled for the meal.

8. Remember that appetite decreases as the rate of growth slows down during the second, third, and fourth years of life. The toddler may refuse certain foods at this time in trying to assert his independence; don't make too much of this.

### SCHOOL FOOD SERVICES

The participation in the school lunch program has increased greatly, but too many children still do not avail themselves of the opportunity for this meal. In many schools breakfast programs are also available. The type A school lunch furnishes about one third of the recommended daily allowances. It includes:

½ pt fluid whole, low fat, or skim milk

Protein-rich food: 2 oz meat, fish, poultry, or cheese; 1 egg; ½ cup cooked beans or peas; or 4 tablespoons peanut butter

2 servings or more (at least ¾ cup) of vegetables and fruit (this must include a rich source of ascorbic acid daily and a rich source of vitamin A at least twice a week)

1 slice whole-grain or enriched bread or rolls, muffin, corn bread, or biscuits

2 teaspoons butter or fortified margarine

The school lunch does more than feed the child. The program helps the child to learn to like nutritious foods and to become familiar with food selection of an adequate diet. It gives an opportunity to strengthen nutrition education in the classroom. (See Fig. 14–4.)

The American Medical Association, the American Dietetic Association, and the National Congress of Parents and Teachers oppose the sale of candy and soft drinks within the schools. These foods contribute little to the nutritional needs of the child, and may divert the child from spending his money for the school lunch.

## Preadolescent and Adolescent Youth

### NUTRITIONAL NEEDS

The caloric needs of boys and girls are somewhat higher than those for men and women, with corresponding higher allowances for thiamine, riboflavin, and niacin. The protein allowances do not differ significantly from those for adults, but the calcium allowance is 1200 mg, which is 50 per cent greater than that for adults. Boys should have an intake of

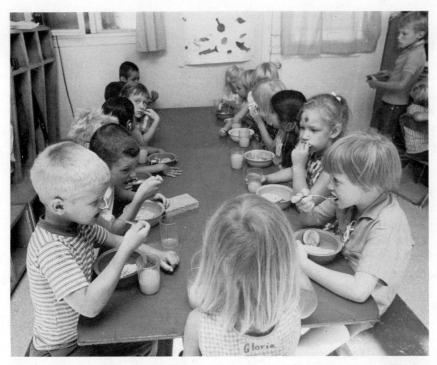

FIGURE 14–4 Child feeding programs of the U.S. Department of Agriculture enable these children of migrant farm workers to eat a nutritious breakfast and other meals at a day-care center. (*Courtesy, Mr. Jack Schneider and U.S. Department of Agriculture, Washington, D.C.*)

18 mg iron through 18 years of age, while girls should continue this level of intake throughout the childbearing years. Iodized salt will meet the increased requirement for iodine.

An allowance of 1000 R.E. (5000 I.U.) vitamin A is recommended for boys and of 800 R.E. (4000 I.U.) for girls. Up to 23 years of age 400 I.U. vitamin D should be included daily. The recommended allowance for ascorbic acid is the same as for adults, namely 45 mg. See Table 4–1 for other recommended allowances.

The teen-age girl frequently becomes pregnant at a time when her own body is still maturing. The mother-to-be needs to increase her already high nutritive allowances by the amounts of nutrients needed for successful pregnancy. (See Chap. 13.)

## FOOD SELECTION AND HABITS

The impression is sometimes gained that all teen-agers are poorly nour-ished and always eat great quantities of empty-calorie snacks. In fact, many teen-agers have good food habits, are well nourished, and might serve as good examples for others in their age group who need to improve their food habits. Perhaps we have not sufficiently appealed to the teen-ager himself in terms of his needs for better nutrition. Girls express a particular need for a good figure, a healthy skin, and beautiful hair. They need to understand the patterns of normal maturing of the body so that they do not indulge in bizarre reducing diets. Although a good diet is essential to a healthy skin, they also need to understand that skin problems arise when rapid changes in hormone production are taking place.

Boys are more likely to be interested in tall stature, muscular development, and athletic vigor and stamina. They too have skin problems about which they are concerned. The large appetite of boys helps to ensure an increased intake of needed nutrients along with the foods that are supplying calories.

The diets of boys and girls most frequently fail to meet the recommended allowances for calcium, vitamin A, and ascorbic acid. In addition, girls often do not get enough iron.

Of the food groups, milk requires special emphasis because of the great calcium need. If dark-green leafy and deep-yellow vegetables and citrus fruits were more adequately consumed, the vitamin A and ascorbic acid intakes would be substantially improved.

Among the particular problems during adolescence are these:

1. *Skipped meals.* Many high school students keep late hours, get up too late in the morning to eat breakfast, eat a hurried lunch at school, and never quite make up during the rest of the day for their nutritional requirements.

2. *Overweight.* The pattern of overweight is often set in earlier childhood through a continuing excessive food intake. Active participation in sports rather than watching others engage in sports is important. Weight control should begin in childhood and during adolescence and not be delayed to middle age.

3. *Snacks.* Boys and girls, as a rule, need some snacks, but their selection should be substantially from the Four Food Groups. A correlation has been established between the excessive intake of sweets, especially those that are sticky, and the amount of tooth decay. This is not to say that any foods are altogether forbidden. Rather, if there is an adequate intake of foods from the Four Food Groups the amounts of empty-calorie foods to satisfy the appetite will be correspondingly reduced.

## REVIEW QUESTIONS AND PROBLEMS

1. Visit a food market to determine the kinds of formulas available for infant feeding. Read the labels to see what kind of information is provided.

2. Compare the recommended allowances for calories, protein, calcium, iron, vitamin A, ascorbic acid, and thiamine for the infant at 12 months, the child of two years, the school child of eight years. List the conclusions you can make from these comparisons.

3. Write a schedule for a day for a seven-month-old infant, indicating the kinds and approximate amounts of foods to include at this time.

4. A baby eats one third of the contents of a can of strained fruit. What would you do with the rest of it?

5. Why is egg white not given until toward the end of the first year?

6. What is meant by a Type A lunch? Why is the school lunch program of such importance for the child? Plan a packed lunch for a 12-year-old boy who attends a school where there is no lunch program.

7. Develop suggestions for helping teen-agers to improve their food habits.

8. What nutrients require special emphasis during adolescence? What foods will meet these needs?

9. Write a menu for one day for adults. Modify this menu so that it is suitable for a 3-year-old, an 8-year-old, and a 15-year-old boy. Include plans for snacks.

## REFERENCES

Children's Bureau, U.S. Department of Health, Education, and Welfare, Washington, D.C.: *The Adolescent in Your Family*, 1964; *Food for Your Baby's First Year*, 1969; *Foods for the Preschool Child*, 1969; *Infant Care*, 1963; *Your Child from One to Three*, 1967; *Your Child from Six to Twelve*, 1966.

*Current Practices in Infant Feeding*. Fremont, Mich.: Gerber Products Company.

Hicks, C. B.: "Eat! Says Fat Little Johnny's Mother," *Today's Health*, 48:48, February 1970.

Jernigan, A. K.: "Suggestions for Feeding Hospitalized Children," *Hospitals*, 44:86–89, May 16, 1970.

Murdaugh, Sr. A., and Miller, L. E.: "Helping the Breast-Feeding Mother," *Am. J. Nurs.*, 72:1420–22, 1972.

O'Grady, R. S.: "Feeding Behavior in Infants," *Am. J. Nurs.*, 71:736–39, 1971.

Robinson, C. H.: *Normal and Therapeutic Nutrition*, 14th ed. New York: Macmillan Publishing Co., Inc., 1972, Chaps. 22 and 23.

Safran, C.: "Parents: Experts Tell You What to Do About Balky Vegetable Eaters," *Today's Health*, 51:54, November 1973.

# FOOD ACCEPTANCE, CULTURAL FOOD PATTERNS, AND FOOD HABITS

*Hunger* is the urge to eat and is accompanied by a number of unpleasant sensations. It follows a period when one has been deprived of food, and is generally associated with contraction of the stomach. The individual begins to feel irritable, uneasy, and tired. If a blood sample is taken at this time, the blood sugar level is somewhat low. When food is taken, the individual begins to feel better almost immediately.

*Appetite* is the anticipation of and the desire to eat palatable food.

People eat not only to satisfy hunger, but also because food has many meanings for them. Good or bad food habits result from the interaction of social, emotional, and cultural factors. In order to help improve your own food habits and to help other people improve theirs, you need to appreciate and understand the variations people have in their likes and dislikes and their attitudes toward food.

Some people have good food habits because they have been fortunate in their early home and school environment. Other people through education have seen the need for change and have been willing to work to modify their habits. Are you one of these?

Many people remain indifferent and ignorant concerning nutrition. They are willing to believe only that which pleases them, and they often use childhood experiences as excuses for being finicky.

## Factors Affecting Food Acceptance

### PHYSIOLOGIC VARIATIONS

Young children have many more taste buds on the tongue and in the cheek, and therefore they have a keener sense of taste than older individuals. Babies and young children prefer bland foods, whereas teenagers begin to like foods that are more spicy and highly flavored. The number of taste buds diminishes later in life, and old people often lose a sense of taste for certain foods.

The sense of taste varies widely from one individual to another. Some people notice slight differences in taste, and others do not. Some persons like much salt, others only a little; some like very sweet foods, others do not; some like spicy foods, and others prefer bland foods. From day to day, the senses of taste and smell also vary. Smelling food too long at a time, or having a steady diet of certain foods, reduces the response of the sense organs.

The feel of foods is also important. A baby learns about food by feeling it as well as tasting it. We all react favorably to velvety ice cream, crisp rolls, fluffy mashed potatoes, but we are likely to object to sugary fudge, greasy meat, lumpy mashed potatoes, and stringy string beans. Young children don't like very hot or cold foods, but adults usually demand that their foods be piping hot or well chilled.

### FAMILY CUSTOMS AND SOCIAL PATTERNS

The family environment has much influence on food habits. Food is more likely to be well accepted when the entire family is together for meals in a happy, relaxed atmosphere. If the homemaker prepares only a few well-liked dishes over and over again, the family members will encounter some difficulty in adapting to other situations. Within the family some allowances may be made for individual likes and dislikes without preparing many separate dishes. If the homemaker selects a variety of foods and prepares them in different ways from time to time, the individual's food experiences are enriched.

Negative attitudes to food may be developed in the home. Children are quick to imitate their parents, who do not eat certain foods. They rapidly note signs of worry, dislike, or anger on the part of the parents and develop antagonisms toward particular foods. They dawdle when they learn it is a way to gain attention. Parents sometimes punish by refusing to give dessert to a child who hasn't finished his meal or bribe and reward with a favorite food like candy if a meal is finished. (See Fig. 15–1.)

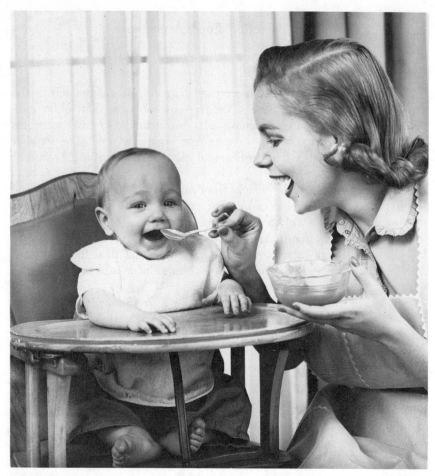

FIGURE 15–1 Good food habits are established during infancy. The environment should be pleasant, secure, and relaxed. (*Courtesy, Gerber Products Company, Fremont, Michigan.*)

Foods are often classed as being for babies, young children, or adults. Milk, cut-up food, peanut-butter-and-jelly sandwiches are looked upon as children's foods; hamburgers, pizza, and large sandwiches are teen-age fare; tea and coffee are for adults.

Meat, potatoes, and pie are typical of masculine meals, whereas soufflés, salads, and light desserts are more characteristic of feminine foods.

Some foods have more prestige value than others, and we use them as company foods to honor or impress our friends. They cost more, are hard to get, take a lot of time to prepare, or are unusual. Examples of such status foods are filet mignon, wild rice, baked Alaska, and a fine imported wine. Other foods are sometimes considered to be only for those with low incomes; ground meat, margarine, dry skim milk, dry beans, and fish, for example. Yet any of the latter foods are just as nutritious and can be prepared in as many delicious ways as more expensive foods.

## FOOD AND THE EMOTIONS

Did you ever go to a soda fountain for a fancy sundae after taking an examination? Or have you sometimes rewarded yourself for finishing a difficult job with an especially good meal in a restaurant? Do you recall with pleasure certain meals at birthday parties or holidays? Food is often used in one way or another to express or to cover up our feelings of happiness, love, security, worry, grief, loneliness, and so on.

The baby who is held when he is fed associates his food with warmth and security. But a child who is scolded for being messy may associate certain foods with unhappiness. Some teen-agers overeat to compensate for a poor record in school or unpopularity with their classmates. Elderly persons living along often eat far too little, because they are lonely and unhappy. People who are grieving or who can't face the problems that beset them are known to gain excessive weight in some instances, because they find relief in eating excessive quantities of food.

## RELIGION AND DIETARY PATTERNS

Various foods have symbolic meanings in religion. Likewise, most religions place certain restrictions upon the use of food. The regulations for fasting placed upon Roman Catholics have been liberalized, but many Catholics still abstain from meat on fast days; to them fish and cheese may be associated with denial and penitence. Muslims abstain from eating pork, whereas Buddhists are vegetarians and will not eat the flesh of any animal. Seventh Day Adventists are lacto-ovo-vegetarians; that is, they do not eat meat but they use eggs, milk, nuts, and legumes as sources of protein.

*Orthodox Jews* adhere to dietary laws based upon tradition and the Bible. Animals and poultry are slaughtered according to ritual, and the meat is soaked in water, salted to remove the blood, and washed. This is known as *koshering.* Pork and shellfish are prohibited.

Milk, sour cream, cottage cheese, and cream cheese are widely used, but no dairy foods are served at a meal with meat. Usually two meals each day are dairy meals, and one meal is a meat meal. Separate utensils are used for the cookery of meat and dairy products. Fish, eggs, vegetables, fruits, cereals, and bread may be used at all meals; however, no milk or butter may be used with these foods if they are included in the meat meal.

No food preparation takes place on the Sabbath, and an Orthodox Jew refuses to eat food that has been freshly cooked on the Sabbath. Religious festivals are celebrated with special dishes, and much symbolism is attached to food. For example, only unleavened bread is eaten during the Passover. Separate sets of dishes are used during the Passover week. On Yom Kippur (Day of Atonement), the most solemn day of the religious year, no food or drink is taken for 24 hours.

Among the widely used foods by Jewish people are *borsch* (a soup), *gefullte fish, blintzes* (thin rolled pancakes filled with cottage cheese or ground beef), *knishes* (pastry with ground meat), *challah* (a braided white bread), *bagel* (doughnut-shaped hard yeast roll), *kuchen* (coffee cake), *leckach* (honey cake served especially at Rosh Hashana, the New Year), and *strudel* (fruit-filled pastry).

## REGIONAL PATTERNS IN THE UNITED STATES

Food habits result from the foods that have been available in the various parts of the world. People everywhere tend to like the foods with which they are familiar. Even before tasting a food they will look with suspicion and dislike on something that is unfamiliar. The ease with which people travel from one part of the world to another is doing much to widen our food experiences and to make us more appreciative of other cultures.

Some regional differences still exist in the United States, but for the most part, these are exceptions rather than major departures from the diet. One is likely to associate New England with clam chowder, codfish cakes, Boston baked beans, and lobster; Pennsylvania Dutch, with seven sweets and sours, scrapple, German-type sausage, and shoofly pie; the South, with corn bread, hominy, fried chicken, hot biscuits, turnip and other greens, and sweet potatoes; Louisiana, with French and Creole cookery; the Southwest, with Mexican dishes; the Midwest, with its abundance of dairy products, eggs, and meat and the traditions of Scandinavian, Polish, and German cookery; the Far West, with its luscious fruits and vegetables, salmon, and the influences of the Orient.

## Cultural Food Patterns

Although people of the United States come from nationality backgrounds from all over the world, the differences in their diets are evident primarily on holidays and family celebrations. Those who adhere more closely to national patterns can readily adapt to the varied supplies of foods in our markets when taught how to do so. A few of the more outstanding examples of some dietary patterns are described briefly below.

## BLACK AMERICAN

The dietary pattern for black Americans is often described in terms of foods used in the South. However, the foods that are selected by black Americans, as with any group of people, are modified by the geographic location of the community, the neighborhoods in which people live—that is, integrated or largely made up of a single group, the availability of foods in the local markets, and changes in income. For example, some black families living in the North use dietary patterns that differ little if at all from those used by white families who have always lived in the North; other black families have retained the food patterns brought from the South and use them with pride.

"Soul food" is a term recently used to denote foods of the black culture, with particular reference to foods of the black South. Many of these foods originated with the slaves of pre-Civil War days, and continued to be used by poor people in the South, both black and white. At one time such foods lacked status; now they have become fashionable in many places. Some of the typical foods are these:

Meat from every part of the pig: pork chops, ham hocks, bacon, salt pork, spareribs (often barbecued), chitterlings (lining of pig stomach, usually boiled and then fried), and pig's feet, tail, and ears
Fried chicken, fried fish, catfish stew
Wild game when available: coon, possum, beaver
Greens—turnip, mustard, collard, dandelion, kale—boiled in salt water with ham hocks, bacon, or bits of salt pork; "pot likker" is consumed as well as the greens
Stewed okra, corn, tomatoes
Cornbread in many ways: hoecakes, crackling bread, spoon bread, hush puppies; baking powder biscuits, served hot
Black-eyed peas with molasses and bacon or salt pork
Grits, rice, sweet potatoes, sweet potato pie

Black people do not consume much milk. Recently this has been explained by the fact that a high percentage of adult blacks have an intolerance to lactose, the carbohydrate in milk. The intolerance is probably a hereditary defect in which there is a deficiency or a lack of lactase, the enzyme in intestinal juice that splits up lactose. Milk should not be excluded from the diet of black children, but an awareness of intolerance should be considered.

## PUERTO RICAN

Many Puerto Ricans have come recently to the large cities of the eastern United States. They are frequently poor, lack employment skills, and live in crowded, often unsanitary, quarters. Because of difficulty in speaking and understanding English, they are likely to patronize small food stores that are owned by Spanish-speaking people. They usually pay much more for the foods they purchase than they would in a supermarket. These and other factors account for a high level of malnutrition, especially among children.

Their staple foods include rice, chick peas, kidney beans, and other legumes, and a variety of *viandas* or starchy vegetables, such as plantain, green bananas, white sweet potato, and others. Dried codfish is often used. Although milk, chicken, and pork are well liked, they are infrequently used because of cost. Fruits and vegetables have always been available to them in abundance, but they have made limited use of them.

Rice (*arroz*) is eaten once or twice a day and may be combined with a little codfish, legumes, and occasionally chicken (*arroz con pollo*) or pork. The legumes are usually cooked and dressed with a highly seasoned tomato sauce (*sofrito*). The starchy vegetables are boiled and served with oil, oil and vinegar, or some dried codfish.

### MEXICAN

The staple foods of Mexicans include corn, pinto or calico beans, and chili peppers; wheat is now replacing some of the corn. Milk is seldom used, and meat and eggs appear on the menu only two or three times a week. Mexican dishes are seasoned liberally with red chili powder, garlic, onion, and spices.

Dried corn is heated and soaked in lime water, washed, and pounded to a puttylike dough called *masa*. Thin cakes rolled from the masa and baked on a hot griddle are known as *tortillas*. Cheese and ground meat with onion and lettuce may be used to fill tortillas in preparations known as *enchiladas*. Tamales consist of highly seasoned ground meat and masa wrapped in corn husks, steamed, and served with chili sauce. (See Fig. 15–2.)

### ITALIAN

Pastas such as spaghetti, macaroni, and noodles in many sizes and shapes are characteristic of the Italian diet. Crusty Italian bread is widely used. Chicken, lamb, pork, and veal and a variety of cold cuts are popular but eaten less frequently than in typical American diets. Milk is not used much, but many varieties of Italian cheeses are favored. Vegetables boiled and dressed with oil or oil and vinegar are well liked. Salads and fruits are important parts of the day's meals.

Noodle doughs may be filled with meat, cheese, and vegetable mixtures for such dishes, as *lasagne, ravioli,* and *pizza.* Chick peas, split peas, kidney

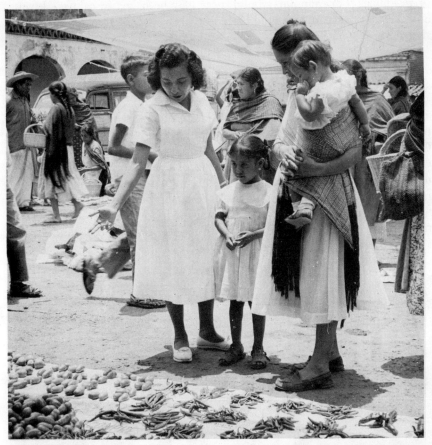

FIGURE 15–2 A community nurse in Mexico points out the importance of selecting fruits and vegetables for the family's meals. (*Courtesy, UNICEF.*)

beans, and lentils are used in such substantial soups as *minestrone*. *Polenta* is a thick cornmeal mush often served plain or with tomato sauce and cheese.

### NEAR EAST

Round, flat loaves of bread are the staff of life at every meal. Cracked parboiled whole wheat (bulgur) and rice are staple foods eaten as such or with vegetables and meat. Fermented milk (yogurt) is preferred to plain milk. Fresh fruits are widely used. Eggplant, zucchini, onions, peppers, okra, cabbage, and cauliflower are favorite vegetables.

Lamb and mutton are preferred, although other meats and poultry are also eaten. Meat is often ground or cut and cooked with wheat, rice, or vegetables. For example, ground meat may be baked in cabbage leaves, and pieces of cut lamb may be placed on skewers with tomato and onion slices for *shashlik*.

### ORIENTAL

Rice, wheat, and millet are staple cereals providing most of the calories and protein for people of the Orient. The Chinese use soybeans and soybean sprouts in many dishes. Finely sliced vegetables are cooked by the Chinese for a short time in a little oil and retain their color and crispness. Chicken, pork, eggs, fish, and shellfish serve as the foundation for many delicious dishes, such as shrimp egg rolls, sweet and sour pork, and chow mein, an American adaptation. Milk, cheese, and beef are not widely used. Sesame oil, peanut oil, and lard are much used. Soy sauce at almost every meal contributes to a high salt intake. Almonds, sesame seeds, and ginger are popular seasonings. (See Fig. 15–3.)

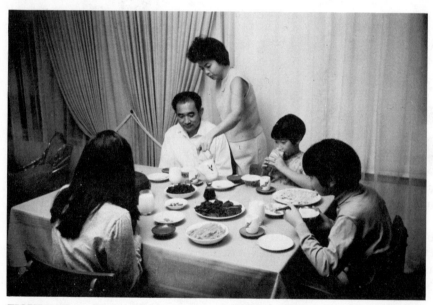

FIGURE 15–3 Dietitians and nurses are more effective in helping people to improve their food habits when they appreciate and understand the food patterns of various cultural groups. (*Courtesy, National Dairy Council, Chicago.*)

## Some Techniques for Changing Food Habits

Good food habits are easily acquired in youth, and it is more difficult to change the habits of people later in life. Perhaps you have found some of your food habits should be improved, or maybe you can help someone in your family or a friend to improve his. The following suggestions may be helpful.

1. A change in food habits is indicated only if the present habits lead to poor nutrition. Remember that persons who have good food habits need not like every nutritious food. Also, it is not necessary to omit all foods that are poor sources of the nutrients.

2. Find out what reasons are most likely to appeal to the individual. Boys are often motivated on the basis of growth in stature, physical vigor, and ability in sports. The teen-age girl, on the other hand, desires a slim figure to be in the latest fashion, or a clear skin and glossy hair. Neither boys nor girls are likely to be interested in the promise of health or of a good old age, but they might like to impress their friends with their cosmopolitan tastes in food. Older people, on the other hand, are interested in weight control from the standpoint of health or for diet control of some disease problems.

3. Look at the whole diet pattern—not just at one meal pattern or the snacks. List the good points of the diet as well as the weaknesses. Start with the good points for building a better pattern.

4. Be realistic in what can be accomplished. Expect only small changes at the time. Make allowances for strong likes and dislikes. Don't suggest foods that are too expensive, hard to get, or contrary to one's beliefs.

5. Encourage the individual to become adventurous in trying new foods at home or when eating out.

6. Provide practical suggestions for preparing foods in attractive ways.

Specific techniques for the development of good food habits in infants and children are listed in Chapter 14.

### REVIEW QUESTIONS AND PROBLEMS

1. A young man away from home for the first time writes that the food he is getting is not to his liking. List as many reasons as you can that affect his food acceptance.

2. What nationality food patterns are found in your community? Write a menu for one day that would be well liked by one nationality group.

3. If possible, visit a food market that caters to a particular nationality group. What foods do you find that are not often seen in supermarkets?

4. A 14-year-old girl is 15 lb overweight. She skips breakfast and drinks little milk, eats no bread, and does not like vegetables. In what ways could you approach her to improve her food habits?

### REFERENCES

Berkowitz, P., and Berkowitz, N. S.: "The Jewish Patient in the Hospital," *Am. J. Nurs.*, 67:2335, 1967.

Chappelle, M. L.: "The Language of Food," *Am. J. Nurs.*, **72**:1294, 1972.

Kight, M. A., *et al.*: "Nutritional Influences of Mexican-American Foods in Arizona," *J. Am. Diet. Assoc.*, **55**:557, 1969.

Register, U. D., and Sonnenberg, L. M.: "The Vegetarian Diet. Scientific and Practical Considerations," *J. Am. Diet. Assoc.*, **62**:253, 1973.

Robinson, C. H.: *Normal and Therapeutic Nutrition*, 14th ed. New York: Macmillan Publishing Co., Inc., 1972, Chaps. 14 and 15.

Sakr, A. H.: "Dietary Regulations and Food Habits of Muslims," *J. Am. Diet. Assoc.*, **58**:123, 1971.

Soulsby, T.: "Russian-American Food Habits," *J. Nutr. Educ.*, **4**:170, February 1972.

*Understanding Food Patterns in the United States*. Leaflet. Chicago: American Dietetic Association, 1969.

Wauneka, A. D.: "Helping a People to Understand," *Am. J. Nurs.*, **62**:88, July 1962.

# SAFEGUARDING THE FOOD SUPPLY

Food is the nation's biggest business. Each American consumes from 1200 to 1500 pounds of food in a year. Considering the number of people involved in growing, processing, and selling this large amount of food, the record of safety is excellent. In fact, the food supply is as safe, wholesome, and nutritious as any in the world. This is so because of many interrelated factors: (1) an agriculture dependent upon scientific methods and controls; (2) a system of rapid transport to market under controlled conditions of temperature and sanitation; (3) a highly developed food technology that enables processing of food under high standards of quality control; (4) a rapid turnover in the market place; and (5) intelligent handling by the consumer whether in the home or institution. Each step in the chain from farm to consumer is protected by legislation to ensure compliance to high standards (see Chap. 17).

Although the overall record is excellent, there is no room for careless handling of the food supply. Death from botulin poisoning is rare, but its dramatic occurrence provides headlines in the news. Milder illness from food poisoning occurs to millions every year, but for the most part such illness goes unnoticed and unreported. Only when such illness strikes infants or an institution where many elderly people are living is there concern; these people may, in fact, die from the infections that would be only mild to healthy adults.

161

## Illness Caused by Food

### BACTERIAL INFECTIONS

The presence of large numbers of certain organisms in food may cause bacterial infection. The bacteria grow in the favorable intestinal environment and in 12 to 36 hours produce symptoms such as fever, vomiting, distention, cramping, and diarrhea. The illness is usually mild, lasts for two or three days, and is not usually reported to public health authorities. The dehydration and electrolyte imbalance that sometimes occur are poorly withstood by infants and elderly people.

*Salmonella* account for a high incidence of bacterial infections. Meat, poultry, fish, eggs, and dairy products that are eaten raw or inadequately heated are frequently the source of infection. For example, raw egg in an eggnog may be the source; or a butcher block, kitchen counter, or utensil that has been in contact with raw meat or poultry could contaminate another food placed upon it.

Typhoid fever is caused by a species of Salmonella. It is usually transmitted to water, milk, or other food by a food handler who is a carrier. The illness is not confined to the gastrointestinal tract, but affects other organs such as the liver, gallbladder, spleen, and kidney. This infection was a major public health problem at the beginning of this century. Today the illness is uncommon because of the greater safety of water and milk supplies. Antibiotics are effective in treatment and shorten the length of the disease.

*Clostridium perfringens,* also known as the gas gangrene organism, appears normally in the soil, in sewage, and in the intestinal tract of man. The bacteria are readily destroyed by heat, but the spores survive even after five or six hours of heating. If a cooked food such as meat or gravy is allowed to stand at room temperature for several hours, the spores germinate and produce tremendous numbers of bacteria. If the food so grossly contaminated is eaten, it produces the typical gastrointestinal upsets. Such infections do not occur when food is eaten immediately after cooking. Nor do they occur if food is refrigerated promptly after cooking so that the spores do not germinate. However, if large masses of foods are refrigerated, considerable growth of bacteria can occur before the center of the food mass is adequately chilled; therefore, such foods should be spread out in thin pans for rapid cooling.

### BACTERIAL INTOXICATIONS

Some bacteria produce a toxin that causes the illness. The symptoms, which are mild to severe, appear much more rapidly than in bacterial infections—usually in one to six hours after the meal.

*Staphylococcal poisoning* occurs after eating food that has been contaminated with staphylococci and kept at temperatures ranging between 10° and 60° C (50° and 140° F) for three or four hours. Custards, cream fillings in pastries, cream puffs, cream sauces, chicken salad, croquettes, potato salad, poultry dressing, ice cream, ground meat, and stews are some of the foods that provide the ideal medium for rapid growth of the bacteria. During growth the bacteria produce the toxin that leads to the illness.

The staphylococci are present in infected cuts of the skin, in pimples, and in the nose and throat of persons handling food. Failure to wash hands or bringing a cut finger in contact with food is sufficient to contaminate the food. High heat destroys the bacteria, but does not destroy the toxin that has already been produced. The foods that are most frequently contaminated are not heated sufficiently to destroy the bacteria and are subsequently not refrigerated promptly.

**Botulism.** *Clostridium botulinum* is an organism found in soils all over the world, and therefore infects vegetables grown on them. The bacteria produce spores that germinate under anaerobic (without air) conditions. As the bacteria grow, they produce the deadly poison *botulin.*

Botulism is rare but about two thirds of all cases are fatal. The toxin affects the nervous system, leading to dizziness, headache, double vision, and paralysis of the muscles leading to respiratory and cardiac failure.

Botulism is traced to canned products, especially home-canned foods, that have been insufficiently sterilized. The spores germinate in the can, and the bacteria in turn produce the toxin. Nonacid foods such as meat, corn, peas, green beans, asparagus, mushrooms, and beets are good media for growth. Acid foods such as tomatoes and certain fruits are not favorable for growth. Boiling a food for at least 10 minutes destroys the toxin. The contents of any can with bulging ends should be discarded without even tasting the food.

### PARASITE INFESTATIONS

*Trichinella spiralis* is a worm that becomes embedded in the muscle tissue of pork. Trichinosis in humans results when infected pork that has been insufficiently cooked is eaten. The larvae develop in the intestinal tract and grow to adult size in a few days. They invade the blood and lymph circulation and involve the muscles of the abdominal wall, the diaphragm, the thorax, the biceps, and the tongue. Muscular pain, chills, and fever result.

Trichinella are destroyed by cooking pork until no trace of pink is present. The organisms are killed at about 60° C (140° F) but the recommended temperature for cooking pork is 77° C (170° F). Trichinella are also destroyed by freezing at −18° C (0° F).

*Endamoeba histolytica* is a protozoa that is transmitted by food handlers who are carriers of the organism, or by contaminated water supplies. The illness, amebic dysentery, is acute, chronic, or intermittent. The diarrhea may be profuse and bloody with erosion of the intestinal mucosa. Abscesses of the liver, lung, brain, and other tissues sometimes occur. The infestation is more common in tropical areas.

### NATURAL TOXICANTS

Many natural constituents of foods produce intoxication when those foods are eaten. Some examples of these are:

Rhubarb leaves, extremely high in oxalic acid

Green part of sprouting potatoes: solanine, an alkaloid, causes pain, vomiting, jaundice, diarrhea; when peeling potatoes the green part should be completely removed

Certain species of mushrooms and toadstools contain deadly poisons

Monkshood, foxglove, deadly nightshade, wild parsnip, and hemlock are poisonous plants

Raw soybeans contain a factor that inhibits the activity of the digestive enzyme trypsin; cooking destroys the tryspin inhibitor

Cottonseed contains a toxic pigment gossypol; processing removes this pigment

Mycotoxins are toxins produced by molds growing on grains and nuts. Aflatoxins are produced by a mold growth on Brazil nuts and peanuts. The problem is important especially in African countries where peanuts often mold on the ground. Discarding nuts with broken shells and discolored, shriveled nut kernels removes the danger

### CHEMICAL POISONING

Food may be accidentally contaminated by poisonous chemicals. Lead poisoning can occur if food is exposed to dust containing lead or if food is kept in containers in which solders, alloys, or enamel containing lead have been used.

Pesticides have sometimes been accidentally mistaken for a food ingredient, or have been ingested by children who had access to them. Pesticides used in excess of regulations are a potential hazard to fruits and vegetables. Careful washing of foods before their use reduces this hazard.

### RADIOACTIVE FALLOUT

Nuclear testing has increased the amount of strontium 90 and iodine 131 in the atmosphere and consequently in the soil. Cattle may transmit strontium 90 from the grasses they eat to their milk, and plants grown on such soils may also contain radioactive elements. The absorption of large quantities of iodine 131 by the body increases the possibility of thyroid cancer. About four fifths of the strontium 90 is excreted in the urine, but some is deposited in the bones and gonads. A liberal intake of calcium appears to be protective against excessive deposit of strontium 90. The Atomic Energy Commission and the United States Public Health Service measure the amounts of radioactive fallout in food supplies from time to time. Presently, the amounts are well below any danger levels.

## Preservation of Foods

### CAUSES OF FOOD SPOILAGE

Bacteria and parasites in food may lead to illness; yeasts produce fermentation, as in cider and fruit juices; molds attack wet berries, citrus fruits, bread, jellies and jams, and other foods. Chemical and physical changes also occur in food; enzyme activity leads to softening of the food, development of off flavors, and loss of some nutrients; in a few hours sunlight destroys much of the riboflavin in milk and changes the flavor; exposure to air leads to darkening of peeled fruit and to rancidity of fats.

Foods are contaminated by any of the following ways:

1. Preparation by persons whose hands have not been washed after each use of the handkerchief, toilet, or contact with other source of dirt and filth.

2. Exposure to dust, flies, insects, and nasal sprays of persons who cough or sneeze.

3. Use of equipment and dishes that are poorly cleaned and rinsed.

4. Failure to refrigerate fresh or cooked food promptly, thus speeding up the action of bacteria, molds, yeasts, and enzymes.

### OBJECTIVES FOR FOOD PRESERVATION

Food preservation aims (1) to destroy microorganisms as by heat, or (2) to retard their growth by removal of moisture or the use of cold temperatures. Chemical changes are minimized by avoiding exposure to air and light, by reducing the environmental temperature, and by destroying enzymes. Some losses in nutritive value, especially ascorbic acid and thiamine, are unavoidable. However, commercial techniques now ensure processed foods with a greater proportion of all nutrients still present.

### DEHYDRATION

Drying is one of the oldest methods of food preservation. Modern techniques have made many of these foods attractive in terms of their ease of preparation, the variety they lend to the diet, and the fact that they can be stored at room temperature. Instant dry milk, instant potatoes, mixes for breads, cakes, cookies, and puddings, instant coffee, beverage powders, and mixes for soups, as well as dried fruit, are among the products we now take for granted.

### COLD TEMPERATURES

*Refrigeration.* Perishable foods are now transported from coast to coast under refrigeration, are kept cold in the market until sold, and remain high in quality for several days to a week in the home refrigerator.

*Freezing* of food has been employed for centuries in cold regions of the world, but the advent of quick freezing of food in the 1930s has revolutionized the food industry. Foods are rapidly frozen at $-37°$ C ($-35°$ F) and may be stored in the home freezer at $-18°$ C ($0°$ F) for several weeks or months (depending upon the product) with minimum changes in texture, color, flavor, or nutritive value. Bacteria and enzymes are not destroyed at freezing temperatures, but they are inactive. Once food is thawed, however, spoilage occurs more rapidly because the cell walls have been broken by the tiny ice crystals. Thawed food should be used promptly and not refrozen.

*Freeze-drying* consists in quickly freezing the food product, such as brewed coffee, drying it in a vacuum, and finally packaging it in the presence of an inert gas such as nitrogen. The food retains its original shape, and can be readily rehydrated with water. It is light in weight and requires no refrigeration. The method is not extensively used for products for home use at the present time.

### HEAT PRESERVATION

*Cookery.* The boiling of food leads to destruction of microorganisms and of enzymes. Lower temperatures, such as those attained in a double boiler, are not sufficient to destroy certain organisms, such as *Salmonella* in eggs. *Trichinella* in pork is destroyed only when the meat is cooked so that no tinge of pink color remains. Some spores of bacteria and some toxins are not destroyed by the heat used in ordinary cooking methods.

*Pasteurization* is the application of heat to destroy pathogenic organisms, but it does not sterilize the product. In the high-temperature, short-time process now widely used, milk is held at 160° F for at least 15 seconds. Undoubtedly, the pasteurization of milk is the major reason why disease now rarely results from the drinking of milk. Milk and cream for the manufacture of cheese, ice cream, and butter are usually pasteurized.

*Canning* is still the primary means used to preserve foods for long periods of time. Commercial canning is done by steam under pressure;

thus at 15 lb pressure the temperature is 250° F. Home canning is far less frequent than at one time. Meat, poultry, and nonacid vegetables, such as corn, peas, and green beans, should be canned only with a pressure cooker to ensure destruction of the spores of *Cl. botulinum.*

### CHEMICAL PRESERVATION

Sugar has a preservative effect when used in high concentrations for jams, jellies, and preserves. Molds will grow on the surfaces of such products, however, unless they are protected from the air. Brine is used for pickles, sauerkraut, and pickled fish. Sodium benzoate may be used in a limited number of products, including margarine. Sulfur dioxide prevents the darkening of apples and apricots during dehydration. The growth of molds is retarded in bread with the use of calcium propionate and in cheese by using wrappings to which sorbic acid has been added.

## Additives

### INTENTIONAL ADDITIVES

An intentional additive is any substance of known composition that is added to a food to serve some useful purpose. Some additives improve nutritional values, such as iodine in salt, vitamin D in milk, vitamin A in margarine, and thiamine, riboflavin, niacin, and iron in enriched flours and cereals. Other additives enhance the keeping qualities of a food; for example, calcium propionate which retards molding of bread, BHT and BHA which are abbreviations for chemicals that maintain freshness of cereals, and salt as a preservative for pickles, sauerkraut, and dried meats and fish. Some additives have emulsifying properties; they help to maintain the smooth texture in cheese, ice cream, peanut butter and other foods. Antioxidants such as ascorbic acid prevent the darkening of fruits, and tocopherols keep oils from becoming rancid. Artificial sweeteners, flavorings, and colorings improve the taste or appearance of foods. It is unlawful to use additives to mask faulty processing or handling, or to cover up inferior ingredients, or to deceive the consumer in any way.

### INCIDENTAL ADDITIVES

Some chemicals gain entrance to foods from contact during growing or processing, or from the package itself. Since such incidental additives cannot be completely eliminated, it is essential that safe pesticides be used within the allowed levels; that all processing be carried on under the strictest controls of safety and sanitation; and that packaging be rigidly tested for its safety. Federal and state laws determine the maximum levels of such incidental additives that will be tolerated in a product.

## REVIEW QUESTIONS AND PROBLEMS

**1.** Visit a local market or restaurant to observe the practices in the handling of food. List the good practices and any that require improvement.

**2.** What would you do if you opened a can of food that appeared to be spoiled?

**3.** Following a picnic many people became ill from eating chicken salad. What organism probably caused the illness? How did it probably gain entrance to the food? Give several rules for avoiding such illness.

**4.** What is meant by botulism? Trichinosis? How can they be avoided?

**5.** Read the labels on the following packaged foods and list the additives contained in them: hydrogenated fat, breakfast cereal, bread, gelatin dessert powder, cake mix, process cheese, and canned soup. List the reasons for as many of these additives as you can.

## REFERENCES

Earl, H. G.: "Food Poisoning: The Sneaky Attacker," *Today's Health*, **43**:64, October 1965.

Editorial: "Botulism: Still a Tragedy," *JAMA*, **210**:338, 1969.

*Food Additives: What They Are. How They Are Used.* Manufacturing Chemists Association, 1825 Connecticut Ave., N.W., Washington, D.C., 1972.

Foster, E. M.: "Microbial Problems in Today's Foods," *J. Am. Diet. Assoc.*, **52**:485–89, 1968.

*Keeping Food Safe to Eat*, Home and Garden No. 162. Washington, D.C.: U.S. Department of Agriculture.

Martin, R.: "What You Don't See Can Hurt You," *Today's Health*, **43**:42, Nov. 1965.

Olcott, H. S.: "Mercury, DDT, and PCBs in Aquatic Food Resources," *J. Nutr. Educ.*, **4**:156–57, Fall 1972.

Oser, B. L.: "How Safe Are the Chemicals in Our Food?" *Today's Health*, **44**:61, March 1966.

Rensberger, B., and Roueché, B.: "When Americans Are a Swallow Away from Death," *Today's Health*, **49**:41, September 1971.

Taylor, A., Jr.: "Botulism and Its Control," *Am. J. Nurs.*, **73**:1380–82, 1973.

Tschirley, F. H.: "Pesticides: Relation to Environmental Quality," *JAMA*, **224**:1157, 1973.

Werrin, M., and Kronick, D.: "Salmonella Control in Hospitals," *Am. J. Nurs.*, **66**:528–31, 1966.

# FOOD LEGISLATION, LABELING, AND SELECTION

## CONSUMER CHALLENGES

Many persons spend more money for food than for any other item. Today's consumer faces great challenges in selecting food from the thousands of items available in any supermarket. Dietitians and nurses in their daily work and also in their neighborly contacts within their own communities are constantly asked about the comparative values of foods.

The tremendous rise in food costs in recent years means that the homemaker tries to be much more selective in her food marketing. She is anxious to know how one product compares with another not only in quantity per unit price but also in nutritive values. Many people are concerned about the additives in foods and want to know what protection they have that these additives are indeed safe and serve a useful purpose. Other individuals require modified diets. For example, someone who is allergic to wheat and eggs needs to be able to identify the products that are wheat-free and egg-free. Another person whose physician has prescribed a cholesterol-restricted fat-controlled diet (see Chap. 24) is interested in the cholesterol and fat content of foods.

These and many other consumer problems are answered through knowledge of legislation that protects the quality of the food supply as well as the honesty of claims made for the product. Recent sweeping new regulations for labeling will help consumers to make wise choices for nutritional values as well as ingredients. Finally, consumers need information concerning good choices within the several food groups.

169

## Food Protection Through Legislation

### FOOD, DRUG, AND COSMETIC ACT

The first federal food and drug law was passed in 1906 and was replaced in 1938 by a more comprehensive Federal Food, Drug, and Cosmetic Act— also known as the "Pure Food and Drug Law." This law pertains to food, other than meat and poultry products, sold in interstate commerce and imported and exported foods. It requires that foods be pure, wholesome, and honestly labeled.

*Amendments.* Several amendments to the law have been enacted. The Miller Pesticide Amendment of 1954 enables the establishment of safe tolerances of pesticides that may remain in foods after they have been harvested. The Additives Amendment of 1958 provides that an additive may be used in a food product only if it can be shown to improve the nutritive quality, appearance, or keeping properties of a food and not to cover up the use of an inferior food. The amendment requires the manufacturer to submit evidence from experimental work on animals that an additive is safe before it may be included in a food product for sale. The Food and Drug Administration examines the evidence, seeks further proof if necessary, and then issues or refuses a permit for the use of the additive, depending upon its findings. The Color Additive Amendment of 1960 provides for the establishment of safe tolerance levels for all colors used in foods. The Fair Packaging and Labeling Act passed by Congress in 1966 authorizes the FDA to set up regulations for packaging and labeling that avoids deceptive practices.

*Enforcement.* The food and drug law, together with its amendments, is enforced by the Food and Drug Administration of the Department of Health, Education, and Welfare. Under the law, factories and warehouses may be inspected to ascertain that the raw materials together with processing, packaging, and storage facilities are sanitary. (See Fig. 17–1.) Adulterated and misbranded products may be seized by inspectors and destroyed or relabeled, depending upon the nature of the offense. Flagrant violations may result in the imposition of fines or imprisonment by the courts.

*Interpretation of the law.* A food is *adulterated* if it contains dirt, filth, or decomposed material or any substance harmful to health; if it is prepared, packaged, or stored under unsanitary conditions; if it is made from diseased animals; if it contains additives that conceal the poor quality of the food; if it contains unsafe additives, uncertified food colors, or pesticide residues in excess of tolerances; if the packaging material contains substances harmful to health.

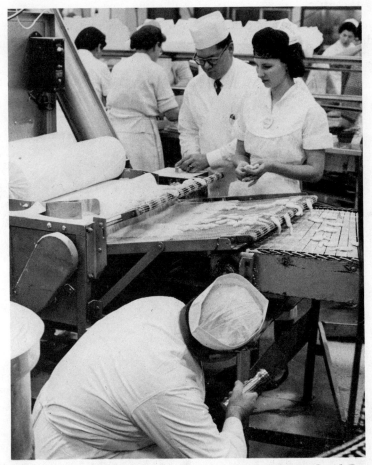

FIGURE 17–1 Plant inspection is one of the activities of the Food and Drug Administration authorized by federal legislation. *(FDA photo.)*

*Misbranded food* is that which has a false, misleading label; a package that fails to specify the weight, measure, or count of the food; a package that is of misleading size, so that the consumer thinks he is getting more than he actually is; a label that does not clearly state the use of imitations, including artificial color, flavorings, and preservatives; a label that fails to list the name of the manufacturer, packer, or distributor; a label that does not list the amounts of nutrients in products for which a nutritional claim is made.

The Food and Drug Administration also establishes what a product actually is by setting standards of *identity, quality,* and *fill.* Foods for which an official standard has been set must contain amounts of ingredients not below the prescribed minimum nor above the legal maximum.

(See Fig. 17–2.) This regulation applies also to the addition of required amounts of nutrients for enrichment and fortification. For nonstandardized products the ingredients are listed in order from the greatest amount to

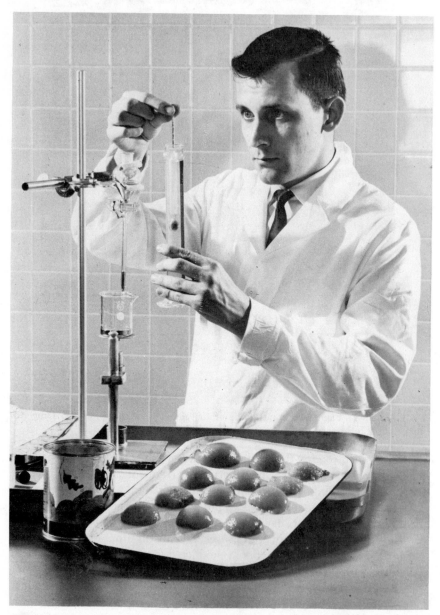

FIGURE 17–2 The Food and Drug Administration conducts numerous laboratory studies that determine whether food products comply with standards of labeling, identity, quality, and fill. (*FDA photo.*)

the least. Standards of quality for canned vegetables, fruits, and meats, and other products pertain to the color, flavor, and freedom from defects. Standards of fill specify how full a container must be.

## MEAT AND POULTRY INSPECTION

The Meat Inspection Act of 1906 and its amendments of 1967 and the Poultry Inspection Act of 1957 accomplish the objectives of the pure food law for meat and poultry. The Bureau of Animal Husbandry of the U.S. Department of Agriculture is charged with the enforcement of these acts. The acts provide for the inspection of premises for processing animals and poultry, the live animals, and the carcasses. Meat that is inspected and is fit for consumption is labeled "U.S. Inspected and Passed," and that which is unfit for human consumption is labeled "Inspected and Condemned." (See Fig. 17–3.) The Act also applies to manufactured meat products and provides for the proper use of additives, the correct labeling of the product, and the maintenance of standards of identity.

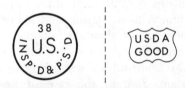

FIGURE 17–3 The round inspection stamp on meat indicates that the meat is wholesome. The shield indicates the grade of meat; grading of meat is not required by law. (*Courtesy, U.S. Department of Agriculture, Washington, D.C.*)

## FEDERAL TRADE COMMISSION

Advertising for products that are involved in interstate commerce is regulated by the Federal Trade Commission. In recent years some of the food supplements such as vitamins and so-called health foods were seized because false claims were made for nutritive values or for cures for disease.

## STATE AND LOCAL LEGISLATION

Because federal legislation applies only to foods sold in interstate commerce, the individual states have passed laws that are similar to the federal laws. The state and local ordinances for the protection and pasteurization of milk, and the regulations for public eating establishments, have usually been patterned after the codes set up by the United States Public Health Service.

The United States Department of Agriculture maintains a voluntary grading service for the quality of livestock, poultry, dairy products, fruits, and vegetables. Many state departments of agriculture cooperate with the federal government in the training of state inspectors and in setting up comparable standards for intrastate products.

## Read the Label

### SOME DEFINITIONS

In order to interpret labels consumers need to have a clear understanding of several descriptions of foods.

*Restored* applies to the addition of nutrients to a processed food so that it has the same value as the original food. For example, suppose the original food contained 5.0 mg iron per pound, and lost 1.0 mg in processing; the addition of 1.0 mg iron restores it to the original value.

*Fortification* is the addition of one or more nutrients that may or may not have been present in the original food; for example, the addition of vitamin D to milk, vitamin A to margarine, and iodine to salt.

*Enrichment* is the addition of thiamine, riboflavin, niacin, and iron to flours and cereals according to specified standards set by the Food and Drug Administration. This constitutes a restoration of nutrients removed in the processing of grain, and, in the case of iron, fortification as well.

A *dietary supplement* is a product specially formulated to furnish additional nutrients to a regular diet. It includes vitamins, minerals, and/or protein in the form of foods, capsules, tablets, pills, powders, or liquids. The Food and Drug Administration has set up regulations that would limit these preparations to amounts ranging between 50 and 150 per cent of the U.S. RDA (see Table 17–1). A product that exceeds 150 per cent of the U.S. RDA cannot be sold as a food or dietary supplement, but must be labeled and sold as a drug. These regulations, as of the time of this writing, are subject to further hearings before they are finally adopted.

*Engineered, formulated,* or *fabricated* foods are products developed by manufacturers from one or more ingredients. They are termed *analogs* when they simulate another food; for example, textured vegetable protein made from soybeans may simulate a pork chop or sausage or other meat product. Several breakfast drinks have been developed for use in place of orange juice, and are similar in color, flavor, and nutrient content. One of the important points to be aware of in choosing a fabricated food is that it furnishes the same amount and variety of nutrients that are contained in the food it replaces.

TABLE 17–1   U.S. RECOMMENDED DIETARY ALLOWANCES (U.S. RDA)
FOR ADULTS AND CHILDREN OVER 4 YEARS

| Required | | Optional | |
|---|---|---|---|
| Protein | 65 gm * | Vitamin D | 400 I.U. |
| Vitamin A | 5000 I.U. | Vitamin E | 30 I.U. |
| Vitamin C | 60 mg | Vitamin $B_6$ | 2.0 mg |
| Thiamine | 1.5 mg | Folacin | 0.4 mg |
| Riboflavin | 1.7 mg | Vitamin $B_{12}$ | 6 mcg |
| Niacin | 20 mg | Phosphorus | 1.0 gm |
| Calcium | 1.0 gm | Iodine | 150 mcg |
| Iron | 18 mg | Magnesium | 400 mg |
| | | Zinc | 15 mg |
| | | Copper | 2 mg |
| | | Biotin | 0.3 mg |
| | | Pantothenic Acid | 10 mg |

* If the protein efficiency ratio of protein is equal to or better than that of casein, U.S. RDA is 45 gm.

## FOOD LABELING

The principal display panel for a packaged or canned food product must include (1) the common name of the product, (2) the net weight in ounces, including the liquids used for packing as well as the solids, and (3) the name and address of the manufacturer, packer, or distributor. A description of the product is also given; for example, "condensed" for soups that are to be diluted when used; "cream style" for corn; whole, halves, pieces, etc., for fruits.

The ingredients for nonstandardized products must be listed in the order of their predominance; that is, the ingredient in the largest amount listed first, the second largest next, and so on. This listing includes the common names of ingredients. The common names of additives are chemical terms that have little meaning to most consumers. Nevertheless, their listing represents a protection to the consumer.

More than 300 products are manufactured under a standard of identity. Manufacturers are not required to list the ingredients for these products, since they are formulated according to standard recipes set by the Food and Drug Administration. However, manufacturers are now being urged to list ingredients in these products so that consumers can be better informed.

## NUTRITIONAL LABELING

The Food and Drug Administration has adopted regulations pertaining to the labeling of processed foods for nutritional information. This labeling will permit consumers to compare the nutritive values of one product with another; to count calories; to learn which foods contribute substantial amounts of nutrients and which foods contain few nutrients; to compare new food products with familiar ones; and to select appropriate foods for modified diets.

Nutritional labeling is voluntary on the part of manufacturers for most foods, but it is hoped that food processors will generally provide such information. Full nutritional labeling is required for (1) any product for which a claim of nutritional value is made in labeling or advertising, and (2) any product that contains one or more added nutrients, such as foods that are restored, fortified, or enriched.

**Labeling standard.** The U.S. Recommended Dietary Allowances (U.S. RDA) replaces the Minimum Daily Requirements (MDR) which is now outdated. Although the standard is based upon the Recommended Dietary Allowances (Table 4–1, p. 32), the two tables must not be confused and used interchangeably. For example the RDA has 17 categories for age, sex, pregnancy, and lactation, while the U.S. RDA includes only 3 groupings. The listing for adults (Table 17–1) will apply generally to foods, while the standards set for infants and children under 4 years, and for pregnant and lactating women will apply to products intended especially for these groups.

When nutrition information is provided, it must follow the format and order set by the Food and Drug Administration. The percentages of U.S. RDA are required for protein and seven vitamins and minerals; the manufacturer may list percentages for twelve additional vitamins and minerals. (See Table 17–1 and Fig. 17–4.)

## LABELING FOR SPECIAL DIETARY USES

Any product sold for a special dietary use must contain full nutritional labeling and use the U.S. RDA for adults, for infants, or for pregnant and lactating women. Five prohibitions apply to the labeling of products:

1. No claim can be made that the product in itself prevents, treats, or cures disease.

2. The label cannot claim or imply that a diet of ordinary foods cannot furnish adequate nutrients.

3. No claim can be made that inadequate diet is due to the soil on which the foods are grown.

4. No claim can be made that transportation, storage, or cooking of foods may result in an inadequate diet.

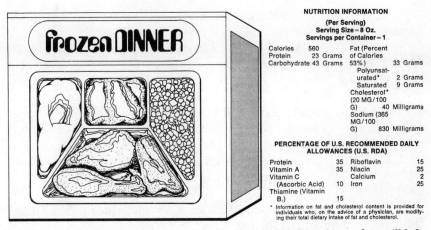

**NUTRITION INFORMATION**

(Per Serving)
Serving Size = 8 Oz.
Servings per Container = 1

| Calories | 560 | Fat (Percent | |
| Protein | 23 Grams | of Calories | |
| Carbohydrate | 43 Grams | 53%) | 33 Grams |
| | | Polyunsat- | |
| | | urated* | 2 Grams |
| | | Saturated | 9 Grams |
| | | Cholesterol* | |
| | | (20 MG/100 | |
| | | G) | 40 Milligrams |
| | | Sodium (365 | |
| | | MG/100 | |
| | | G) | 830 Milligrams |

**PERCENTAGE OF U.S. RECOMMENDED DAILY ALLOWANCES (U.S. RDA)**

| Protein | 35 | Riboflavin | 15 |
| Vitamin A | 35 | Niacin | 25 |
| Vitamin C | | Calcium | 2 |
| (Ascorbic Acid) | 10 | Iron | 25 |
| Thiamine (Vitamin | | | |
| B₁) | 15 | | |

\* Information on fat and cholesterol content is provided for individuals who, on the advice of a physician, are modifying their total dietary intake of fat and cholesterol.

**FIGURE 17-4** Nutrition information such as that provided for this product will help consumers to compare food products and also to determine whether a product is appropriate for a given modified diet. (*Courtesy, Food and Drug Administration, Rockville, Maryland.*)

5. No nutritional claim can be made that nonnutritive ingredients such as inositol, paraminobenzoic acid, or bioflavinoids have nutritional value.

*Cholesterol and fat.* Any product that is labeled for cholesterol must state the amount of cholesterol in milligrams per serving and per 100 grams of food. The fatty acid content of food may be stated if the total fat content is more than 2 gm per serving. It should include the grams of total fat, grams of fat from saturated fatty acids, grams of fat from polyunsaturated fatty acids, and per cent of calories from fat. When information on cholesterol and fatty acids is included in labeling, the following statement must also appear on the label: "Information on fat (and/or cholesterol) content is provided for individuals who, on the advice of a physician, are modifying their total dietary intake of fat (and/or cholesterol)."

## Selection by Food Groups

### GENERAL RULES FOR ECONOMY

1. Read food columns in newspapers to learn which foods are plentiful and lower in cost. Take advantage of advertised specials in newspapers.

2. Plan menus in advance and prepare a market order. Be prepared to modify your plans if when you get to the market you find that some foods are too expensive or are not available.

3. Avoid buying foods on impulse.

4. Read labels and compare prices, weights, grades, and nutritional values of different brands.

5. Buy fresh foods in season. Fresh foods out of season are usually more costly than canned or frozen foods.

6. Compare cost of convenience and home-prepared foods. Many canned and dried products and some frozen products are about as low in cost as home-prepared foods and save considerable time for the home-maker. Highly perishable convenience foods, such as salad mixes of fruits or vegetables and bakery foods, are likely to be much more expensive.

7. Consider the nutritive value of the snack foods—popcorn, candy, pretzels, soft drinks, and others. Is too much of your food budget spent for these?

8. Purchase only the amounts that are likely to be used by the family. Use leftovers promptly. (See Fig. 17–5.)

### MILK GROUP

Of fluid milks, fresh milk costs most, and skim milk made from nonfat dry milk costs least. Fresh milk is available in many variations, all of which are pasteurized; whole; homogenized; 2 per cent milk; fortified with vitamin D; multivitamin fortified; chocolate; skim; and buttermilk. Fresh pasteurized milk is usually fortified with vitamin D. Fresh milk purchased in a supermarket is less expensive than having it delivered to the home. Half-gallon and gallon containers are economical for families who require large amounts of milk.

Evaporated milk and nonfat dry milk are much less expensive than fresh milk. Evaporated milk is double-strength whole milk and is fortified with vitamin D. It has the same nutritive value as fresh milk when an equal amount of water is mixed with it. It may be used in any cooked dishes that require milk. For a recipe that calls for 1 cup milk, use ½ cup evaporated milk plus ½ cup water. Evaporated milk may be whipped for desserts and may be used on cereals and as cream in coffee.

Nonfat dry milk has the same nutritive value as the fresh skim milk from which it was made. People who must drink skim milk because of special dietary needs find the milk from nonfat dry milk to be just as acceptable as the fresh skim milk. It should be prepared several hours before serving and chilled thoroughly. It may be mixed half and half with whole milk for a very palatable beverage. Nonfat dry milk may be used in any recipe that requires milk. The directions on any package state the proportions to use.

Cream, yogurt, cream cheese, and ice cream are more expensive dairy products and should be used infrequently when the budget is limited. Half-and-half contains about 12 per cent fat, coffee and cultured sour cream about 18 per cent fat, and whipping cream 30 to 40 per cent fat.

Cottage cheese, American cheddar and Swiss cheese, and process

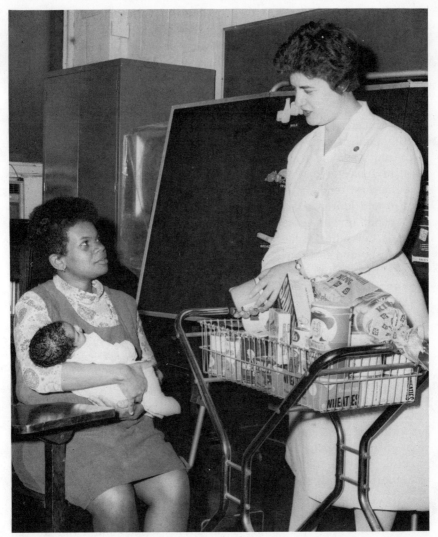

FIGURE 17-5 A market basket is used to illustrate the nutritive and economic values of foods. (*Courtesy, School of Nursing, Thomas Jefferson University, Philadelphia.*)

cheeses are inexpensive sources of protein, and provide good occasional substitutes for a meat meal. Imported cheeses, such as Roquefort, Gouda, Camembert, Edam, Gorgonzola, and many others are more expensive.

## MEAT GROUP

*Meat, poultry, fish.* It is difficult to provide firm rules for the purchase of meats because the relative cost of one variety as compared with another depends upon the market supply. Beef, for example, may be more or less expensive than lamb. Lean beef, lamb, pork, veal, poultry, and fish are similar in nutritive value. Therefore a selection of the meat that is least expensive per pound of lean will save money.

Meat that bears the round purple stamp of the Meat Inspection Board is safe and wholesome, but this stamp is no indication of quality. The cost of meat depends upon the grade, with U.S. Choice, Good, Standard, and Commercial grades being most common. Prime grade is seldom seen on the retail market. Choice grades of meat come from the younger animals and are more tender than the cuts from older animals. The lean meat of choice grade is well marbled with streaks of fat. Such meat will give the most tender steaks, chops, and oven roasts.

Rib and loin cuts of meat, such as steaks, chops, and rib roasts, are tender and usually more expensive than cuts from the more exercised parts of the animal, such as the flank, the shoulder used for pot roasts, Swiss steak, and meat loaf. Less tender cuts are very flavorful if properly cooked. Beef, lamb, and pork liver are much less expensive than calves' liver and just as nutritious.

When comparing the costs of meat, one should note the amount of fat, bone, and gristle in relation to the lean. Some lower-priced cuts of meat are sometimes more expensive because there is so little lean. One pound of lean meat, such as ground beef or round steak, will serve three to four persons. Steak and chops, because of the amount of bone and fat, will usually require 1 lb for two persons. Meat with much fat and bone, such as brisket and short ribs, will serve only one to two persons per pound.

Chicken and turkey have been good buys in recent times. The relative proportion of bone and skin to lean meat is somewhat higher than in the meat of larger animals.

Fish, whether fresh, canned, or frozen, is likely to be less expensive than meat. Shellfish, such as oysters, lobsters, shrimp, and crabs, are luxury items except where locally available.

**Eggs.** Eggs are priced according to quality and size. Top-quality eggs, grade AA and A, have a strong, clean, unbroken shell and a tiny air cell (less than ⅛ in.) when the egg is exposed to light in the candling process. When the egg is broken, the white is thick and gelatinous, and the yolk is round, high, and does not break easily. Such eggs are good for poaching, cooking in the shell, and frying. Grade B and C eggs will show a somewhat larger air cell on candling and will have thinner whites and flatter yolks when broken. Such eggs are suitable for cooking and baking. They have a somewhat less delicate flavor for table use.

Eggs are sorted according to size, based on weight per dozen: extra large, 27 oz.; large, 24 oz; medium 21 oz; and small, 18 oz. Medium and small eggs are usually a good buy in the fall, whereas large eggs may be a good buy in the spring. Medium eggs are a better buy than large eggs if their cost is at least one eighth less per dozen. White and brown eggs are equally good. Always buy refrigerated eggs.

**Legumes.** Legumes are a good protein source when the budget is limited, and they lend themselves to a variety of uses. Split peas, navy beans, Lima beans, kidney beans, lentils, soybeans, chick peas, and peanuts are among the varieties available. Peanut butter is a good buy. Dried legumes require soaking and a longer cooking time.

Textured vegetable protein (TVP) is sold under a variety of names. It is prepared from soybeans and is an excellent extender for meats such as hamburgers and meat loaf. When combined with meat the quality and amount of protein is as good as though the dish had been prepared from meat alone.

## VEGETABLE-FRUIT GROUP

Fresh, frozen, dehydrated, and canned fruits and vegetables may be purchased. Fresh fruits and vegetables, especially those locally grown, are often less expensive in season. Canned or frozen fruits and vegetables are likely to be better buys at other times of the year. Frozen orange juice is less expensive than freshly squeezed juice, but usually costs a little more than canned juice. Frozen vegetables prepared with butter or cream sauces are appreciably higher in cost than plain vegetables that would be seasoned at the time of cooking.

Fruits should be ripe, firm, free from decay spots, and not soft or with mold spots. Vegetables should be firm, crisp, and clean—not wilted or bruised. Overripe fruits or too mature vegetables are not good economy even though the price may be somewhat lower.

A canned product should be selected for its use; for example, whole fruit may be desired when it is to be served as a dessert, but fruit pieces are just as good for a mixed salad or for pastries. Likewise, grade A peas may be preferred for buttered peas, but grade B peas would be suitable for a casserole dish.

## BREAD-CEREAL GROUP

Enriched or whole-grain breads, cereals, pastas, and flours should be purchased. Enriched white bread is the least expensive way to purchase bread. Day-old bread, when available, is somewhat reduced in price. Many specialty breads that contain butter, stone-ground flour, honey, raisins, or other flavor ingredients and sweet breads and rolls are considerably more expensive. Many homemakers today find much satisfaction in baking their own breads and rolls.

Cooked breakfast cereals are usually less expensive than dry breakfast cereals. For variety, some of each should be used. Sugar-coated cereals and those containing dried fruit are more expensive than their plain counterparts. Precooked rice is more expensive than uncooked rice. To compare the cost of cereals, watch for unit prices.

### FATS

Butter and margarine are of equal nutritive value and are comparable in flavor. Margarine is much less costly, but there are considerable differences in price from brand to brand. Lard and hydrogenated fats are inexpensive cooking fats. With the current emphasis on vegetable oils, corn, cottonseed, and soybean oils will be found to be just as satisfactory as the more expensive oils sometimes advertised.

### SWEETS AND CONDIMENTS

Cane and beet sugars are inexpensive, whereas brown and confectioners' sugars are somewhat higher in cost. Molasses is a good buy, because it contains iron as well as carbohydrates. It can be used for many dishes, such as baked beans, gingerbread, cookies, puddings, and sometimes in a glass of milk for children. Honey, maple sugar and syrup, and candies represent expensive ways to buy sweets.

Spices, flavoring extracts, and herbs are important additions, because they enhance the flavors of food so much. Flavors are rapidly lost to the air, and only small containers of infrequently used seasonings should be purchased. Coffee, tea, catsup, meat sauces, pickles, and relishes add interest to meals. Depending upon the choices made, these food adjuncts may increase the food expenditure appreciably.

### REVIEW QUESTIONS AND PROBLEMS

1. Visit a supermarket and examine carefully the labeling for a can of fruit, a package of cereal, a package of biscuit mix, a frozen dinner, a brand of soft margarine, a loaf of bread, and a package of some dietetic food. What information do you find on the label of each? How would you evaluate this information for the nutritional importance of the product?

2. What national laws protect the food supply?

3. When is labeling for nutritional information required for a food product?

4. List four practices that would lead a product to be adulterated.

5. List four ways in which a product would be seized because it was misbranded.

6. Examine the labeling for two brands of instant potatoes. Are they fortified with vitamin C? How much per serving? How does this compare with the vitamin C content of one serving of fresh potatoes?

7. Compare the cost of a pound of round steak, short ribs, chuck roast, and rib roast. How many servings per pound of each?

8. A homemaker tells you that she cannot afford to buy enough milk for her family including herself, her husband, and four children ages 6, 8, 11, and 14. How much milk should she include each day? Show how much money she could save by using half of the day's allowance as whole milk and half as nonfat dry milk, as compared with all fresh milk.

## REFERENCES

Bauman, H. E.: "What Does the Consumer Know About Nutrition?" *JAMA*, **225**:61–62, 1973.

Council on Foods and Nutrition: "Improvement of the Nutritive Quality of Foods," *JAMA*, **225**:116–18, 1973.

Deutsch, R.: "Where You Should Be Shopping for Your Family," *Today's Health*, **50**:16, April 1972.

Food and Drug Administration, Washington, D.C.: *We Want You to Know About Nutrition Labels on Foods*, Pub. No. 74–2039; *We Want You to Know About Labels on Foods*, Pub. No. 73–2043; *How the FDA Works for You*, Pub. No. 1.

Moore, J. L., and Wendt, P. F.: "Nutrition Labeling—A Summary and Evaluation," *J. Nutr. Educ.*, **5**:121–25, April 1973.

Moore, M. L.: "When Families Must Eat More for Less," *Nurs. Outlook*, **14**:66–69, April 1966.

"The Syndrome of Poverty," *Am. J. Nurs.*, **66**:1749–61, 1966.

# NUTRITION AND DIET FOR
# THE PATIENT

## ILLNESS AND NUTRITION

Illness has many effects on the body's ability to use nutrients and upon the specific requirements. Lack of appetite, vomiting, and pain often prevent the intake of a sufficient amount of food. In severe diarrhea the absorption of all nutrients is poor, so that loss of weight, dehydration, and signs of malnutrition may be found. A fever increases the rate of metabolism, thus increasing the need for calories, protein, and vitamins. In metabolic diseases nutrients are not utilized fully; for example, the untreated diabetic patient will not make adequate use of carbohydrate. The patient who must remain in bed or in a wheelchair for a long time usually loses increased amounts of nitrogen and calcium from his body. As the student continues her study of diet therapy and becomes more experienced in the care of patients, she will undoubtedly find numerous examples of the effects of illness upon nutrition.

## ILLNESS AND FOOD ACCEPTANCE

The many physiologic, cultural, economic, and emotional factors affecting food acceptance have been discussed in Chapter 15. The person who is ill must face added problems related to his meals. Diet is related to both the comfort and the treatment of the patient, but sometimes it is necessary to take therapeutic measures that may distress rather than provide immediate comfort. The nurse plays an essential role in helping to bridge this gap. (See Fig. 18–1.)

187

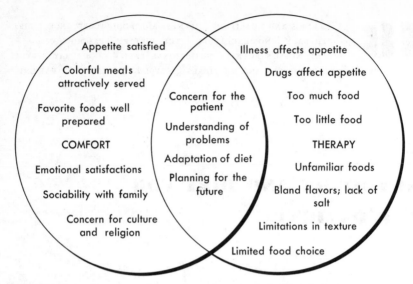

FIGURE 18–1 Patients seek comfort through food. Modified diets may present many problems. The nurse must help the patient to solve these problems.

Illness itself often reduces interest in food because of anorexia, gastrointestinal distention, or discomfort following meals. Inactivity and some drugs also reduce the desire for food.

The patient in a hospital may be away from home for the first time. He probably misses his family and the sociability of family meals. He finds that the food pattern in the hospital and the time for meals differ, more or less, from his usual pattern. He finds it difficult to manage a tray in bed. His food intake is affected by his worries about mounting hospital bills, about return to work, or about the extent of his return to full health.

If the diet is modified, the patient may be getting less or more food than he normally eats. The change in flavor or texture of some diets is not appealing. He may be unwilling to accept any change, worried about how he will get the new foods for his diet at home, or bothered about the inconvenience of sticking to a diet that is different from that of his family or friends. His modified diet may make him feel that he is deprived and punished.

In his illness the patient often becomes more self-centered, and he reacts by being irritable or even angry. He may complain incessantly about his food in order to get more attention, or he may be quite indifferent to his diet, eat poorly, and ignore the suggestions made by doctors, nurses, or dietitians.

## DIET THERAPY

An appropriate diet is essential in the total-care plan developed for every patient. Usually it supplements medical and surgical care; sometimes it is the specific treatment for disease. Diet therapy accomplishes one or more of these aims: (1) maintains normal nutrition; (2) corrects nutritional deficiency, for example, high-protein diet; (3) changes body weight, as with low- or high-calorie diets; (4) adjusts to the body's ability to use one or more nutrients, for example, diabetic diet; (5) permits maximum rest to the body or an organ, as with a soft, low-calorie diet in six feedings.

The normal diet may be modified for (1) consistency and texture; (2) flavor; (3) energy value; (4) nutrient levels such as fat, protein, carbohydrate, sodium, and others; or (5) food categories such as types of fats or elimination diets for allergies.

Often a combination of modifications is required; for example, 500-mg sodium, 1200-calorie, soft diet. In planning modified diets the normal diet should always be used as the frame of reference. The aim should always be to keep as many characteristics of the normal diet as possible.

## NOMENCLATURE

Diets that are changed from the normal are referred to as *modified* or *therapeutic*; the term "special diet" has little meaning, and should be avoided. Diets should be described exactly in terms of the change made in consistency, flavor, and the level of nutrients. The words "high" and "low" have meaning only when they are used with reference to the normal diet or when a given diet manual specifies the nutritive level. For example, a low-calorie diet might mean 800 kcal to one individual, 1200 kcal to another, and 1800 kcal to a man whose normal requirement is 2600 kcal per day. Diets should not be named for persons or for diseases; the latter practice is likely to be a continual reminder to the patient of his condition.

## THE DIETARY PRESCRIPTION

The physician orders the appropriate diet for each patient, just as he orders medications and other therapy. A given diet cannot arbitrarily and inflexibly be prescribed for a given disease condition. Each prescription is the result of an evaluation of the patient's symptoms, laboratory tests if they have been done, and his nutritional needs. In some instances priority must be given to one aspect of diet, while other requirements are deferred for a later time. For example, a very low-residue diet is lacking in some vitamins, but it might be essential for an acute gastrointestinal disorder or prior to surgery; after a few days the nutritional lack can usually be taken care of by a more liberal diet.

## THE NURSE'S ROLE IN NUTRITIONAL CARE

All people responsible for care should consider each patient as a person and should recognize his physical, psychologic, cultural, and emotional needs. Thinking only in terms of treating a specific disease is inexcusable, for it denies to each patient the right to be an individual. A correct, nutritious, attractive, and well-prepared meal for the patient requires the teamwork of the medical, nursing, and dietary services. In the hospital the dietitian translates the diet prescription into a menu and supervises the food preparation and service to the patient. The nurse has the most continual direct contract with the patient and makes certain that he receives and consumes his meals under the best circumstances.

If a selective menu is used, the dietary technician or nurse may help the patient to select his meals according to his diet prescription. As a nurse you would expect to prepare the patient for his meals so that his tray can be served as soon as it arrives. Perhaps you may need to feed him. Helping the patient to accept his diet by giving encouragement and praise is a decided contribution. This also means that you avoid criticism if he is not eating well, or pity because the diet is one you would not like very much.

Observing, listening, and reporting are three important functions performed by the nurse in nutritional care. How well the patient eats his food, what kinds and amounts of food are refused, and the patient's attitude toward his food are readily determined. You are more likely than anyone else to observe problems such as these: poorly fitting dentures and inability to chew; a sore mouth and pain when acid juices are taken; arthritic fingers that make it difficult to cut up food; portions that are too large for some elderly persons or too small for teen-agers; difficulty in breathing so that eating a large meal at one time is not possible; between-meal feedings interfering with the appetite for the meals; fatigue and poor appetite at the end of the day; and many others.

By listening you show your general interest in and your understanding of the patient, and help him to express his feelings and perhaps to "blow off steam." You begin to learn that some foods are favorites, others are thoroughly disliked, and still others cannot be eaten because of religious beliefs. You become aware of what food means to the patient, and what concerns the patient may have about the diet he will have when at home.

Acting upon your information is essential to the best care of the patient. Sometimes it is direct action on your part. More often it involves reporting to the nursing supervisor, dietitian, or physician, depending upon the circumstances.

As a nurse you have opportunity for some informal teaching. Patients often ask questions about their diets. Some of these you will be able to answer, but if you are not certain of the correct reply you should consult with the dietitian. When the patient has been given instructions for the diet to be used at home, you may be able to reinforce this by helping the patient to review his diet. For example, the lists of foods for a diet might seem very confusing at first. As you help the patient to see that foods on his tray correspond to these lists, you help him to become familiar with planning for the diet when he goes home. Patients often ask about food fads, meal planning, the kinds of foods needed for good health, tips for buying and preparing foods, and so on. Such questions give you an opportunity to emphasize the essentials of food nutrition.

## GOOD TRAY SERVICE

Meals are often the high point of the day for patients. An attractive tray of well-prepared food presented cheerfully to a patient who is ready for his meal goes a long way toward ensuring acceptance. (See Fig. 18–2.) The essentials of good tray service are:

1. A tray of sufficient size for uncrowded arrangement of dishes.
2. An immaculately clean, unwrinkled tray cover and napkin of linen or good quality paper.
3. An attractive pattern of spotless china without chips or cracks; sparkling glassware; and shining silverware.
4. Convenient orderly arrangement of all items on the tray so that the patient can easily reach everything.
5. Portions of food suitable for the patient's appetite.
6. Food attractively arranged with appropriate garnishes.
7. Meals served on time.
8. Hot foods served on warm plates and kept warm with a food cover; cold foods served on chilled dishes.
9. Trays promptly served to the patient so that food is at its best.

## THE PATIENT AND HIS MEALS

A pleasant cheerful environment is essential to the greatest enjoyment of food. Before the tray is served the nurse should make every effort to provide surroundings that are clean, orderly, and well ventilated. Activities not associated with meal service should be avoided as far as possible while patients are eating. If an interruption in a meal is unavoidable because of a doctor's visit, or if there is a delay because of a laboratory test, arrangements should be made to keep food hot (or chilled, as the case may be) in a nearby kitchen.

Before the trays arrive the patient's hands should be washed, and if the patient is in bed, he should be positioned so that he is comfortable

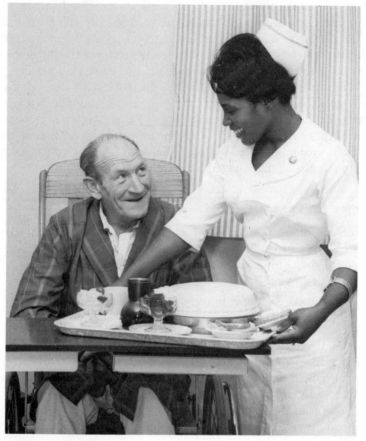

FIGURE 18–2 A meal that is colorful and varied in textures and flavors helps to make mealtime more enjoyable. The patient senses the genuine interest of the nurse in his welfare. (*Courtesy, School of Nursing, Thomas Jefferson University Hospital, Philadelphia.*)

and able to feed himself. The tray should be checked as soon as it reaches the patient's room to be certain that everything needed is there and is convenient for the patient. Sometimes it is necessary to butter the bread, open food containers, or cut the meat. The patient should be encouraged to eat, but should not be made to feel that he must hurry. Trays should be removed promptly when the patient has finished his meal.

### FEEDING THE HELPLESS PATIENT

Acutely ill and elderly infirm patients often must be fed. Feeding a patient requires patience and understanding, especially if the patient eats slowly. If you can imagine how you would want someone fed who is very dear to you, you could probably set up a good guide. Here are some suggestions:

Before starting to feed the patient, make certain that you have everything you need. If the patient eats very slowly, it is a good idea to keep food hot by placing the plate over a hot-water container. Sit, rather than stand, so that you and the patient will be more comfortable and relaxed. If the patient is blind, give an attractive description of the food you are about to feed him. Offer small amounts of food at a time, and encourage the patient to chew his food well. Alternate one food with another, as the individual would normally do if he were feeding himself. Offer a beverage as seems indicated or as the patient requests it.

Focus upon the patient, rather than on the feeding process. Avoid giving the impression that the feeding is a bother to you and that you must hurry. Talk to the patient about pleasant things, and also give him a chance to talk. Listen thoughtfully and with interest to what he has to say. Explain the reasons for any change in his diet, and give encouragement when he makes progress. (See Fig. 18–3.)

## REVIEW QUESTIONS AND PROBLEMS

**1.** List some changes that occur in illness and that affect the nutrition of the patient.

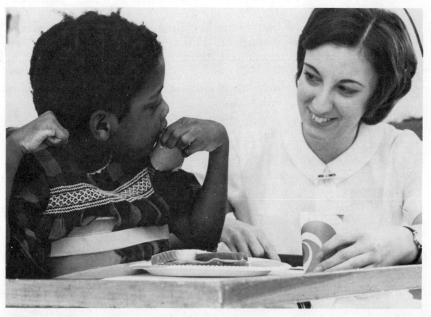

**FIGURE 18–3** A nurse provides assistance and encouragement to a handicapped child at mealtime. (*Courtesy, Handicapped Children's Unit, St. Christopher's Hospital for Children, Philadelphia.*)

2. Keep a record for a few days of the things that annoy you about food service. Also list the comments about food made by your friends and by patients. What reasons can you assign for these complaints? How would you as a nurse help the patient to better acceptance of his diet?

3. Become familiar with the arrangement of trays in your hospital. Arrange a tray for meals so that it is attractive and convenient.

4. What is meant by *diet therapy?* What purposes can be served by diet therapy?

5. Why are the following names for diet undesirable: cardiac diet, Meulengracht diet, ulcer discharge diet, low-salt diet?

6. Prepare a detailed list of ways in which you, as a nurse, can assist the patient with his nutrition.

7. Observe the meals served to patients for whom a house diet has been prescribed. How do they differ from normal diets with which you are familiar? Explain any differences you have noted.

## REFERENCES

Coulter, P. P., and Brower, M. J.: "Parallel Experience: An Interview Technique," *Am. J. Nurs.*, **69**:1028–30, 1969.

Dawson, M. J.: "New Patients Dine with the Nurse," *Am. J. Nurs.*, **66**:287–89, 1966.

Etzwiler, D. D.: "The Patient Is a Member of the Medical Team," *J. Am. Diet. Assoc.*, **61**:421–23, 1972.

Johnson, D.: "Effective Diet Counseling Begins Early in Hospitalization," *Hospitals*, **41**:94–100, January 16, 1967.

MacGregor, F. C.: "Uncooperative Patients: Some Cultural Interpretations," *Am. J. Nurs.*, **67**:88–91, 1967.

Mason, M. A.: *Basic Medical-Surgical Nursing*, 3rd ed. New York: Macmillan Publishing Co., Inc., 1974, Chap. 1.

Morris, E.: "How Does a Nurse Teach Nutrition to Patients?" *Am. J. Nurs.*, **60**:67–70, January 1960.

Robinson, C. H.: "Updating Clinical Dietetics: Terminology," *J. Am. Diet. Assoc.*, **62**:645–48, 1973.

Smith, D. W.: "Patienthood and Its Threat to Privacy," *Am. J. Nurs.*, **69**:508–13, 1969.

Tarnower, W.: "Psychological Needs of the Hospitalized Patient," *Nurs. Outlook*, **13**:28–30, July 1965.

# **19**

# MODIFICATIONS OF THE NORMAL DIET FOR TEXTURE

*Normal, Fluid, and Soft Fiber-Restricted Diets*

## NORMAL DIET AND ITS MODIFICATIONS

The normal, regular, general, or house diet is the most frequently used of all diets. A normal diet, like a modified diet, is of great importance in a therapeutic sense. With satisfactory food intake the body's tissues are continuously maintained, and there is opportunity for repair from the effects of illness. On the other hand, the patient's failure to eat a normal diet could lead to loss of body tissue and a prolonged convalescence.

The normal diet in hospital usage follows the principles outlined in the preceding units, and is planned to provide the Recommended Dietary Allowances. The Four Food Groups offer a convenient basis for menu planning, and diets in this section will be arranged according to these groups. The normal diet in the hospital requires no restrictions upon food choice. Strongly flavored vegetables, fried foods, cakes, pies, pastries, spicy foods, and relishes all have a place on the menu, but they should be used with discretion.

## Liquid Diets

### CLEAR-FLUID DIET

This is an allowance of tea, coffee or coffee substitute, and fat-free broth. Ginger ale, fruit juices, flavored gelatin, fruit ices, and water gruels are sometimes given. Small amounts of fluid are offered every hour or two to the patient. The diet is used for 24 to 48 hours following acute vomiting, diarrhea, or surgery.

The primary purpose of this diet is to relieve thirst and to help maintain water balance. Broth provides some sodium, and broth and fruit juices contribute potassium. Carbonated beverages, sugar, and fruit juices, when used, furnish a small amount of carbohydrate.

## FULL-FLUID DIET

This is a nutritionally adequate diet consisting of liquids and foods that liquefy at body temperature. It is used for acute infections and fever of short duration and for patients who are too ill to chew. It may be ordered as the first progression from the clear-fluid diet following surgery or in the treatment of acute gastrointestinal upsets.

The diet is offered in six feedings or more. Initially, amounts smaller that those represented by the plan below are given. To increase the caloric intake, 1 pt light cream may be substituted for 1 pt milk. The protein level of the full-fluid diet may be increased approximately 30 gm by including 80 gm (1⅓ cups) nonfat dry milk each day. This may be added to fresh milk, to cream soups, to cereal gruels, or to custards. Strained meats may be added to broth or to hot tomato juice. Raw eggs are sometimes a source of *Salmonella* infection. Therefore, only commercially pasteurized eggnogs or beverages prepared from pasteurized dried egg powder should be used.

### FULL-FLUID DIET

#### Food Allowance for One Day

6 cups milk
2 eggs
1–2 oz strained meat
1 cup strained citrus juice
½ cup tomato juice
½ cup vegetable purée
½ cup strained cereal
2 servings dessert: soft custard, Junket, plain ice cream, sherbert, or plain gelatin
2 tablespoons sugar
1 tablespoon butter

Protein: 85 gm
Calories: 1950

#### Sample Menu

*Breakfast*
Grapefruit juice
Strained oatmeal with butter, hot milk, and sugar
Milk
Coffee with cream and sugar

*Midmorning*
Orange juice
Soft custard

*Luncheon*
Broth with strained beef
Tomato juice
Vanilla ice cream
Milk

*Midafternoon*
Milk

*Sample Menu*

*Dinner*

Cream of asparagus soup
Eggnog, commercial, pasteurized
Strawberry gelatin with whipped cream
Tea with lemon and sugar

*Bedtime*

Chocolate malted milk

## Soft Diets

### MECHANICAL SOFT DIET

The Mechanical Soft Diet differs from the normal diet only in that it is limited to soft foods for those who have difficulty in chewing because of no teeth or poorly fitting dentures. No restriction is made upon the diet for seasonings or method of food preparation.

The normal diet is modified in the following ways:

1. Meat and poultry are minced or ground; fish usually is sufficiently tender without further treatment.

2. Vegetables are cooked. They may be cooked a little longer than usual to be sure they are soft, and may be diced or chopped; for example, diced beets, chopped spinach, and so on.

3. Chopped raw tomatoes, chopped lettuce, and finely chopped cabbage may sometimes be used.

4. Soft raw fruits: banana, citrus sections, diced soft pear, peach, apple, apricots, melons, berries. All canned and frozen fruits.

5. Soft rolls, bread, and biscuits instead of crisp rolls, crusty breads, and toast.

6. All desserts on a normal diet that are soft, including pies with tender crusts, cakes, puddings. Nuts and dried fruits are used only if they are finely chopped.

### SOFT FIBER-RESTRICTED DIET

The Soft Fiber-Restricted Diet is a nutritionally adequate diet that differs from the normal diet in being reduced in fiber content and soft in consistency. It is used intermediately between the Full-Fluid Diet and the normal diet following surgery, in acute infections and fevers, and in gastrointestinal disturbances.

The food allowances and a sample menu for the Soft Fiber-Restricted Diet is shown in Table 19–1. Note the following changes from the normal diet:

| Food Allowances | Sample Menu * |
|---|---|
| *Beverages*—coffee, tea, carbonated | **Breakfast** |
| *Bread*—white, fine whole-wheat, rye without seeds; white crackers | Orange sections<br>Oatmeal<br>Milk |
| *Cereal foods*—dry, such as cornflakes, Puffed Rice, rice flakes; fine-cooked, such as corn meal, farina, hominy grits, macaroni, noodles, rice, spaghetti; strained coarse, such as oatmeal, Pettijohn's, whole-wheat | Sugar<br>Soft-cooked egg<br>Whole-wheat toast<br>Butter or margarine<br>Coffee with cream, sugar |
| *Cheese*—mild, soft, such as cottage and cream; Cheddar; Swiss | **Luncheon** |
| *Desserts*—plain cake, cookies; custards; plain gelatin or with allowed fruit; Junket; plain ice cream, ices, sherbets; plain puddings, such as bread, cornstarch, rice, tapioca | Tomato bouillon<br>Melba toast<br>Roast chicken<br>Buttered rice |
| *Eggs*—all except fried | Asparagus tips<br>Parkerhouse roll |
| *Fats*—butter, cream, margarine, vegetable oils and fats in cooking | Butter or margarine<br>Golden cake with fluffy<br>  white icing |
| *Fruits*—raw: ripe avocado, banana, grapefruit or orange sections without membrane; canned or cooked: apples, apricots, fruit cocktail, peaches, pears, plums—all without skins; Royal Anne cherries; strained prunes and other fruits with skins; all juices | Milk; tea, if desired<br><br>**Dinner**<br>Grapefruit juice<br>Small club steak |
| *Meat*—very tender, minced, or ground; baked, broiled, creamed, roast, or stewed: beef, lamb, veal, poultry, fish, bacon, liver, sweetbreads | Baked potato without skin, butter<br>Buttered julienne green beans |
| *Milk*—in any form | Dinner roll with butter |
| *Soups*—broth, strained cream or vegetable | Apple crisp |
| *Sweets*—all sugars, syrup, jelly, honey, plain sugar candy without fruit or nuts, molasses<br>Use in moderation | Milk<br>Tea or coffee, if desired |
| *Vegetables*—white or sweet potato without skin, any way except fried; young and tender asparagus, beets, carrots, peas, pumpkin, squash without seeds; tender chopped greens; strained cooked vegetables if not tender; tomato juice | |
| *Miscellaneous*—salt, seasonings and spices in moderation, gravy, cream sauces | |

* May be given in six feedings by saving part of the food from the preceding meal.

1. Tender, minced, or ground meats.

2. Elimination of sharp cheeses; most raw fruits and vegetables; fibrous foods; hot seasonings and spices; fried foods; rich pastries, pies, and desserts.

## REVIEW QUESTIONS AND PROBLEMS

1. What foods are usually allowed on a clear-fluid diet? What nutrients are supplied by this diet? When is it used?

2. Keep a record of the normal diet served to a patient for one day. What changes would you make in this menu so that it would be suitable for a patient who has no teeth?

3. Modify the normal diet recorded for question 2 so that it is suitable for a patient who has an infection, with an order for a soft diet.

4. List four situations when a soft diet might be used.

# DIETARY CALCULATIONS WITH FOOD EXCHANGE LISTS

### NEED FOR CALCULATED DIETS

A number of conditions require control of the quantities of one or more constituents of the diet: obesity, diabetes mellitus, hyperinsulinism, and others. A daily calculation for the specific foods of the menu would be extremely time consuming and impractical. As a matter of fact, even the detailed calculation would give only an approximate value for the actual intake because no two samples of the same kind of food are completely identical in their composition. Furthermore, people vary considerably in their metabolism from day to day.

### FOOD EXCHANGE LISTS

This chapter describes a practical, rapid method for planning diets by using average values for groups of foods. The Food Exchange Lists (Table A–2, p. 329) were prepared some years ago by a joint committee of the American Dietetic Association, American Diabetes Association, and Diabetes Section of the United States Public Health Service. Initially intended for simplification of diabetic diets (Chap. 22), the lists soon found wide use in the planning of low-calorie diets (Chap. 21). More recently fat-controlled diets (Chap. 24) and sodium-restricted diets (Chap. 25) have been developed with the use of food lists.

An *exchange* list is a grouping of foods in which the carbohydrate, protein, and fat values are about equal for the items listed. For example, any fruit in List 3, in the amounts stated, will supply 10 gm carbohydrate:

one small apple, or one-half grapefruit, or two prunes, or one-half small banana, and so on. From List 4, Bread Exchanges, ½ cup cooked rice, or one small potato, or ¾ cup cornflakes could be exchanged for one slice bread. The six exchange lists include milk, vegetables—groups A and B, fruit, bread, meat, and fat. A seventh list includes items of negligible food value such as lemon juice, bouillon, and dill pickles that may be used as desired. (See Figs. 20–1, 20–2, 20–3, and 20–4.)

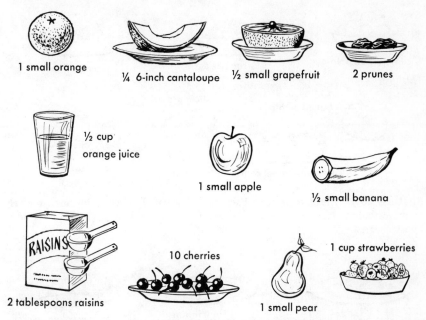

1 small orange

¼ 6-inch cantaloupe    ½ small grapefruit    2 prunes

½ cup orange juice

1 small apple

½ small banana

2 tablespoons raisins

10 cherries

1 cup strawberries

1 small pear

FIGURE 20–1 Fruit exchanges. Each exchange supplies 10 gm carbohydrate and negligible protein and fat. See List 3 of Table A–2 (p. 330) for additional choices.

## METHOD FOR DIETARY CALCULATIONS

A physician prescribes the amounts of carbohydrate, protein, and fat that are to be used in measured diets. Using the values for the exchange lists, the dietitian, dietetic technician, or nurse calculates the number of exchanges to be furnished by the diet.

The steps in planning the measured diet are listed below. A sample calculation in Table 20–1 illustrates the procedure for a diet prescribed to furnish 150 gm carbohydrate, 70 gm protein, and 70 gm fat.

1. Become familiar with the patient's usual pattern of meals, the food likes and dislikes, and so on. Whether the patient eats at home, carries lunches, or eats in a restaurant will affect the planning. The amount of money that can be spent, the preparation facilities, and the cultural patterns must be considered.

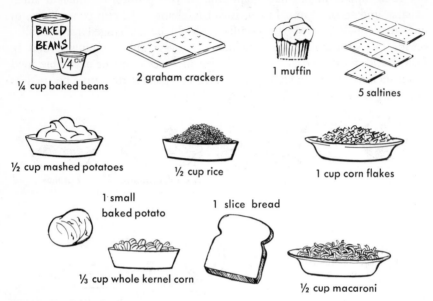

**FIGURE 20–2 Bread exchanges.** Each food illustrated above yields approximately 15 gm carbohydrate, and 2 gm protein. See List 4 of Table A–2 (p. 331) for additional choices.

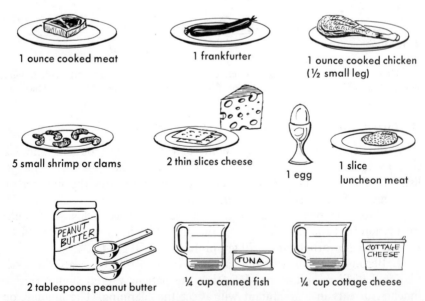

**FIGURE 20–3 Meat exchanges.** Each exchange provides 7 gm protein and 5 gm fat. About 3 exchanges are used for an average dinner serving of cooked meat; use 4 oz raw, lean meat to equal 3 oz cooked. See List 5 in Table A–2 (p. 331) for additional choices.

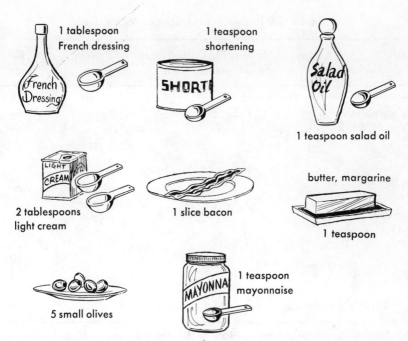

1 tablespoon
French dressing

1 teaspoon
shortening

1 teaspoon salad oil

2 tablespoons
light cream

1 slice bacon

butter, margarine

1 teaspoon

5 small olives

1 teaspoon
mayonnaise

FIGURE 20–4  Fat exchanges. Each of the foods illustrated above provides approximately 5 gm fat per exchange. See List 6 in Table A–2 (p. 332) for additional choices.

2. Include basic foods to ensure adequate levels of minerals and vitamins: 2 cups milk (3 or more for children); 5 exchanges meat; two servings vegetables; two servings fruit; breads and cereals.

3. List the carbohydrate, protein, and fat values for the milk, vegetables, and fruit.

4. Subtract the carbohydrate value of these foods (61 in the example) from the carbohydrate level prescribed (150 gm). Divide the difference by 15 to determine the number of bread exchanges (6 in the example).

5. Total the protein values of the milk, vegetables, and bread exchanges (30 in the example). Subtract from the protein prescribed (70). Divide the difference by 7 to determine the number of meat exchanges (6 in the example).

6. Total the fat values for milk and meat (50 in the example) and subtract from the total fat prescribed (70). Divide the difference by 5 to determine the number of fat exchanges (4 in the example).

7. Check the calculations to be certain that they are correct. It is not a good idea to split the fruit, bread, and meat exchanges into half. The calculations for carbohydrate should be within 7 gm of the prescribed level, and those for protein within 3 gm of the prescribed level.

8. Divide the total exchanges for the day into meal patterns according to the physician's diet order and the patient's preference. A meal pattern and sample menu illustrate the diet calculated in Table 20–1.

### TABLE 20-1 SAMPLE CALCULATION OF DIET

| Exchange List | Number of Exchanges | Carbohydrate gm | Protein gm | Fat gm |
|---|---|---|---|---|
| Milk | 2 | 24 | 16 | 20 |
| Vegetables A | 1–2 | — | — | — |
| Vegetables B | 1 | 7 | 2 | — |
| Fruit | 3 | 30 | — | — |
| | | (61) * | | |
| Bread | 6 | 90 | 12 | — |
| | | | (30) † | |
| Meat | 6 | — | 42 | 30 |
| | | | | (50) ‡ |
| Fat | 4 | — | — | 20 |
| Totals for the day | | 151 | 72 | 70 |

\* 150 − 61 = 89 gm carbohydrate to be supplied from bread exchanges
   1 bread exchange = 15 gm carbohydrate
   89 ÷ 15 = 6 bread exchanges
† 70 − 30 = 40 gm protein to be supplied from meat exchanges
   1 exchange meat = 7 gm protein
   40 ÷ 7 = 6 meat exchanges
‡ 70 − 50 = 20 gm fat to be supplied from the fat exchanges
   1 fat exchange = 5 gm fat
   20 ÷ 5 = 4 fat exchanges

| Meal Pattern | Sample Menu |
|---|---|
| **Breakfast** | |
| Milk—1 exchange | Milk—1 cup |
| Fruit—1 exchange | Cantaloupe—¼ medium |
| Bread—2 exchanges | Wheat flakes—¾ cup |
| | Toast—1 slice |
| Meat—1 exchange | Egg—1 |
| Fat—2 exchanges | Butter—1 teaspoon |
| | Cream, light—2 tablespoons |
| **Luncheon** | |
| Milk—1 exchange | Milk—1 cup |
| Vegetable, group A | Radishes and celery sticks |
| Fruit—1 exchange | Apple—1 small |
| | Sandwich |
| Bread—2 exchanges |    Bread—2 slices |
| Meat—2 exchanges |    Roast beef—2 oz |
| Fat—1 exchange |    Mayonnaise—1 teaspoon |

|                  Meal Pattern                  |                  Sample Menu                   |

*Meal Pattern*                 *Sample Menu*

*Dinner*

| Meal Pattern | Sample Menu |
|---|---|
| Vegetable, group A | Asparagus tips |
| Vegetable, group B—1 exchange | Baked acorn squash—½ |
| Fruit—1 exchange | Pears, water-packed—2 halves |
| Bread—2 exchanges | Potato, baked—1 small |
|  | Roll, dinner—1 |
| Meat—3 exchanges | Roast pork, lean—3 oz |
| Fat—1 exchange | Butter on potato—1 teaspoon |

## REVIEW QUESTIONS AND PROBLEMS

1. List the foods in the vegetable group A that are especially rich in vitamin A; in ascorbic acid.

2. Which vegetables are included in the bread list?

3. Plan a breakfast that includes the following exchanges: milk, 1; fruit, 1; bread, 2; meat, 1; fat, 3.

4. Calculate the carbohydrate, protein, and fat value of the following day's allowance: milk, 2; vegetable, group A, 1; vegetable, group B, 1; fruit, 3; bread, 4; meat, 7; fats, 5.

5. Arrange the day's allowance from question 4 into three meals. Write a sample menu for the pattern you have set up.

# PROBLEMS OF WEIGHT CONTROL

*Low- and High-Calorie Diets*

## HAZARDS OF OVERWEIGHT AND UNDERWEIGHT

Obesity or excessive fatness of the body is a hazard to health. Imagine your reaction if you were told to carry a 25-lb package with you wherever you went! That is exactly what the overweight person must do—10, 25, 50 lb or whatever the excess may be. It goes with him whether he walks upstairs, or ties a shoelace, or tries to hurry for a train. The extra weight makes demands upon his heart, his blood circulation, his back, his feet, and so on. It is no surprise that obese people more often have heart disease; they also have gallbladder disease, diabetes, and other chronic diseases more frequently. They face an extra risk if they require surgery. The obese pregnant woman is more likely to have complications than the woman of normal weight.

Underweight, though less emphasized, also presents dangers to health. Underweight persons are more likely to have infections and disturbances of the gastrointestinal tract. Tuberculosis is more frequent among young, underweight people.

## BALANCING ONE'S WEIGHT

The degree of obesity or undernutrition is most often judged by comparing what one weighs with a height-weight table (see Table A–3, p. 333). If one weighs 10 to 19 per cent more than is desirable for his height and body frame, he is *overweight*; if he weighs 20 per cent or more over desirable weight, he is *obese*. People who are 15 per cent or more below normal weight are *underweight*. The degree of body fatness may also be determined by measuring the thickness of skin folds of the upper arm or abdomen with a caliper. (See Fig. 21–1.)

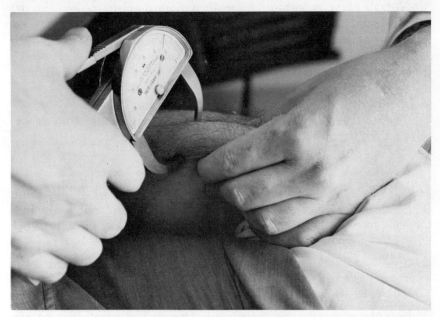

**FIGURE 21–1** The degree of body fatness is determined by measuring the thickness of a skinfold with a caliper. (*Courtesy,* Roche Medical Image, *Hoffmann-LaRoche, Inc.*)

Gaining or losing weight is simply a question of balancing food calories with the body's need for calories. One kilogram of fat is equal to about 7500 kcal. Thus, if you have 500 kcal every day above what your body needs, you will gain about ½ kg (1 lb) in a week. If your intake is 500 kcal below your needs, you will lose about ½ kg in a week.

Let us take another example. Suppose you need 2000 kcal a day, but your daily diet averages 2100 kcal. In 30 days this excess adds up to 3000 kcal. You would gain about 0.4 kg or 0.9 lb in that month ($3000 \div 7500 = 0.4$). Perhaps this does not seem like very much gain, but in one year it amounts to 5 kg (11 lb).

To keep in balance you would need to eliminate the surplus calories from your diet. You could also avoid gaining weight by increasing your activity. By walking a mile a day the average adult uses about 100 to 125 calories; so this increase in exercise would help to avoid weight gain.

## CAUSES OF OVEREATING AND UNDEREATING

Too often we assume that obese people simply eat tremendous amounts of food. In fact, however, obesity more often results because of the little extras day by day; perhaps an extra pat of butter, a second roll, a snack, a second piece of candy, or a rich dessert each day rather than a low-calorie dessert.

Not all obese people eat more than normal-weight people. Several recent studies have shown that many obese boys and girls actually eat less than normal-weight boys and girls. However, they were found to be much less active. Failure to get enough exercise meant that their diets, which seemed quite normal, furnished too many calories for them. Likewise, many adults probably do not eat large amounts of food, but they are so inactive that their intakes are excessive for them.

The following list presents some of the factors that might be responsible for failing to balance one's calories with body weight.

| *Some Reasons for Calorie Intake in Excess of Needs* | *Some Reasons for Inadequate Calorie Intake* |
|---|---|
| 1. Family patterns of rich, high-calorie foods; mother often has reputation of being a good cook | 1. Family pattern places emphasis upon low-calorie foods; few rich desserts, for example |
| 2. Good appetite; likes to eat; likes many rich foods; may dislike fruits and vegetables | 2. Small appetite; has little interest in eating; has many dislikes; unpalatable therapeutic diets |
| 3. Ignorance of calorie value of foods | 3. Ignorance of essentials of an adequate diet |
| 4. Skips breakfast; is a frequent nibbler; coffee breaks with high-calorie snacks | 4. Skips meals; seldom makes up for skipped meals; rarely nibbles |
| 5. Pattern of living<br>  a. Sedentary occupation; idleness<br>  b. Riding to work or school<br>  c. Little exercise during leisure<br>  d. Often sleeps more as he becomes older. | 5. Pattern of living<br>  a. Often tense<br>  b. Overactive<br>  c. Not enough sleep and rest |
| 6. Emotional outlet: eats to overcome worry, boredom, loneliness, grief | 6. Emotional outlet: unhappy, worried, grieving, but refuses to eat |
| 7. Many social events with rich foods; frequent eating in restaurants | 7. Often lives alone; misses sociability; doesn't like to eat alone |
| 8. Lower metabolism with increasing age, but failure to reduce intake | 8. Illness and infection; fever, diarrhea; hyperthyroidism |
| 9. Influenced by pressures of advertising for many high-calorie foods | 9. Affected by claims for fad diets; may get inadequate diet |

## PREVENTION OF OBESITY

To avoid obesity one must first understand fully the reasons for excessive calorie intake as described in the preceding section. But there must also be the will to take prompt measures when the first few extra pounds appear. It is much easier to prevent obesity than to treat it. Prevention is most effective when patterns of diet and exercise are established early in life. Mothers need to know that the fat baby is not necessarily the healthiest baby, and that they should not force the infant to eat every last bit of food. Preschool children should not be bribed or rewarded with food; they should have a variety of activities so that they do not depend too much upon food for pleasure.

In families where one or both parents are obese, children are very likely to become obese and remain so throughout life. This can be prevented by changing the eating patterns so that fewer calorie-rich foods are eaten. Use fruits for desserts often and cakes, pies, or pastries seldom; broil, stew, or roast meats instead of frying; put less butter and cream on vegetables and learn to use other flavorings.

Children should be urged to get more exercise and should be expected to perform some chores requiring daily physical activity. Family recreation needs to include more participation in physical activity and somewhat less of the quiet pastimes such as watching television and riding about in automobiles.

## Diets for Obesity

### PLANNING FOR WEIGHT LOSS

Any program of weight loss of more than a few pounds should be directed by a physician. If a weight-losing program is to be successful, the individual must be convinced of the rewards that will come: better health, a slimmer figure, more pep, and perhaps a longer life. Although a low-calorie diet is used only so long as weight needs to be lost, each obese person must be convinced that he needs to modify his lifetime eating habits. If he fails to do this, he will gain back all the pounds he has lost.

It is important to set a reasonable goal. A weekly weight loss of ½ to 1 kg (1 to 2 lb) is better than a crash program that leaves one tired and unwilling to continue. If one needs to lose 25 kg (55 lb), six to nine months is not an unreasonable time allowance.

Keeping a weekly weight chart is a good idea. The person should weigh at the same time every week on the same scale and with the same amount of clothing. He needs to know that the scales might not show any weight loss for the first week or two because, in some instances, water is temporarily held in the tissues when people are placed on reducing diets. After a while this water will be released from the tissues, and the weight loss will show up.

Exercise has its place in a weight-reduction program. Walking is one of the best exercises. People can walk a few extra blocks to work or make it a practice to see a little more of the outdoors on foot rather than from an automobile window. Moderate exercise does not increase the appetite as some claim. For very obese persons, or those who have been ill, the recommendation for exercise by the physician should be followed closely. It is never a good idea for a person who has been sedentary to suddenly engage in violent exercise.

### THE LOW-CALORIE DIET

Women usually lose satisfactorily on diets restricted to 1000 to 1500 kcal, whereas men lose satisfactorily on diets furnishing 1200 to 1800 kcal. Bed patients, such as those with heart disease, are often placed on diets restricted to 800 to 1000 kcal, and sometimes less.

The daily food allowances for the 1000-, 1200-, and 1500-kcal diets are somewhat higher in protein. (See Table 21-1.) This is desirable, because it provides most people with a feeling of satisfaction. Also, it helps to correct the greater losses of muscle tissue that occur during reducing. The extra protein is provided from the meat group, with some restriction of the bread-cereal group.

TABLE 21–1   LOW-CALORIE DIETS BASED ON FOOD EXCHANGE LISTS *

| | | 1000 kcal | 1200 kcal | 1500 kcal |
|---|---|---|---|---|
| Milk, skim | Cups | 2 | 2 | 3 |
| Vegetables, group A | | As desired | As desired | As desired |
| group B | Cups | ½ | ½ | ½ |
| Fruit | Exchanges | 3 | 3 | 3 |
| Bread | Exchanges | 2 | 2 | 4 |
| Meat | Exchanges | 8 | 9 | 9 |
| Fat | Exchanges | 0 | 2 | 4 |
| | Protein, gm | 78 | 85 | 97 |
| | Fat, gm | 40 | 55 | 65 |
| | Carbohydrate, gm | 91 | 91 | 133 |
| | Kilocalories | 1036 | 1199 | 1505 |

* Food choices are listed in Table A–2 (p. 329).

The food exchange lists are used for planning the daily food choices for the low-calorie diets. The patient with a little practice becomes familiar with the kinds of foods included, the correct size of portions, and the methods of food preparation. For example, if he is allowed one exchange fruit for breakfast, he may have two prunes, not five or six; or one-half banana, not a whole banana. If his diet permits four meat exchanges for dinner, he may have 4 oz of steak, not 8 oz as many men prefer. Since the 1000-kcal diet allows no fat exchanges, he would eat his roll or bread without butter, and substitute lemon juice or herbs for the flavoring of vegetables.

Usually the food allowances are divided into three approximately equal meals. Skipping breakfast is not a good idea. Some people prefer to have a midafternoon or bedtime snack, and these may be included by saving some milk or fruit from the meal. Of course, tea or coffee without cream or sugar, and bouillon may also be used.

Meals on a low-calorie diet should be attractive and palatable. Herbs and spices may be used to lend variety to vegetables and meat preparation. Meats, fish, and poultry should be lean, and prepared by broiling, roasting, or stewing. Fresh fruits or canned unsweetened fruits are used. Group A vegetables may be used in salads for variety in texture and flavor, and add bulk to the diet. Low-calorie salad dressings are available commercially or may be prepared at home.

Low-calorie diets would not include alcoholic beverages, sweetened carbonated beverages, cakes, candy, cookies, cream, fried foods, sweetened fruits, pastries, pies, potato chips, pretzels, puddings, and so on. One needs to be especially conscious of the little extras not included in the diet such as a teaspoon of butter, a tablespoon of cream, or a little gravy. Of course, even occasionally eating a piece of pie or cake will wreck the efforts that may have been made toward dieting all day!

A sample menu for a 1200-kcal diet is shown in Table 21–2.

### FAD DIETS

People who are overweight do not always remember that they did not become so in just a few days, and yet they often expect to return to normal weight in a short time. They are frequently misled by advertising as well as articles in magazines or newspapers that promise spectacular losses in a few days; for example, "Lose 9 pounds in 9 days." Some fad diets do not supply the protein, minerals, and vitamins needed by the person who is reducing. As a result, such diets lead to weakness and ill health if they are used for a long time. Other fad diets are based upon bizarre food combinations or unusual proportions of carbohydrate, fat, and protein. No specific food or combination of foods has any special ability to increase the rate of weight loss, nor does the proportion of carbohydrate to fat or

## Table 21–2 Sample Menus for Low- and High-Calorie Diets

| 1200-kcal Diet | High-Calorie Diet (3000–3200 kcal) |
|---|---|
| *Breakfast* | |
| Half grapefruit | Half grapefruit |
| Soft cooked egg—1 | Dry cereal—1 cup |
| Toast—1 slice | Milk, whole—1 cup |
| Butter—1 teaspoon | Soft cooked egg—1 |
| Coffee—no cream or sugar | Toast—1 slice |
| | Butter—2 teaspoons |
| | Sugar for cereal and coffee—2 teaspoons |
| | Cream for coffee—2 tablespoons |
| | Coffee |
| *Luncheon* | |
| Salad plate: | Cream of mushroom soup—1 cup |
| Whole tomato stuffed with | Saltines—2 |
| Tuna fish—2 oz | Salad plate: |
| Diced celery | Whole tomato stuffed with |
| French dressing—1 tablespoon | Tuna fish—2 oz |
| Lettuce | Diced celery |
| Sliced hard-cooked egg | French dressing—1 tablespoon |
| Muffin, plain—1 | Lettuce |
| Milk, skim—1 cup | Sliced hard-cooked egg |
| Plums, unsweetened—2 | Muffin, plain—1 |
| | Butter—2 teaspoons |
| | Jelly—1 tablespoon |
| | Milk, whole—1 cup |
| | Plums in syrup—3 |
| | Sugar cookie—1 |
| *Dinner* | |
| Roast leg of lamb, lean—4 oz | Roast leg of lamb, lean—4 oz |
| Broccoli with lemon | Mashed potato—⅔ cup |
| Carrots | Broccoli, buttered |
| Milk, skim—1 cup | Dinner roll—1 |
| Tea with lemon | Butter, on vegetables and for roll—2 pats |
| | Milk, whole—1 cup |
| | Cherry pie |
| *Bedtime* | |
| Apple—1 small | Milk, whole—1 cup |
| Cheese—1 oz | Chicken sandwich: |
| | Bread—2 slices |
| | Mayonnaise—1 teaspoon |
| | Butter—1 pat |
| | Chicken—1½ oz |

protein make any difference. Among the fad diets that come and go and that are not recommended are the nine-day diet; the low-carbohydrate, high-fat, high-protein diet such as the drinking man's diet and others; "Air Force" diet (the U.S. Air Force did *not* recommend this diet); the egg diet (also known as the "Mayo diet" although the Mayo Clinic did *not* subscribe to it); banana–skim milk diet; grapefruit diet; grape juice diet; meat and fat diet.

Formula diets are widely used, and people often ask about their value. Unlike most fad diets the formulas include all the nutritional essentials; they are convenient to use; and they take away the problems of dietary planning. An important disadvantage is that they do not retrain the individual to a new pattern of eating once the weight has been lost. If used exclusively, the formula diets provide little bulk, and constipation may be a problem. Formula diets are probably most useful for individuals who substitute them for one meal a day and who need to lose only a few pounds.

Reducing candies and pills of various kinds have no place in the reducing program. They are a waste of money and may be dangerous. Some pills cause diarrhea and increased excretion of water by the kidney—a temporary weight loss that is soon replaced; it is fat, not water, that one should lose. Other pills lead to overactivity of the thyroid, increase in metabolism, and increase in heart rate; the results could be disastrous. Obesity is rarely caused by endocrine disturbances.

## Diet for Underweight

### INDICATIONS FOR HIGH-CALORIE DIET

Long illness not infrequently leads to much weight loss because of nausea, lack of appetite, and inability to eat. In some individuals vomiting and diarrhea lead to failure to absorb all nutrients, so that weight loss and undernutrition become severe. Moreover, the individual with an upset gastrointestinal tract is often so uncomfortable that he is reluctant to eat.

Other patients with a high fever lose much weight, because each degree Fahrenheit rise in body temperature increases the rate of metabolism by about 7 per cent. Thus a temperature of 102° or 103° would considerably increase the calorie needs. Occasionally, an individual has a very high metabolic rate because of an overactive thyroid. Although hyperthyroidism is usually treated by drugs or surgery, many individuals have lost much weight before they sought medical advice.

## THE HIGH-CALORIE DIET

About 500 kcal daily above the normal caloric requirements are needed in order to gain 0.4 kg (1 lb) per week. Ordinarily, a 3000- to 3500-kilocalorie diet is considered to be high in calories for the adult. In some cases of marked weight loss and greatly increased metabolism, 4000 to 4500 kcal are indicated. A sample menu for a high-calorie diet is shown in Table 21–2. Note that the menu items used in the low- and high-calorie diets were, for the most part, the same. The increase in calories was brought about by substituting a high-calorie dessert and adding butter, sugar, jelly, bread, soup, and so on.

Weight loss is often accompanied by loss of protein tissue as well as fat tissue. Therefore it is necessary to provide a liberal protein allowance—usually 100 gm per day. When the undernutrition is severe, the physician may prescribe supplements to correct vitamin and mineral deficiencies.

Weight gain for some people is just as difficult as weight loss is for others. Usually the person who requires 3000 kcal will be found to be consuming only half as many calories. To suddenly place before him a tray loaded with food can only result in further loss of appetite and reluctance to eat. The high-calorie diet, then, must begin with the patient's present intake. Perhaps some changes are first made to a menu selection that is somewhat higher in calories but that does not contain much extra bulk. The increase in the amount of food is usually achieved gradually.

All the following foods rapidly increase the calorie content of the diet: light or coffee cream on fruit or on cereal, sour cream for baked potato or in salad dressings, whipping cream, half milk and half cream, ice cream; butter, margarine, mayonnaise, and other salad dressings; jelly, jam, marmalade, honey, sugar, candy; cake, cookies, puddings, pie, and pastry.

Many persons find an excess of fats or sugars to be nauseating, so it is important that the above foods be used with care. On the other hand, one should avoid filling up the patient on too many bulky low-calorie foods, such as vegetables and fruits.

Three meals a day plus a bedtime snack are, as a rule, preferable to three meals plus midmorning and midnafternoon feedings. Often the between-meal feedings take the edge off the appetite, so that the meals are less well eaten. However, such quickly digested and absorbed foods as fruit juice with crackers and cookies increase the calorie intake without interfering with the appetite. Three examples of calorie-rich bedtime snacks are:

| | | |
|---|---|---|
| Chicken salad sandwich | Chocolate milk shake | Strawberry ice cream |
| Milk | Plain sugar cookies | Angel food cake |

# REVIEW QUESTIONS AND PROBLEMS

1. What are the effects of obesity on health?

2. A patient is 12 kg (26 lb) overweight. If he needs 1800 kcal a day but eats a diet that provides 1200 kcal a day, how long would it take him to lose this weight?

3. List eight factors in the American way of life that make it easy to gain weight.

4. Plan menus for three days for a man on a 1500-kilocalorie diet, using the food allowances in Table 21–1.

5. Visit a supermarket and make a list of five products that are claimed to be low in calories. Read the label information. What conclusions do you reach?

6. If a person eats all his meals in a restaurant, what are some suggestions you could give him so that he does not gain weight?

7. Plan five bedtime snacks for a person who is trying to gain weight. Be certain that these snacks also provide a good supply of nutrients.

8. Discuss ways by which you might improve the food intake of a patient who has a very poor appetite and for whom a high-calorie diet has been ordered.

# REFERENCES

Consumer and Food Economics Research Division: *Calories and Weight: the USDA Pocket Guide.* HG # 153. Washington, D.C.: U.S. Department of Agriculture, 1970.

*A Girl and Her Figure and You: A Workbook.* Chicago: National Dairy Council, 1970.

Leverton, R. M.: *Food Becomes You,* 3rd ed. Ames: Iowa State University Press, 1965, Chaps. 6 and 7.

Krupp, G. R.: "Why Some Mothers Fatten Their Children," *Today's Health,* 45:56, November 1967.

Mayer, J.: "Obesity Control," *Am. J. Nurs.,* 65:112–13, June 1965.

Peckos, P. S., and Spargo, J. A.: "For Overweight Teenage Girls," *Am. J. Nurs.,* 64:85–87, May 1964.

Sherrill, R.: "Before You Believe Those Exercise and Diet Ads," *Today's Health,* 49:34, August 1971.

Singer, S.: "When They Start Telling You It's Easy to Lose Weight," *Today's Health,* 50:47, November 1972.

Stokes, S. A.: "Fasting for Obesity," *Am. J. Nurs.,* 69:796–99, 1969.

*Weight Control Source Book.* Chicago: National Dairy Council, 1966.

Weisenger, M.: "How to Stick to Your Diet," *Today's Health,* 51:30, July 1973.

White, P. L.: "Which Diets Work—Which Don't," *Today's Health,* 49:59, September 1971.

# 22

# DIABETES MELLITUS

## Diet Controlled for Carbohydrate, Protein, and Fat

Diabetes mellitus is a metabolic disease that affects the endocrine system of the body and the use of carbohydrate, fat, and protein. Specifically, there is not enough insulin available for the body's needs. In some patients the islands of Langerhans of the pancreas do not produce enough insulin; in others the pancreas requires some stimulation to manufacture enough insulin; and in still others the insulin that is produced cannot, for some reason, be used by the tissues.

### INCIDENCE

Between 4 and 5 million persons in the United States have diabetes, although almost half of them are unaware that they are diabetic. Persons who have a family history of diabetes and who are overweight are more likely to have diabetes. It has been estimated that there are as many as 50 million persons who are diabetic carriers. Obviously, the campaigns to detect diabetes in the population should be vigorously supported. Two types of diabetes are recognized.

**Maturity-onset,** or adult-type, diabetes accounts for most patients with the disease. About 80 per cent of all diabetics are 40 years of age or over. Of this group 85 per cent are obese. The disease is usually mild, stable, and can be regulated by diet alone or by oral compounds.

**Juvenile diabetes** occurs from birth through adolescence. Only 5 per cent of all diabetic patients are under 15 years of age. This type of diabetes is of sudden onset, severe, requires insulin and a carefully regulated diet, and is difficult to manage. The patients often fluctuate widely between insulin shock and diabetic coma. Some adults who have so-called *brittle* diabetes are also difficult to control.

### SYMPTOMS AND LABORATORY FINDINGS

Diabetes in adults is often so mild that it is detected only by blood and urine tests. Other patients show many of the typical symptoms described below.

Because the blood glucose cannot be used by the tissues, the level of sugar in the blood rises (hyperglycemia). After a night's fast the blood sugar is quite a bit above the normal level of 70 to 90 mg per 100 ml. If a *glucose tolerance test* is made, the diabetic patient shows a sugar curve that begins at a higher level and stays higher than the curve for a normal person. The curve comes down slowly for the diabetic person, but sharply for the normal person. (See Fig. 22–1.)

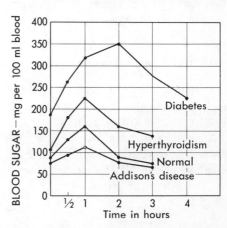

FIGURE 22–1 The glucose tolerance test shows the differences in various disorders of carbohydrate metabolism.

As the blood sugar increases, some sugar is excreted in the urine (glycosuria). To excrete the sugar, water is taken from the tissues. Thus, the patient complains of frequent urination (polyuria) and increased thirst (polydipsia). The appetite is often increased (polyphagia) because the patient is not fully utilizing the food he normally eats.

When the body is unable to use carbohydrate, it oxidizes more and more fat to supply energy. The liver breaks down the fatty acids to ketones (acetone, beta-hydroxybutyric acid, acetoacetic acid). Normally, the ketones are further broken down to yield energy and the end products carbon dioxide and water. However, in diabetes the breakdown of fatty acids is more rapid than the body can care for. Some of the ketones are excreted in the urine (ketonuria, acetonuria). The ketones are acid products. When they accumulate in the blood the pH of the blood is lowered; the patient then has symptoms of acidosis or diabetic coma.

In addition to the symptoms described above, patients often complain of poor healing of cuts and scratches; boils; itching; cold feet; numbness and tingling of the extremities; and blurring of vision. Cardiovascular disease, renal diseases, and blindness are complications in patients who have had diabetes for many years.

## ESSENTIALS OF TREATMENT

The goals of treatment are (1) to relieve symptoms; (2) to enable the patient to lead a normal life; and (3) to prevent or delay the onset of complications. The following are crucial requirements if these goals are to be met: (1) maintenance of normal weight; (2) regular spacing of meals; (3) normal nutritional requirements with normal proportions of carbohydrate, fat, and protein; (4) possibly restriction of cholesterol and modification of the type of fat; (5) use of oral compounds or insulin, if not controlled by diet alone; (6) regulation of physical activity; and (7) attention to body hygiene.

## THE DIET PRESCRIPTION

*Energy.* Weight control is the single most important objective of dietary management. An overweight patient is initially placed on a diet that permits a loss of ¾ to 1 kg (1½ to 2 lb) each week. From 1000 to 1200 kcal is suitable for obese women and 1200 to 1500 kcal for obese men. The diets described on page 210 are suitable without further calculation of the diet for protein, fat, and carbohydrate.

Individuals of normal weight are given sufficient calories to maintain weight:

| | |
|---|---|
| In bed | 25 kcal per kg (11 kcal per lb) |
| Sedentary | 30 kcal per kg (14 kcal per lb) |
| Moderately active | 35 kcal per kg (16 kcal per lb) |

*Protein.* About 1 to 1½ gm protein per kg body weight (½ to ⅔ gm per lb) permits an intake typical of American diets.

*Carbohydrate.* Severe restriction of carbohydrate is no longer recommended. Diets that provide more liberal intake of carbohydrate do not proportionately increase the hyperglycemia or the need for insulin or oral compounds. About 45 per cent of the total calories for the day from carbohydrate is suitable; this proportion is typical of normal American diets.

*Fat.* After subtracting the calories provided by carbohydrate and protein, the remaining calories are furnished by fat. Let us suppose that a diet is being planned for a sedentary individual weighing 60 kg who needs 1800 kcal and is to be given 75 gm protein.

$0.45 \times 1800$ kcal $= 810$ kcal from carbohydrate
$810 \div 4 = 202.5$ gm carbohydrate
$75 \times 4$ kcal $= 300$ kcal from protein
$810$ kcal $+ 300$ kcal $= 1110$ kcal from carbohydrate and protein
$1800 - 1110 = 690$ kcal to be supplied from fat
$690 \div 9 = 77$ gm fat

The prescription would be rounded off to the nearest 5 gm: carbohydrate, 205 gm; protein, 75 gm; fat, 75 gm.

*Modified fat diets.* Many diabetic patients have elevated levels of cholesterol and triglycerides in the blood. These are factors that increase the risk to atherosclerosis, cardiovascular disease, and renal disease. Many physicians now recommend that the cholesterol be restricted to not more than 300 mg per day, and that the fats should be selected from foods high in polyunsaturated fatty acids, rather than those high in saturated fatty acids. These changes require the following modification of the exchange lists: skim milk instead of whole milk; lean meat with more frequent use of fish and poultry; not more than 3 eggs per week; vegetable oils (safflower, corn, cottonseed, soybean) or salad dressings or soft margarines made from these oils; no butter, hydrogenated fats, or cream.

## DIETARY PLANNING

The patient's economic status, time and place for meals, food preparation facilities, and cultural and religious preferences must be considered when planning the daily meals. The diet is calculated by using the method described for exchange lists in Chapter 20. One way in which the prescription above might be calculated is shown in Table 22–1.

*Meal distribution of carbohydrate.* The division of carbohydrate at mealtime depends upon whether the patient is taking insulin or not, the type of insulin that is used, and the results of urine sugar tests. For example, the 206 gm carbohydrate in the calculation shown in Table 22–1 might be divided as follows:

| Breakfast | Lunch | Dinner | Bedtime | |
|---|---|---|---|---|
| 68 (1/3) | 68 (1/3) | 68 (1/3) | | No insulin; oral compounds |
| 29 (1/7) | 58 (2/7) | 87 (3/7) | 29 (1/7) | Small breakfast; long-acting insulin such as protamine zinc insulin |
| 58 (2/7) | 58 (2/7) | 58 (2/7) | 29 (1/7) | Intermediate and long-acting insulin such as NPH, lente |

TABLE 22–1 SAMPLE CALCULATION FOR DIET: CARBOHYDRATE 205 GM, PROTEIN 75 GM, FAT 75 GM

|  | Exchanges | Carbohydrate gm | Protein gm | Fat gm |
|---|---|---|---|---|
| Milk, skim | 2 | 24 | 16 | — |
| Vegetable, 2 A | as desired | — | — | — |
| Vegetable, 2 B | 1 | 7 | 2 | — |
| Fruit | 4 | 40 | — | — |
|  |  | (71) |  |  |
| Bread | 9 | 135 | 18 | — |
|  |  |  | (36) |  |
| Meat | 6 | — | 42 | 30 |
|  |  |  |  | (30) |
| Fat | 9 | — | — | 45 |
| Totals |  | 206 | 78 | 75 |

**FOOD PREPARATION AND SERVICE**

All foods for the diet are measured according to the amounts in the food exchange lists. Level measures with standard measuring cups and spoons are used. When purchasing meat, for 3 oz of cooked meat allow:

4 oz raw lean meat or fish, if there is no waste;
5 oz raw meat, fish, or poultry, if there is a small amount of bone or fat to be trimmed off;
6 oz raw meat, fish, or poultry, if there is much waste.

Foods are prepared using only those allowed on the meal pattern. No extra flour, bread crumbs, butter, or other foods may be used. Many recipes are available from diabetic cookbooks and can be adapted to the patient's prescription.

Meats may be broiled, baked, roasted, or stewed. If they are fried, some of the fat allowance must be used.

Water-packed fruits (canned without sugar) are available in most food markets and may be used according to the exchange lists. Frozen or canned fruits packed with sugar must be avoided. It is important to read labels carefully. (See Fig. 22–2.)

Snacks are permitted only if they are calculated in the diet plan. They are necessary with the long-acting insulins. The patient may have coffee, tea, fat-free broth, unsweetened gelatin, and vegetables from the 2A group at any time, without calculating them.

## Dietetic Peaches

Packed in water without added sugar

PROXIMATE ANALYSIS
(including liquid in this can)

| | | | |
|---|---|---|---|
| Protein | 0.6% | Milligrams sodium per | |
| Fat | 0.03% | 100 grams | 6 |
| Crude fiber | 0.4% | Milligrams sodium per | |
| Ash | 0.3% | 4 ounce serving | 7 |
| Moisture | 92% | Calories per 100 grams | 31 |
| Available carbohydrate | 6.7% | Calories per ounce | 9 |

**FIGURE 22–2** Foods intended for therapeutic diets must be labeled with the information concerning their nutritive values.

Each patient's tray is a teaching aid. The patient should be instructed to become visually accustomed to the size of portions. He should learn to relate the specific foods on his tray to the exchange lists. (See Fig. 22–3.)

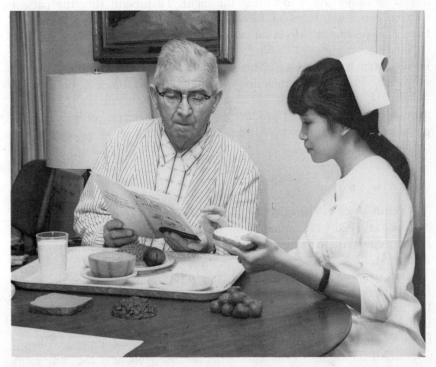

**FIGURE 22–3** With the aid of plastic food models a nurse helps a patient become familiar with the Food Exchange Lists in his instruction booklet. (*Courtesy, School of Nursing, Thomas Jefferson University Hospital, Philadelphia.*)

As a nurse you should consistently check the patient's tray after each meal to know how well he is eating. If he is taking insulin and refuses food, an arrangement is made for a substitution so that he will not go into insulin shock.

A typical meal pattern and sample menu for the diet calculated on page 220 is shown in Table 22–2. Note that the pattern provides three meals of approximately equal carbohydrate value plus a bedtime meal.

## INSULIN AND ORAL COMPOUNDS

Patients with maturity-onset diabetes can almost always be managed successfully with diet alone or with diet and oral compounds. Those with juvenile-type diabetes always require insulin, and oral compounds are not appropriate.

Insulin must be given by injection, because it would be digested and made inactive if given by mouth. The amount and kind of insulin are determined by the physician. Most insulins now used are long-acting, which means that one injection a day is usually needed. For some insulins, the action is delayed so that a small breakfast is preferred. There is some danger of insulin reaction during the night. To prevent this, the patient is given a bedtime snack of carbohydrate food, also including some protein. This feeding is calculated as part of the diet. (See Table 22–2.)

Oral agents are used by adult patients with mild diabetes who cannot be regulated by diet alone. These compounds are not insulin. The sulfonylurea compounds, including tolbutamide (Orinase), tolazamide (Tolinase), chlorpropamide (Diabinese), and acetohexamide (Dymelor), stimulate the pancreas to produce insulin. Another type of preparation, phenformin (DBI), increases the peripheral utilization of glucose in the muscle.

## INSULIN SHOCK

Insulin shock is the effect of too much insulin. It occurs because the patient has failed to eat some of his food; he has increased his activity; or he has a gastrointestinal upset so that the nutrients are not being normally absorbed.

The symptoms of insulin shock result from the marked lowering of the blood glucose. The patient becomes weak, nervous, pale, and hungry. He trembles, perspires, complains of headache, and may become irrational in behavior as if intoxicated. If he is not given carbohydrate promptly he becomes drowsy, disoriented, and eventually unconscious. Prolonged hypoglycemia is damaging to the brain cells because glucose is the only form of energy used by nervous tissue.

TABLE 22-2 TYPICAL MEAL PATTERN AND SAMPLE MENU

| Meal Pattern | Exchanges | Carbohydrate gm | Sample Menu |
|---|---|---|---|
| **Breakfast** | | | |
| Fruit | 1 | 10 | Orange, sliced—1 small |
| Bread | 2 | 30 | Dry cereal—¾ cup |
| | | | Toast—1 slice |
| Milk, skim | 1 | 12 | Milk, skim—1 cup |
| Fat | 2 | | Margarine—2 teaspoons |
| | | — | Coffee or tea as desired; no |
| | | 52 | sugar |
| | | | |
| **Luncheon** | | | *Packed Lunch* |
| Meat | 2 * | | Sandwiches—1½ |
| Bread | 3 | 45 | Bread—3 slices |
| Fat | 3 | | Sliced turkey—2 oz |
| | | | Mayonnaise—1 teaspoon |
| | | | Margarine—2 teaspoons |
| | | | Lettuce |
| Vegetable, A | 1 | | Whole tomato |
| Fruit | 2 | 20 | Banana—1 small |
| | | — | Coffee or tea, if desired |
| | | 65 | |
| | | | |
| **Dinner** | | | |
| Meat | 4 * | | Lean roast beef—4 oz |
| Vegetable, A | 1 | | Tossed green salad |
| Vegetable, B | 1 | 7 | Peas—½ cup |
| Bread | 3 | 45 | Potato, baked—1 medium |
| | | | Dinner roll—1 small |
| Fat | 3 | | French dressing—1 table- |
| | | | spoon |
| | | | Margarine—2 teaspoons |
| Fruit | 1 | 10 | Strawberries—1 cup fresh |
| | | — | |
| | | 62 | |
| | | | |
| **Bedtime** | | | |
| Milk, skim | 1 | 12 | Milk, skim—1 cup |
| Bread | 1 | 15 | Graham crackers—2 |
| Fat | 1 | | Margarine—1 |

* The above plan is low in cholesterol, and with the use of oils and special margarines is high in polyunsaturated fatty acids. An egg may be included 3 to 4 times a week by reducing the meat by one exchange at lunch or dinner.

Patients who take insulin should always carry some lump sugar or hard candy in case they feel the signs of a reaction. Orange juice or other fruit juice or tea with sugar may be given to the patient who has signs of insulin shock. When the patient is unconscious glucose is given intravenously.

## DIABETIC COMA (ACIDOSIS)

Diabetic coma is caused by inadequate insulin to meet body needs. The patient may have failed to follow his diet, or to take the prescribed insulin, or may have an infection.

When the insulin supply to the body is inadequate, the blood sugar rises and glycosuria occurs. A rapid increase of incompletely metabolized fatty acids in the blood leads to a low blood pH. The patient may complain of thirst, headache, frequent urination, fatigue, and drowsiness. His face becomes red, his skin is hot and dry, and his breath has a sweetish (acetone) odor. Nausea and vomiting sometimes occur. The respirations become rapid and the pulse is fast. Finally, the patient lapses into unconsciousness.

Immediate medical attention is required for the patient who goes into diabetic coma. Treatment includes insulin and fluid therapy.

## SOME FALLACIES AND FACTS

1. *Fallacy.* A patient who has an infection and who is eating poorly should stop taking his insulin.

*Fact.* The insulin requirement is usually higher in fevers and infections. The patient should take his insulin and take fluids supplying carbohydrate if he cannot eat solid foods. He should continue to test his urine, and should alert his physician.

2. *Fallacy.* A "free" diet means the patient can eat anything he wants.

*Fact.* Patients permitted to eat so-called "free" diets must observe regular meal hours and must eat foods that meet their nutritional requirements. They are generally told not to eat concentrated sweets such as sugar, candy, jelly, cake, and cookies. The single and double sugars are rapidly absorbed thus causing the blood sugar to become sharply elevated and making control more difficult.

3. *Fallacy.* Honey can be used in place of cane sugar.

*Fact.* Honey is about 80 per cent carbohydrate, chiefly fructose. The fructose is eventually used as glucose, thereby requiring insulin. Therefore, the use of honey is not desirable.

4. *Fallacy.* Dietetic foods may be used as desired by diabetic patients.

*Fact.* Dietetic foods contain some carbohydrate, protein, and fat. Their use is seldom justified, and these foods are relatively expensive. If they are used, the patient should check with the dietitian or physician so that the value can be calculated into the diet.

## REVIEW QUESTIONS AND PROBLEMS

1. What is the cause of diabetes mellitus?

2. What symptoms are seen in patients with diabetes?

3. What tests are used to determine whether an individual has diabetes?

4. A diabetic diet is essentially a normal diet. How does the diet differ from the normal pattern?

5. The menu for a family dinner is beef stew with potatoes, carrots, onions; tossed salad with Russian dressing; rolls and butter; lemon meringue pie; milk. Tell exactly how you would adapt this menu for a patient who is allowed the following exchanges: milk, 1; group B vegetables, 2; fruit, 1; meat, 3; fat, 2.

6. Why is a bedtime feeding ordinarily used for patients who are taking insulin?

7. List ten foods that diabetic patients usually should avoid.

8. Why must insulin be given by injection? What is meant by *oral compound*?

9. What symptoms would lead you to suspect that a patient is having an insulin shock? What would you do?

## REFERENCES

Editorial: "Diabetic Diet—1971," *JAMA*, **218**:1939, 1971.

Garnet, J. D.: "Pregnancy in Women with Diabetes," *Am. J. Nurs.*, **69**:1900–1902, 1969.

Leiner, M. S., and Rahmer, A. E.: "The Juvenile Diabetic and the Visiting Nurse," *Am. J. Nurs.*, **68**:106–108, 1968.

McFarlane, J.: "Children with Diabetes: Special Needs During Growth Years," *Am. J. Nurs.*, **73**:1360–62, 1973.

McFarlane, J., and Hames, C. C.: "Children with Diabetes: Learning Self-Care in Camp," *Am. J. Nurs.*, **73**:1362–65, 1973.

Martin, M. M.: "Diabetes Mellitus: Current Concepts," *Am. J. Nurs.*, **66**:510–14, 1966.

Martin, M. M.: "Insulin Reactions," *Am. J. Nurs.*, **67**:328–31, 1967.

Mason, M. A.: *Basic Medical-Surgical Nursing*, 3rd ed. New York: Macmillan Publishing Co., Inc., 1974, Chap. 15, pp. 341–52.

Nickerson, D.: "Teaching the Hospitalized Diabetic," *Am. J. Nurs.*, **72**:935–38, 1972.

Porter, A. L., *et al.*: "Giving Diabetics Control of Their Own Lives," *Nursing '73*, **3**:44–99, September 1973.

Rosenthal, A.: "Learning to Lead Not-So-Normal Lives," *Today's Health*, **48**:56, April 1970.

Stuart, S.: "Day-to-Day Living with Diabetes," *Am. J. Nurs.*, **71**:1548–50, 1971.

Walker, E.: *Diabetes Guide for Nurses*. Public Health Service Pub. No. 861. Washington, D.C.: U.S. Department of Health, Education, and Welfare, 1969.

Zitnik, R.: "First, You Take a Grapefruit," *Am. J. Nurs.*, **68**:1285–86, 1968.

## 23

Endocrine Disorders | HYPERTHYROIDISM | HYPOGLYCEMIA |
ADDISON'S DISEASE · Enzyme Deficiencies | PHENYLKETONURIA |
GALACTOSEMIA · Bone and Joint Diseases | ARTHRITIS |
GOUT | OSTEOPOROSIS

# VARIOUS METABOLIC DISORDERS

## Endocrine Disorders

### HYPERTHYROIDISM

*Clinical findings.* Excessive secretion by the thyroid gland leads to an increase in the metabolic rate by as much as 50 per cent. Some of the symptoms are weight loss, nervousness, increased appetite, prominent eyes, and enlarged thyroid gland. The increased metabolic rate leads to rapid loss of glycogen from the liver and some tissue wasting. Calcium and phosphorus excretion is often increased, resulting in osteoporosis (see p. 231). In some patients surgery is required, while others are treated with antithyroid compounds to bring the metabolic rate to normal.

*Dietary management.* If there has been much weight loss a diet supplying 3000 to 4000 kcal and 100 to 125 gm protein is needed. Snacks are provided between meals and at bedtime. Sometimes mineral and vitamin supplements are required. Coffee, tea, and alcohol are usually eliminated because of their stimulating properties.

### HYPOGLYCEMIA

The incidence of hypoglycemia is greatly exaggerated by faddists who claim that most fatigue and anxiety can be explained on this basis. The facts are otherwise, and hypoglycemia can be diagnosed only by determining the fasting blood sugar and a glucose tolerance test.

Hypoglycemia means low blood sugar, and is a symptom of a number of conditions. It occurs when a patient with diabetes mellitus has taken too much insulin or oral compounds or has failed to eat. Similar symptoms occur in some patients who have had a gastrectomy so that food passes through the intestinal tract rapidly. (See Dumping Syndrome, p. 300.) It also occurs in Addison's disease, and is sometimes a functional disorder.

*Functional hypoglycemia (hyperinsulinism).* No organic lesion is present. When the individual eats carbohydrate there is increased production of insulin and the blood sugar drops 2 to 4 hours after meals with typical hypoglycemic symptoms: weakness, hunger, nervousness, trembling, increased perspiration, and occasionally loss of consciousness.

*Dietary management.* The diet is calculated using meal exchange lists as described in Chapter 20. The diet prescription is planned as follows:

1. The calorie level is sufficient to maintain desirable weight.

2. Carbohydrate is restricted to 75 to 100 gm. This reduces the amount of insulin that is produced. The carbohydrate is supplied by milk, fruit and vegetable exchanges; bread exchanges are usually omitted.

3. The protein intake is increased to 100 to 150 gm; about 50 per cent of protein can be metabolized to glucose for the body's needs but the slower rate of absorption does not stimulate the production of insulin.

4. The remaining calories are provided by fat.

5. The daily food allowance is divided so that each meal provides the same amount of protein, fat, and carbohydrate.

## ADDISON'S DISEASE

This is a relatively rare, serious disorder of the adrenal gland in which there is insufficient production of one or more hormones. The patient excretes too much sodium and water, thus becoming dehydrated. Too little potassium is excreted, so that the blood levels are increased and the rhythm of the heart beat is altered. The glycogen reserves of the liver are rapidly depleted. The ingestion of carbohydrate stimulates the production of insulin so that hypoglycemia follows after meals.

Hormone therapy corrects the sodium and potassium metabolism, but not the fault in carbohydrate metabolism. The diet should be high in protein and fat, and somewhat restricted in carbohydrate. Simple sugars, candies, and sweets are omitted because they are absorbed too rapidly. Between-meal and bedtime snacks high in protein are necessary to avoid the episodes of hypoglycemia.

## Enzyme Deficiencies

More than a hundred enzyme deficiencies have been described. These are generally inherited and are sometimes called *inborn errors of metabo-*

*lism.* Many of them are evident shortly after birth and others are acquired later in life. Deficiency of the intestinal enzymes leads to malabsorption, discussed further in Chapter 28.

## PHENYLKETONURIA

*Clinical findings.* Phenylketonuria occurs in about 1 infant of every 10,000. The infant is born without the enzyme necessary to use phenylalanine, one of the essential amino acids. As a result the level of the blood is increased and phenylketones are also excreted in the urine—hence the name phenylketonuria (PKU). The deficiency can be diagnosed shortly after birth by blood and urine tests.

High blood levels of phenylalanine are toxic. The infants are usually blond, blue-eyed, fair, and often have eczema. Untreated infants are hyperactive, irritable, and have an unpleasant personality. They have a persistent musty or gamey body odor caused by the production of the phenylketones. If the disease is not diagnosed in the first months of life, mental retardation is usually severe.

*Dietary management.* Phenylketonuria is successfully treated by a phenylalanine-restricted diet when diagnosis is made in the first months of life. If treatment is delayed, the mental retardation that has occurred cannot be reversed.

The phenylalanine is adjusted to maintain a normal level in the blood. Since this is an essential amino acid, some must be provided to meet normal growth needs. This has been estimated to be 20 to 30 mg per kg. Thus, a 3-month infant weighing 6 kg would need 120 to 180 mg phenylalanine daily.

Proteins contain about 5 per cent phenylalanine. The recommended allowance for protein for a 6 kg infant is about 13 gm. From milk formulas and supplementary foods this would supply 650 mg phenylalanine, which is about 4 to 5 times as much as he should have.

A special formula Lofenalac® is used for these infants.* It supplies just enough phenylalanine for growth and is adequate for all other nutrients. As the infant grows, ordinary foods that are low in phenylalanine are added. Mothers are given detailed food lists for fruits, vegetables, breads, and cereals from which to choose, and careful instructions are needed for measurement. Even low-protein foods such as fruits contain some phenylalanine and must be given in measured amounts. (See Fig. 23–1.)

Successful treatment depends upon dietary adjustment at frequent intervals. Based upon the blood levels of phenylalanine the diet is adjusted so that the amount furnished to the body is neither too low or too

---

* Mead Johnson & Co., Evansville, Indiana.

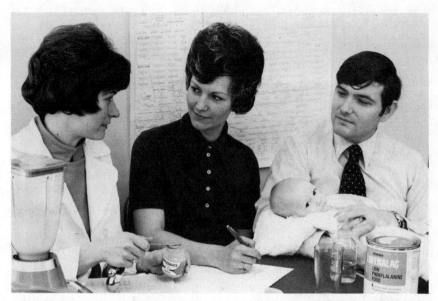

FIGURE 23–1 Detailed counseling is required for successful diet therapy for a child with phenylketonuria or other metabolic errors. The dietitian and nurse will provide follow-up from time to time. (*Courtesy, Handicapped Children's Unit, St. Christopher's Hospital for Children, Philadelphia.*)

high. As the child grows the diet is increased to meet all nutritional requirements. The low-phenylalanine diet is continued throughout the early years of childhood. Whether it needs to be continued indefinitely is not yet known.

## GALACTOSEMIA

*Clinical findings.* From birth infants with this condition lack *transferase*, a liver enzyme that converts galactose to glucose. Galactose is one of the simple sugars resulting when lactose is digested. When the enzyme is absent the levels of galactose in the blood reach toxic levels. A few days after birth the infant has vomiting, diarrhea, drowsiness, edema, liver failure, and hemorrhage. If the infant survives, mental retardation is severe.

*Dietary management.* A galactose-free formula must be started within the first few days of life. Nutramigen ®, Sobee ®, Mul-Soy®, and MBF (Meat-base formula) are suitable.* Since milk is the only food that supplies lactose, other foods are added to the infant's diet as he grows. All

* Nutramigen ® and Sobee ®, Mead Johnson & Co., Evansville, Indiana.
  Mul-Soy ®, Borden Company, New York, N.Y.
  MBF (Meat-base formula), Gerber Products Company, Fremont, Michigan.

milk-containing foods must be rigidly excluded. A list of such foods is given on page 279.

## Bone and Joint Diseases

### ARTHRITIS

The chronic, painful, and disabling nature of arthritis leads many people to try unproved methods of treatment. Each year arthritic patients spend some 300 million dollars on phony diets, drugs, and devices.

There is no diet that will cure arthritis or modify its course. Patients are well advised to eat a normal diet selected from the four food groups. Young patients who have rheumatoid arthritis and who are underweight may need to increase their caloric intake. On the contrary, the older patient with degenerative arthritis is sometimes obese and should lose weight to reduce the burden on weight-bearing joints.

Patients with severe deformities often need the advice of physical and occupational therapists in the use of devices that aid in normal activities; for example, special utensils for feeding, and methods for food preparation adapted to physical limitations.

### GOUT

Gout is an inherited condition of abnormal purine metabolism. Purines are nitrogen-containing compounds that are broken down in the body to uric acid. Normally uric acid is eliminated in the urine. In gout some of the uric acid is deposited as an insoluble salt in the joints and causes pain, especially in the great toe.

Medications have largely replaced the need for a modified diet in gout. Patients are usually advised to avoid foods that are high in purines: liver, kidney, brains, sweetbreads, heart, sardines, anchovies, broth, bouillon, meat soups, and meat gravies.

Some physicians also recommend the omission of all foods moderate in purine content during the acute attacks. Liberal amounts of milk, eggs, and cheese would supply adequate protein in place of the meat, fish, and poultry normally included. When the acute attacks have subsided, small servings of meat, fish, and poultry are added three to four times a week. Excessive intakes of fat and of alcohol are believed to increase the blood uric acid levels.

Many patients with gout are obese. Weight loss increases the blood levels of uric acid and may bring about an acute attack. If recommended, weight loss should be gradual and never rapid. Starvation regimens are prohibited. A low-calorie diet should not be initiated during an acute attack because this could further aggravate the symptoms.

## OSTEOPOROSIS

Osteoporosis is extremely common in older women. The bones contain less bone substance than usual and are more porous. Weight-bearing bones break easily and are hard to repair. Low back pain is frequent, there is gradual loss in height, and the appearance of the "dowager's hump." Osteoporosis occurs in many persons who are immobilized, in diseases of malabsorption such as sprue (see Chap. 28), and is often associated with decreased estrogen production after the menopause. Hormone therapy and mineral supplements are generally recommended.

Osteoporosis occurs less frequently in geographic areas where the water supply is high in fluoride. The disease is less common in persons who have had an adequate intake of calcium throughout life. A high-calcium diet—that is, one containing a quart of milk a day—is often prescribed; it may be of some help in preventing further damage.

## REVIEW QUESTIONS AND PROBLEMS

1. What diet modification is sometimes ordered for a patient with hyperthyroidism? Why?

2. What are some conditions in which hypoglycemia is present?

3. Why is a low-carbohydrate diet recommended for functional hypoglycemia?

4. What is meant by phenylketonuria? Why is early treatment with diet essential?

5. What foods contain large amounts of phenylalanine? Why is some phenylalanine included in the diet for patients with phenylketonuria?

6. A patient with arthritis says he has heard that a low-carbohydrate diet is useful in treating his condition. How would you respond to this?

7. What is meant by a low-purine diet? When is it used? What foods are restricted?

8. Why is weight loss by patients with gout introduced cautiously?

## REFERENCES

Cole, W.: "Hypoglycemia: Shortage of Body Fuel," *Today's Health*, **46**:40, November 1968.

*Diet and Arthritis.* Pub. Health Service Pub. 1857, Diabetes and Arthritis Control Program. Washington, D.C.: U.S. Department of Health, Education, and Welfare, 1969.

Frisch, R. O., *et al.*: "Responses of Children with Phenylketonuria to Dietary Treatment," *J. Am. Diet. Assoc.*, 58:32–37, 1971.

*Gout: Diagnosis and Treatment*. Pub. Health Service Pub. 1606. Bethesda, Md.: National Institute of Arthritis and Metabolic Diseases.

Hamilton, A.: "Good News About Gout," *Today's Health*, 45:16, December 1967.

Herman, I. F., and Smith, R. T.: "Gout and Gouty Arthritis," *Am. J. Nurs.*, 64:111–13, December 1964.

Jay, A. N.: "Hypoglycemia," *Am. J. Nurs.*, 62:77, January 1962.

Lutwak, L.: "Nutritional Aspects of Osteoporosis," *J. Am. Geriatr. Soc.*, 17:115–19, 1969.

*Phenylketonuria: Low Phenylalanine Dietary Management with Lofenalac®*. Evansville, Ind.: Mead Johnson Laboratories, 1969.

Reich, B. H., and Ault, L. P.: "Nursing Care of the Patient with Addison's Disease," *Am. J. Nurs.*, 60:1252–55, 1960.

Soika, C. V.: "Combatting Osteoporosis," *Am. J. Nurs.*, 73:1193–97, 1973.

# ATHEROSCLEROSIS

*Fat-Controlled, Cholesterol-Restricted Diets*

Heart attack, stroke, and other diseases of the heart and blood vessels affect over 27 million Americans, and each year more than one million of these persons die. In 1970 coronary heart diseases alone accounted for 666,000 deaths; 171,000 of these were under 63 years.

### RISK FACTORS

About one fourth of persons who are disabled by heart disease or who die have one or more of these characteristics: hyperlipidemia, hypertension, and cigarette smoking. Many factors increase the risks of atherosclerosis and heart attack: (1) males between the ages of 45 and 64 years are highly susceptible; (2) a family history of heart and blood vessel disease; (3) tension, frustration, emotional stress, meeting deadlines; (4) sedentary occupation and lack of exercise; (5) obesity; (6) diabetes mellitus; (7) diet high in saturated fats and in cholesterol. Even the relative softness of drinking water in some geographic areas and the drinking of excessive amounts of coffee (more than 5 cups daily) have been listed by some researchers as risk factors.

### ATHEROSCLEROSIS

*Atherosclerosis*, the most common form of hardening of the arteries, refers to the thickening of the inner walls (intima) of the blood vessel. It

233

is the most frequent cause of heart attacks and strokes. It can lead to aneurysm (dilation) of the abdominal aorta or gangrene of the leg.

Atherosclerosis develops gradually throughout life. In childhood fatty streaks appear in the inner lining of the blood vessel. These streaks do not lead to any clinical symptoms. In early adult years fatty materials and cholesterol continue to be deposited and are covered with thick fibrous layers of connective tissue. These deposits are known as *atheroma*, or *plaques*. The channel through which the blood flows becomes narrower, and it is increasingly difficult to supply enough blood to the tissues. In later years angina pectoris is a manifestation of this deficiency of blood (ischemia). (See Fig. 24–1.)

The plaques sometimes ulcerate and hemorrhage, or the rough surfaces can initiate blood clotting. If the vessel is blocked by a clot, the tissue served by that vessel dies. Blocking of a coronary vessel, also known as a coronary occlusion, results in myocardial infarction; sudden death occurs if a principal vessel is affected. Occlusion of a vessel to the brain is

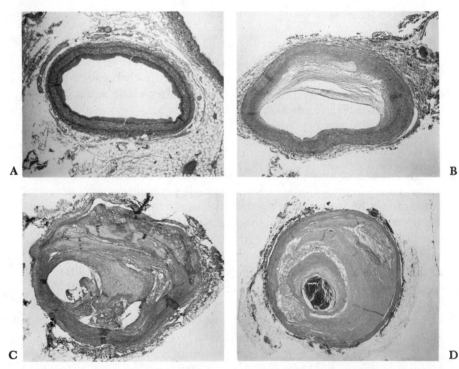

FIGURE 24–1 Gradual development of atherosclerosis in a coronary artery, leading to a heart attack. (A) Normal artery; (B) deposits formed in inner lining of artery; (C) deposits harden; and (D) normal channel is blocked by a blood clot. (*Courtesy, American Heart Association, New York.*)

a stroke (cerebral thrombosis), while blockage of a blood vessel in the leg leads to gangrene.

## HYPERLIPIDEMIAS

*Hyperlipidemia* is an elevation of the blood lipids, and includes cholesterol or triglycerides or both. Cholesterol and triglycerides in the blood are attached to protein molecules; these complex molecules are called lipoproteins, of which there are several classes. In some laboratories measurements are made of the levels of these classes of lipoproteins; an elevation is termed a *hyperlipoproteinemia*. For the purposes of the discussion in this text, these terms may be used interchangeably.

Hyperlipidemias are a high risk for premature atherosclerosis; some of them lead to unsightly skin lesions called xanthoma; and some rare types are associated with pancreatitis and severe abdominal pain.

Hyperlipidemias are often the result of an abnormal diet or an abnormal reaction to a diet, or of some inherited metabolic defect. Obesity, alcoholism, pancreatic disease, and ketosis-resistant diabetes mellitus are examples of these abnormalities. In many instances hyperlipidemias are secondary to other conditions such as the nephrotic syndrome, hypothyroidism, poorly controlled insulin-dependent diabetes mellitus, and multiple myeloma. When the hyperlipidemia is secondary to these diseases, the treatment of the disease condition usually leads to lowering of the blood lipids.

## DIETARY MODIFICATION

Based upon laboratory tests, symptoms, and medical history and examination, the hyperlipidemias may be classified in five groups according to criteria set by Fredrickson.* Diet is the primary therapy for all types. Often no other therapy is required, but drugs are sometimes prescribed. The food allowances for the five types are listed in Table 24–1. Several characteristics apply to all diets.

1. All diets furnish recommended allowances for protein, minerals, and vitamins to maintain satisfactory nutrition for indefinite periods of time.

2. Obesity is a frequent problem. When it is present, any nutritionally balanced low-calorie diet can be used. (See Chap. 21.) Weight loss should approximate ½ to 1 kg (1 to 2 lb) per week. With loss of weight the blood lipid levels are usually lowered, and may even reach normal levels. When desired weight is achieved, the diet is adjusted to provide maintenance

* D. S. Fredrickson *et al.*: *Dietary Management of Hyperlipoproteinemia: A Handbook for Physicians* (Bethesda, Md.: National Heart and Lung Institute, 1970).

TABLE 24–1  FOOD ALLOWANCES FOR DIETS FOR TYPES 1 TO 5 HYPERLIPOPROTEINEMIA AT 1800 KILOCALORIES *

| Food | Type 1 | Type 2 | Type 3 | Type 4 | Type 5 |
|---|---|---|---|---|---|
| Skim milk—cups | 4 | 2 | 2 | 2 | 4 |
| Lean meat, poultry, fish—ounces | 5 | 6–9 † | 6 | ad lib | 6 |
| Egg yolks as substitute for one ounce meat | 3/week | none | none | 3/week | 3/week |
| Breads, cereals—servings | 6+ | 7+ | 7 | 7 | 9 |
| Potato or other starchy vegetable—servings | 1+ | 1+ | 1 | 1 | 1 |
| Vegetables—servings | ⎱ 5 | ⎱ 5 | ad lib | ad lib | ad lib |
| Dark green or leafy, daily | ⎰ | ⎰ | | | |
| Fruit—servings | ⎱ 5 | ⎱ 5 | 3 | 3 | 3 |
| Citrus, daily | ⎰ | ⎰ | | | |
| Fats, teaspoons | none ‡ | 6–9 § | 12 | ad lib | 6 |
| Sugars, sweets | ad lib | ad lib | none | none | none |
| Low-fat dessert | ad lib | ad lib | none | none | none |
| Alcohol | none | with discretion | subst ‖ | subst ‖ | none |

* Adapted from *Dietary Management of Hyperlipoproteinemia: A Handbook for Physicians*, National Heart and Lung Institute, Bethesda, Md., 1970.

† For type 2 diet, restrict pork, ham, beef, and lamb to three 3-ounce portions each week. Use veal, poultry, and fish for remainder of meals.

‡ Medium chain triglycerides may be prescribed by physician to supply additional calories.

§ Use only safflower or corn oil and safflower margarine for type 2 diet.

‖ Substitute 2 servings alcoholic beverages for 2 slices bread. One slice of bread is equal to 1 ounce gin, rum, vodka, or whiskey; 1½ ounces sweet or dessert wine; 2½ ounces dry wine; or 5 ounces beer.

calories, and may be modified for fat, cholesterol, and carbohydrate content if the blood lipid levels indicate a need for this.

3. The cholesterol intake is restricted.

4. The intake of saturated fat is reduced to a minimum. This means that only skim milk, skim-milk cheeses, lean meats, poultry, and fish are used. Butter, regular margarines, solid fats, cream, whole-milk cheeses are avoided. The intake of polyunsaturated fatty acids is increased.

Further recommendations for the specific types are summarized below.

*Types 1 and 5.* These patients have very high levels of blood triglycerides, pancreatitis, and severe abdominal pain, especially when fats are ingested. The triglyceride level is lowered and the pain is alleviated by using a very low-fat diet (10 to 20 per cent of calories). The protein intake is increased to about 20 per cent of calories, but the choices must be from very low-fat protein sources. See food lists, Table 24-2. Of necessity the carbohydrate intake is high—over 60 per cent of calories. Preference should be given to starchy foods rather than simple sugars.

Some patients in the type 5 group are obese; therefore, a low-fat, low-calorie diet should be used until normal weight is achieved. On the other hand, patients in type 1 may be thin and find it difficult to consume enough food to maintain normal weight. For these, the physician may prescribe *medium-chain triglycerides,* an oil that is obtained at a pharmacy; these are well tolerated and increase the caloric intake.

The principal sources of vitamin A in the very low-fat diets are the deep-yellow and dark green leafy vegetables and some yellow fruits. Because of their high cholesterol content, organ meats are omitted and egg yolks are restricted to no more than three per week. The absorption of carotene from plant sources is reduced when the fat intake is low. Therefore, a supplement of vitamin A is usually prescribed if the diet is to be used for a long time.

*Type 2.* The blood cholesterol level is increased in this group, and triglycerides are normal (type 2a) or elevated (type 2b). Overweight is frequent and a low-calorie, low-cholesterol diet is initiated. The diet plans outlined in Chapter 21 may be used, but eggs should be omitted. When the desirable weight has been achieved, the maintenance diet is selected as follows:

1. A diet restricted in fat (20 to 25 per cent of calories) and low in cholesterol (300 mg) should be tried initially. See food lists for type 5, Table 24-1.

2. If the fat-restricted diet does not bring about sufficient lowering of the blood cholesterol and triglycerides, a diet supplying a P/S ratio of 2:1 should be used. This means that the amount of polyunsaturated fatty acids included are twice as high as the saturated fatty acids included. In order to achieve this high ratio it is essential that beef, pork, lamb, and ham be restricted to three meals a week and that eleven meals a week be selected from veal, poultry, fish, and low-fat cheese. In addition, safflower margarine

and safflower and corn oils are the only fats allowed. See food lists, Table 24–2.

*Types 3 and 4.* These hyperlipidemias are characterized by a high serum triglyceride. The blood cholesterol is always high in type 3 and often high in type 4. Obesity is prevalent in both types, and there is a high incidence of cardiovascular disease. Type 3 is rare, while type 4 is common. Many patients with type 4 have an abnormal glucose tolerance or overt diabetes mellitus.

Weight loss is the single most important consideration. If the blood lipids are elevated when the desirable weight is achieved, the maintenance diet should be modified as follows:

1. Cholesterol is restricted to 300 mg daily.

2. Fat intake is planned to 35 per cent of calories. The intake of saturated fats is reduced and fats high in polyunsaturated fatty acids are substituted. However, the emphasis upon the P/S ratio described for type 2 is not important here. Consequently, any lean meats, poultry, and fish may be used in the recommended amounts. (See Table 24–1.)

3. The carbohydrate intake is planned for about 40 per cent of calories. Some clinicians recommend that the carbohydrate be selected from starches rather than simple sugars, since it is believed that simple sugars increase the triglyceride levels. Other clinicians state that the kind of carbohydrate is unimportant so long as the caloric intake does not exceed the needs for maintenance.

4. Alcohol in excessive amounts increases the triglyceride levels. In these diets, up to 2 ounces alcohol may be substituted daily for 2 exchanges of bread.

### MEAL PLANNING AND FOOD LISTS

The nurse or dietitian who helps patients to plan meals for any of the five diets must know which foods are high in saturated fats, in polyunsaturated fats, and in cholesterol. See Table 24–2 for food lists applicable to the five types of diets outlined in Table 24–1. See also pages 329 and 330. Sample menus for the 1800-kilocalorie diets for types 1 and 2 are shown in Table 24–3.

TABLE 24–2  FOOD LISTS FOR DIETS FOR HYPERLIPIDEMIAS *

| Foods to Use | Foods to Avoid |
| --- | --- |
| *Milk list* | |
| Skim milk | Whole milk, homogenized milk, canned |
| Nonfat dry milk | milk |
| Buttermilk, nonfat | Sweet cream, powdered cream |

* Adapted from *Planning Fat-Controlled Meals for 1200 and 1800 Calories,* Revised. New York: American Heart Association, 1966. Also adapted from *Dietary Management of Hyperlipoproteinemia: A Handbook for Physicians.* Bethesda, Md.: National Heart and Lung Institute, 1970.

TABLE 24–2 (*Continued*)

| Foods to Use | Foods to Avoid |
|---|---|
| | Ice cream unless homemade with nonfat dry milk<br>Sour cream<br>Whole-milk buttermilk and yogurt<br>Cheese made from whole milk |

*Vegetables*
See List 2, Table A–2 (p. 329)

*Fruits*
See List 3, Table A–2 (p. 330)  |  Avocado; olives

*Breads, cereals list*
1 slice bread (white, whole-wheat, raisin, rye, pumpernickel, French, Italian, or Boston brown bread)
1 roll (2 to 3 in. across)
1 homemade biscuit or muffin (2 to 3 in. across)
1 square of homemade corn bread (1½ by 1½ in.)
1 griddle cake (4 in. across) made with skim milk and with fat or oil from day's allowance
4 pieces Melba toast (3½ by 1½ by ⅛ in.)
1 piece matzo (5 by 5 in.)
¾ oz bread sticks, rye wafers, or pretzels
1½ cups popcorn (popped at home with fat or oil from day's allowance)
½ cup cooked cereal
¾ cup dry cereal
½ cup cooked rice, grits, hominy, barley, or buckwheat groats
½ cup cooked spaghetti, noodles or macaroni
¼ cup dry bread crumbs
3 tablespoons flour
2½ tablespoons corn meal
½ cup cooked dried peas, beans, lentils, or chickpeas
⅓ cup corn, kernels or cream style
1 ear corn on the cob (4 in. long)
1 small white potato
¼ cup sweet potato, cooked

Foods to Avoid (breads, cereals):
Commercial biscuits, muffins, corn breads, griddle cakes, waffles, cookies, crackers
Mixes for biscuits, muffins, and cakes (except angel food)
Coffee cakes, cakes (except angel food), pies, sweet rolls, doughnuts, and pastries

*Meat, fish, and poultry list*
Selections from this group for 11 of the 14 main meals (type 2 diet)
Poultry without skin: chicken, turkey, Cornish hen, squab
Fish: any kind except shellfish
Veal: any lean cut
Meat substitute: cottage cheese (preferably uncreamed), yogurt from partially skimmed milk, dried peas or

Foods to Avoid (meat, fish, poultry):
Skin of chicken or turkey
Duck or goose
Fish roe; caviar
Fish canned in olive oil
Shellfish (shrimp, crab, lobster, clams)
Note: 2 oz may be used *in place of* 1 egg

TABLE 24–2 (*Continued*)

| Foods to Use | Foods to Avoid |
|---|---|
| beans, peanut butter, nuts (especially walnuts) | Coconut, cashew nuts, macadamia nuts |
| Selections from this group for 3 of the 14 main meals (type 2 diet) | |
| Beef: | Beef high in fat or marbled |
| Hamburger—ground round or chuck | Lamb high in fat |
| Roast, pot roasts, stew meats—sirloin tip, round, rump, chuck, arm | Pork high in fat |
| Steaks—flank, sirloin, T-bone, porter-house, tenderloin, round, cube | Bacon, salt pork, spareribs |
| Soup meats—shank or shin | Frankfurters, sausage, cold cuts |
| Other—dried chipped beef | Canned meats |
| Lamb: | Organ meats such as kidney, brain, sweet-breads, liver |
| Roast or steak—leg | Note: 2 oz liver, sweetbreads, or heart may be substituted for 1 egg |
| Chops, loin, rib, shoulder | Any visible fat on meat |
| Pork: | Commercially fried meats, fish, poultry |
| Roast—loin, center cut ham | Frozen or packaged casseroles or dinners |
| Chops—loin | |
| Tenderloin | |
| Ham: | |
| Baked, center cut steaks, picnic, butt, Canadian bacon | |

*Fat list*

| | |
|---|---|
| Corn oil | Butter |
| Cottonseed oil | Ordinary margarines |
| Safflower oil | Ordinary solid shortenings |
| Sesame seed oil | Lard |
| Soybean oil | Salt pork |
| Sunflower oil | Chicken fat |
| Mayonnaise (1 teaspoon mayonnaise equals 1 teaspoon oil) | Coconut oil |
| French dressing made with allowed oil (1½ teaspoons dressing equals 1 tea-spoon oil) | Olive oil |
| | Chocolate |
| Special margarines | |

*Sugars and sweets list*

White, brown, or maple sugar
Corn syrup or maple syrup
Honey
Molasses
Jelly, jam, or marmalade

*Dessert list* (only for type 1 and type 2)
Each serving listed is equal to
    1 tablespoon sugar—about 50 calories.
    All except sugar cookies are fat-free

| | |
|---|---|
| ¼ cup tapioca or cornstarch pudding made with fruit and fruit juice or with skim milk from milk allowance | Puddings, custards, and ice creams unless homemade with skim milk or nonfat dry milk |
| ¼ cup fruit whip (prune, apricot) | Whipped-cream desserts |
| ⅓ cup gelatin dessert | Cookies unless homemade with allowed fat or oil |
| ¼ cup sherbet (preferably water ice) | |

TABLE 24-2 (Continued)

| Foods to Use | Foods to Avoid |
|---|---|
| ⅓ cup canned or frozen fruit (sweetened fruit equals 1 portion fruit and 1 tablespoon sugar)<br>1 small slice angel food cake<br>2 sugar cookies made with oil from day's allowance<br>3 cornflake or nut meringues<br>¾ cup sweetened carbonated beverage<br>⅔ cup cocoa (not chocolate) made with skim milk from milk allowance<br>Candies: 3 medium or 14 small gum drops; 3 marshmallows; 4 hard fruit drops; or 2 mint patties (not chocolate) | Candies made with chocolate, butter, cream, or coconut |
| *Miscellaneous* (use as desired)<br>Coffee, tea, coffee substitutes<br>Unsweetened carbonated beverages<br>Lemons and lemon juice<br>Egg white<br>Unsweetened gelatin<br>Artificial sweeteners<br>Fat-free consommé or bouillon<br>Pickles, relishes, catsup<br>Vinegar, mustard, seasonings<br>Herbs, spices | Sauces and gravies unless made with allowed fat or oil or made from skimmed stock or nonfat milk<br>Commercially fried foods such as potato chips, French fried potatoes<br>Creamed soups and other creamed dishes<br>Foods made with egg yolk unless counted as part of allowance<br>Commercial popcorn<br>Substitutes for coffee cream |

## FOOD PREPARATION

Booklets for patients for each of the types of diets are available from the National Heart and Lung Institute and the American Heart Association. They provide detailed information on the purpose of the diet, the lists of foods that may be used and those to be avoided, typical meal patterns, how to shop for allowed foods, how to prepare foods, and what to do when eating meals away from home.

*Very low-fat diets* (types 1 and 5). The meats selected must be lean, trimmed of all visible fat. If meats are roasted or broiled, they should be placed on a rack so that the drippings will be removed. If the meat is stewed, it may be cooked a day ahead, cooled in the refrigerator, and the fat skimmed off the top of the liquid. Meats, fish, and poultry may be basted with tomato juice, lemon juice, wine, or bouillon, and baked in aluminum foil.

Since vegetables cannot be dressed with butter, margarine, or sauces, lemon juice, vinegar, and herbs lend variety to them. See suggestions for flavoring vegetables on page 253.

If prescribed by the physician, MCT oil may be used in salad dressings, in cream sauces made with skim milk, and for marinating meat.

TABLE 24–3 SAMPLE MENUS FOR TWO TYPES OF FAT-CONTROLLED DIETS

| Very Low-Fat Diet (Type 1) | Low-Cholesterol Fat-Controlled Diet P/S:2:1 (Type 2) |
|---|---|
| *Breakfast* | *Breakfast* |
| Stewed apricots | Honeydew melon—1 slice |
| Cooked or dry cereal | Dry or cooked cereal—¾ cup |
| Sugar | Sugar—1 teaspoon |
| Toast | Whole-wheat toast—2 slices |
| Jelly | Safflower oil margarine—2 teaspoons |
| Skim milk | Jelly—2 teaspoons |
| Coffee, if desired | Skim milk—1 cup |
| | |
| *Luncheon* | *Luncheon* |
| Salad: | Sandwich: |
|    Cottage cheese, uncreamed— |    Rye bread—2 slices |
|      ½ cup |    Sliced turkey—2 oz |
|    Peach halves, canned |    Mayonnaise—2 teaspoons |
|    Escarole | Cabbage-green pepper salad—½ cup |
| Rolls, soft |    Mayonnaise—1 tablespoon |
| Jelly | Banana—1 small |
| Raspberry sherbet | Skim milk—1 cup |
| Angel food cake | |
| Cocoa made with skim milk, sugar, cocoa | |
| | |
| *Dinner* | *Dinner* |
| Grapefruit sections | Broiled flounder—4 oz |
| Roast leg of veal—3 oz | Safflower or corn oil—1 teaspoon |
| Baked noodles and tomatoes | Parslied potato—1 small *with* |
| Asparagus tips |    Safflower or corn oil—1 teaspoon |
| Dinner roll | Mixed diced carrots and celery—½ cup |
| Jelly | Dinner roll—1 |
| Apple tapioca pudding | Safflower oil margarine—1 teaspoon |
| Coffee or tea, if desired | Tomato aspic on water cress *with* |
| |    French dressing—1 tablespoon |
| | Angel cake—1 small piece |

*Diets with increased amounts of oils* (types 2, 3, and 4). Safflower, and corn oils are used for the type 2 diet; soybean and cottonseed oils are also used with diets for types 3 and 4. Oils may be used in the following ways:

1. As a marinade for meat. Combine the allowed oil with herbs and lemon juice; tomato juice, vinegar, or wine. Brush the meat with oil-herb-juice mixture and allow to stand for several hours or overnight in the refrigerator. Turn the meat often and brush again with the mixture. Drain

off liquid from the meat, wipe dry, and broil or roast. Use the liquid for basting.

2. Pan-fry meat, chicken, fish, eggs, pancakes.

3. Substitute oil for solid fat in muffin, biscuit, pancake, and waffle recipes. Use skim milk instead of whole milk.

4. Mix with a tiny pinch of herbs to flavor vegetables; or add to vegetables with a tablespoon or two of water before cooking, cover tightly and cook until tender but still crisp.

5. Add to mashed potatoes with skim milk.

6. Use in mayonnaise, French dressing, and cooked salad dressings.

7. Use in place of solid fats for making white sauces with skim milk.

8. Use for pie crust and chiffon cakes.

## REVIEW QUESTIONS AND PROBLEMS

1. From the risks listed on page 233, identify those that apply to yourself or someone you know.

2. A patient has a slightly elevated blood cholesterol, and high blood triglyceride. He is 30 pounds overweight, and has an abnormal glucose tolerance. What changes in the diet would be indicated?

3. Write a day's menu for the patient described in question 2. After he has reached desirable weight, what would be a suitable maintenance diet for him?

4. Name five foods that are high in saturated fat.

5. Why are eggs restricted or omitted on these diets?

6. Why are concentrated sweets and alcohol omitted on some diets?

7. Why would a supplement of vitamin A be prescribed for a patient receiving a very low-fat diet?

8. In any cookbook look up the recipes for biscuits, buttered vegetables, creamed chicken, pie crust. How could you change the recipes so that they would be low in saturated fat and high in polyunsaturated fat?

9. Write a menu for one day for a 1200 kcal diet that is low in cholesterol and very low in fat.

## REFERENCES

American Heart Association Publications. *Diet and Coronary Heart Disease*, 1973; *Eat Well But Eat Wisely*, 1969; *Planning Fat-Controlled Meals for 1200 and 1800 Calories*, Revised 1966; *Planning Fat-Controlled Meals for 2000 and 2600 Calories*, Revised 1967; *Programmed Instruction for Fat-Controlled Diet, 1800 Calories*, 1969; *Recipes for Fat-Controlled Low-Cholesterol Meals*, 1968; *The Way to a Man's Heart*, 1968.

Council on Foods and Nutrition: "Diet and Coronary Heart Disease. A Council Statement," *JAMA*, **222**:1647, 1972.

*Dietary Management of Hyperlipoproteinemia*, booklets for patients, Type I, II, III, IV, and V. Bethesda, Md.: National Heart and Lung Institute, 1970.

Eshleman, R., and Winston, M.: *The American Heart Association Cookbook.* New York: David McKay Company, Inc., 1973.

Grollman, A.: "A Common Sense Guide to Cholesterol," *Today's Health,* **44:**3, August 1966.

Kannel, W. B.: "The Disease of Living," *Nutr. Today,* 6:2–11, May 1971.

Robinson, C. H.: *Normal and Therapeutic Nutrition,* 14th ed. New York: Macmillan Publishing Co., Inc., 1972, Chap. 42.

Stamler, J., *et al.*: "Coronary Proneness and Approaches to Preventing Heart Attacks," *Am. J. Nurs.,* 66:1788–93, 1966.

# DISEASES OF THE HEART

## Sodium-Restricted Diets

### TYPES OF CARDIOVASCULAR DISORDERS

*Hypertension* (high blood pressure) is a symptom, not a disease. About
23 million Americans are hypertensive; probably half of these are not even
aware of the condition. High blood pressure is a leading contributor to
heart attack and stroke; it is associated with diseases of the kidney and
toxemias of pregnancy. Hypertension is treated primarily by drugs, not by
diet. However, for the obese there is value in using a low-calorie diet to
effect weight loss. Some physicians also recommend some restriction of
salt intake.

*Angina pectoris* is the sensation of tightness, pressure, and pain usually
in the chest; the pain often spreads to the left shoulder, arm, or hand. It is
a sign that the blood supply to the heart muscle is not adequate. Any
muscle aches when it does not get a sufficient supply of blood. Angina
is brought about as a result of the gradual thickening of the blood vessel
walls, and the narrowing of the lumen through which the blood flows. The
attacks of angina take place after physical exertion, by exposure to a cold
wind, through excitement, or during the digestion of a heavy meal. Loss
of weight, if obese, and meals that are small and easily digested are helpful
measures for these patients.

*Myocardial infarction* is also known as coronary occlusion, coronary
thrombosis, coronary, or heart attack. It refers to the damage to heart tissue
resulting from the blockage of an artery supplying the heart. The tissue
served by that artery is not supplied with the oxygen and nutrients that it
needs, and consequently it dies. When a small artery is blocked the area of

245

tissue damage is small, and recovery is good especially if there is collateral circulation; if a major artery is affected, sudden death follows.

**Congestive heart failure** occurs when the heart is unable to maintain adequate circulation to the tissues. *Decompensation* is said to have taken place. The reduced level of circulation allows sodium to accumulate in the tissues. To hold sodium in solution, fluid also accumulates in the chest cavity, the abdomen, the back, legs, and feet. The fluid accumulation further interferes with heart action.

### NUTRITIONAL PLANNING

The nutritional care of the patient who has sustained a myocardial infarction must be tailored to the individual's needs. It must include planning for the acute illness, the period of convalescence, and following recovery.

Several factors must be considered in planning for the patient's diet, namely shortness of breath, fatigue, abdominal distention, the presence or absence of edema, loss of appetite, and fear of eating. Meals that are large or that are slowly digested necessitate increased circulation to the intestinal tract and therefore place greater strain on the heart. Distention of the stomach causes pressure on the diaphragm and this in turn increases dyspnea.

An essential characteristic of therapy in acute myocardial infarction is rest. (See Fig. 25–1.) A regimen of nutritional care has been described by Christakis and Winston, and is summarized below.*

**Acute illness.** For the first 24 to 48 hours the physician may direct that no food be given by mouth. Then a low-fat liquid diet supplying 500 to 800 kcal (1000 to 1500 ml fluid) is used for two or three days—longer if arrhythmia persists. This diet can include clear soups, weak tea, decaffeinated coffee, ginger ale, fruit juices, and skim milk. Very hot and very cold liquids should be avoided. Only small amounts of liquid are given at one time. The possibility that milk may produce distention because of lactose intolerance should be kept in mind.

Generally it has been considered advisable to feed the acutely ill patient. A recent study, however, has shown that it made little difference whether the patient was fed, or fed himself. Men, especially, preferred to feed themselves.†

Within a few days the patient usually progresses to a soft diet with these characteristics:

* G. Christakis and M. Winston, "Nutritional Therapy in Acute Myocardial Infarction," *J. Am. Diet. Assoc.*, 63:233–38, 1973.
† R. Merkel and C. M. Brown, "Evaluating Feeding Activities in a CCU," *Am. J. Nurs.*, 70:2348–50, 1970.

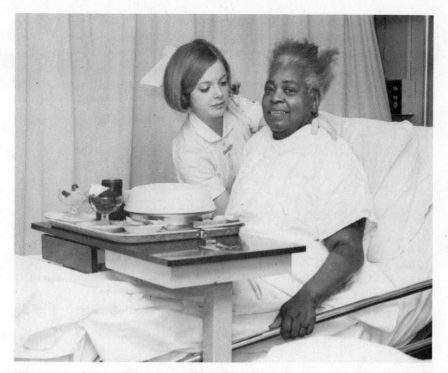

FIGURE 25–1 By adjusting the patient's position, the nurse helps to reduce the energy the patient must exert in eating her meal. (*Courtesy, School of Nursing, Thomas Jefferson University, Philadelphia.*)

1. 1000 to 1200 kcal so that there is minimum circulation required for the digestive-absorptive processes, and to initiate weight loss if obese.

2. Five to six small, easily digested meals, especially if the patient is dyspneic or has angina.

3. Cholesterol restricted to 300 mg.

4. Low in saturated fat with an increased proportion of polyunsaturated fatty acids. See Chapter 24.

5. Restricted in sodium if there is congestive heart failure.

6. Avoidance of distending foods.

When diuretics are given to the patient with congestive heart failure, the potassium loss may be increased. The physician may request the inclusion of more potassium-rich foods such as plums, prunes, orange juice, potatoes, and other vegetables. The use of a potassium salt as medication is a more reliable way to assure compensation for the losses.

*Maintenance diet.* As the patient adjusts once again to a normal pattern of living, his diet is based upon his weight status and the blood lipid levels. Gradual weight loss is indicated if the patient is obese; however, some patients do not respond well, physically or psychologically, to weight-losing regimens. A maintenance diet that is restricted to 300 mg cholesterol and that is reduced in its saturated fatty acid content is useful in reducing the likelihood of a recurrence of the coronary. The selection of the diet to be used on a long-term basis is best determined by the levels of the blood cholesterol and triglycerides about 6 months to a year following the heart attack. See Chapter 24 for diets for hyperlipidemias.

## Sodium-Restricted Diets

### NOMENCLATURE

Normally the daily sodium intake is 3 to 7 gm (3000 to 7000 mg). A sodium-restricted diet is limited to a specified amount of sodium, and ranges from a mild to severe restriction. Terms such as "salt free," "salt poor," and "low salt" are so indefinite that the patient might well receive a diet with much more sodium than he should have or, perhaps, one with less than he could have.

The levels of sodium restriction described in booklets published by the American Heart Association are:

250 mg sodium, Very Low-Sodium Diet. Used primarily for hospital patients.
500 mg sodium, Strict Low-Sodium Diet. Used primarily for hospital patients.
1000 mg sodium, Moderate Sodium-Restricted Diet. Often used as a maintenance diet for patients at home.
Mild Sodium Restriction. Sodium content of this diet may vary from about 2400 to 4500 mg. This is essentially a normal diet that omits salty foods and the use of salt at the table. This is frequently prescribed as a maintenance diet for patients at home.

### SOURCES OF SODIUM

The principal source of sodium in the diet is salt used (1) in numerous ways in food processing; for example, bacon, sauerkraut, dried fish, canned vegetables and meats, and many others; (2) in baking or cooking of foods; and (3) at the table. Salt is about 40 per cent sodium. Thus a teaspoon of salt that weighs about 6 gm would provide 2400 mg sodium. If a recipe requires one teaspoon salt and serves six people, you can see that one serving of that food alone would give 400 mg sodium from the addition of the salt.

All living things, plants as well as animals, require some sodium. Hence one would expect to find some sodium in foods as they naturally occur before they are processed by the manufacturer or cooked in the home. Animal foods are relatively high in sodium, and plant foods, with few exceptions, are low. You will note that 2 cups of milk alone provide almost half the sodium in the calculation of the 500-mg-sodium, 1800-kcal diet (see Table 25-1, p. 251). Meat, fish, and poultry are naturally high in sodium, and their amounts must be controlled on all levels except the mild sodium restriction. Shellfish are higher than meat and poultry and are therefore avoided. Eggs are also high in sodium, one egg containing about 65 mg. Most of the sodium is in the white, so it is possible to omit the white in some preparations and to use only the yolk.

Most vegetables are low in sodium, but several, such as beets and spinach, are "salt-loving" in their growth, and therefore contain too much sodium except for diets permitting 1000 mg or more per day.

Fruits, unsalted cereals, unsalted bread, unsalted butter, and sugar contain small amounts of sodium or none at all, and may be used without restriction as far as sodium is concerned.

Numerous compounds containing sodium are used by the manufacturer or in home preparation to improve the flavor or texture of foods. Among the more common ones are:

| | |
|---|---|
| Baking powder | Sodium benzoate |
| Baking soda | Sodium citrate |
| Monosodium glutamate | Sodium propionate |
| Sodium acetate | Sodium sulfite |
| Sodium alginate | |

It is not important that you know why each of these compounds is added to foods. But it is essential that you form the habit of looking for the words *sodium*, *salt*, and *soda* on any label (see Fig. 25-2). However, the label provides no information for such foods as mayonnaise and catsup, which are standardized according to the regulations of the Food and Drug Administration.

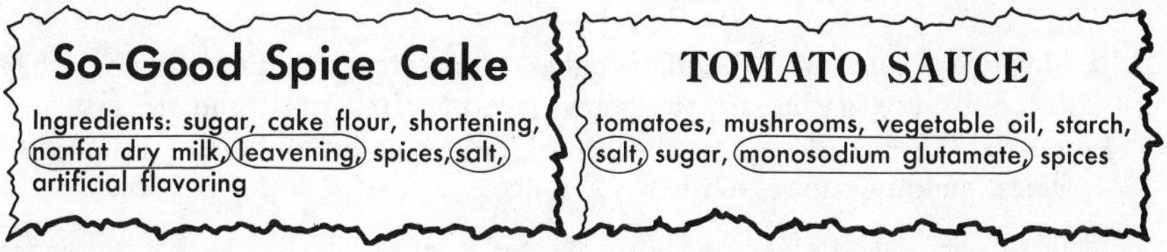

## So-Good Spice Cake

Ingredients: sugar, cake flour, shortening, nonfat dry milk, leavening, spices, salt, artificial flavoring

## TOMATO SAUCE

tomatoes, mushrooms, vegetable oil, starch, salt, sugar, monosodium glutamate, spices

FIGURE 25-2 Watch for the words "salt" and "sodium" when selecting foods for sodium-restricted diets. Leavenings and nonfat dry milk also contribute much sodium.

Some drinking waters are high in sodium, especially if water softeners are used. Many drugs, such as sedatives, laxatives, and alkalizers, contain sodium. The patient needs to be warned against self-medication with baking soda or various antacids.

## FOOD SELECTION

The Food Exchange Lists (see Table A–2, Appendix A) have been adapted by the American Heart Association in its booklets for the sodium-restricted diet. All foods used for these diets must be processed and prepared without salt or other sodium compounds. Canned foods, for example, must be eliminated if they contain salt; canned fruits would be the only exception. Many low-sodium dietetic canned foods are suitable if the labeling indicates that they are no higher in sodium than the fresh product.

Table A–2 may be used for calculating diets, provided that the following foods within each list are avoided.

*List 1, Milk and related products:* avoid buttermilk, soda fountain beverages, ice cream, ice milk, sherbet

*List 2, Vegetables:* avoid beet greens, beets, carrots, celery, chard, dandelion greens, kale, mustard greens, sauerkraut, spinach, white turnips; any canned vegetables unless canned without salt; frozen peas, if salted

*List 3, Fruits:* avoid dried fruit if treated with sodium sulfite; maraschino cherries; glazed fruit

*List 4, Breads and cereals:* avoid any products containing salt, baking powder, or baking soda; regular yeast breads, muffins, rolls; all dry breakfast cereals except puffed wheat, puffed rice, and shredded wheat; quick breads, muffins, pancakes, waffles; quick bread, biscuit, muffin, pancake, waffle mixes; self-rising flour; pretzels; popcorn; potato chips; canned baked beans, corn, or Lima beans; frozen Lima beans

*List 5, Meat:* avoid fresh or canned shellfish, including clams, crabs, lobsters, oysters, scallops, shrimp; all kinds of cheese; canned, dried, or smoked meat, such as bologna, chipped or corned beef, frankfurters, ham, kosher meat, luncheon meat, sausage, smoked tongue; frozen fish fillets; canned, salted, or smoked fish, including anchovies, caviar, salted and dried cod, herring, sardines; canned salmon, tuna; and peanut butter, except low-sodium

*List 6, Fats:* avoid salted butter or margarine; bacon and bacon fat; salt pork; olives; commercial French dressing, mayonnaise, or salad dressing; salted nuts

*Miscellaneous foods:* avoid bouillon cubes, commercial candies, catsup, celery salt, chili sauce, garlic salt, sweetened gelatin mixes, meat and steak sauces, prepared horseradish, prepared mustard, monosodium glutamate, onion salt, pickles, pudding mixes, relishes, soy sauce

## DIETARY PLANS

The selection of foods for three calorie levels of a 500-mg-sodium diet is shown in Table 25–1. The calculations for sodium in the 1800-calorie diet are based on average values assigned to each food list.

TABLE 25-1   500-MG-SODIUM DIET AT THREE CALORIE LEVELS *

| | 1000 kcal Exchanges | 1200 kcal Exchanges | 1800 kcal | |
|---|---|---|---|---|
| Food List | | | Exchanges | Sodium (mg) |
| 1. Milk | 2 skim | 2 skim | 2 whole | 240 |
| 2. Vegetables, A group | 1–2 | 1–2 | 1–2 | 18 |
|     B group | 1 | 1 | 1 | 9 |
| 3. Fruit | 3 | 3 | 3 | 6 |
| 4. Bread | 4 | 4 | 6 | 30 |
| 5. Meat (only 1 egg daily) | 6 | 6 | 7 | 175 |
| 6. Fat | 0 | 4 | 6 | — |
| Sugars and sweets | 0 | 0 | 7 teaspoons | |
| | | | | 478 |

\* *250 mg sodium:* substitute low-sodium milk for regular milk.

*1000 mg sodium:* measure ¼ teaspoon salt into shaker and use on food during the day; *or* use 2 slices regular bread and 2 teaspoons regular butter in place of 2 slices unsalted bread and 2 teaspoons unsalted butter.

*Mild sodium restriction:* food may be lightly salted in cooking. Use regular bread and butter. Omit salt at the table. Omit salty foods, such as potato chips, pretzels, pickles, relishes, meat sauces, salty meats, fish and so on.

*Unrestricted calories:* provide additional calories from fruits, unsalted breads and cereals, unsalted fats, sugars and sweets.

TABLE 25-2   TWO SAMPLE MENUS FOR THE 500-MG SODIUM DIET

| 1000-kcal Soft Diet * (No salt used in cooking) | 1800-kcal Regular Diet (No salt used in cooking) |
|---|---|
| *Breakfast* | *Breakfast* |
| Orange sections | Orange sections |
| Puffed rice | Shredded wheat |
| Skim milk—½ cup | Milk, whole—1 cup |
| No sugar | Sugar—2 teaspoons |
| Toast, unsalted—1 slice | Soft-cooked egg—1 |
| No butter | Toast unsalted—1 slice |
| | Butter, unsalted—1 teaspoon |
| *Luncheon* | |
| Sliced tender chicken (ground, if necessary)—2 oz | *Luncheon* |
| | Salad bowl: |
| Asparagus tips with lemon wedge |     Lettuce, endive, escalore, raw cauli- |
| Roll, unsalted, soft—1 |     flower, green pepper, tomato |
| No butter |     wedges |
| Peaches, unsweetened, canned—2 halves | Sliced chicken strips—2 oz |
| | French dressing, unsalted—1 table- |
| Milk, skim—1 cup |     spoon |

**TABLE 25–2** (*Continued*)

| 1000-kcal Soft Diet * (No salt used in cooking) | 1800-kcal Regular Diet (No salt used in cooking) |
|---|---|
| | Roll, unsalted—1 |
| | Butter, unsalted—1 teaspoon |
| | Marmalade—2 teaspoons |
| | Milk, whole—1 cup |
| | Peaches, fresh, sliced |
| *Dinner* | *Dinner* |
| Tender roast beef (ground, if necessary)—3 oz | Roast beef—4 oz with currant jelly—1 tablespoon |
| Baked potato without skin—1 small | Potato, baked—1 medium with chive butter—2 teaspoons |
| Peas, canned, unsalted | Fresh peas with mushrooms |
| Milk, skim—½ cup | Roll, unsalted—1 |
| Banana—½ | Butter, unsalted—1 teaspoon |
| | Tokay grapes |

\* Give fruit and milk between meals during early stages of recovery.

**PREPARATION OF FOOD**

Patients who have always used much salt at the table are likely to complain bitterly about the flat taste of the food. Others, who prefer foods only lightly salted, find the diet to be more tolerable. In time most patients find that they can adjust to the restriction of sodium by learning to substitute other flavorings. Salt substitutes are useful to some. Because these compounds may be harmful to patients with damaged kidneys, they should be used only with a physician's prescription.

Many flavoring extracts, spices, and herbs may be used to lend interest to the diet. Usually a dash of spices or a small pinch of herbs is sufficient for most family-size recipes. The flavor should be delicate and subtle rather than strong and overpowering. Meats may be marinated in wine, vinegar, low-sodium French dressing, or sprinkled with lemon juice before cooking. A few suggestions for flavor combinations are provided below.\*

MEAT, POULTRY, FISH, EGGS

*Beef:* bay leaf, lemon juice, marjoram, dry mustard, mushrooms, nutmeg, onion, green pepper, pepper, sage, thyme; currant or grape jelly

\* C. H. Robinson, *Proudfit-Robinson's Normal and Therapeutic Nutrition*, 13th ed. (New York: Macmillan, Inc., 1967), pp. 759, 760.

*Chicken or turkey:* basil, bay leaf, lemon juice, marjoram, onion, pepper, rosemary, sage, sesame seeds, thyme; cranberry sauce

*Lamb:* curry, garlic, mint, onion, oregano, parsley, rosemary, thyme; mint jelly, broiled pineapple

*Pork:* garlic, lemon juice, marjoram, sage; applesauce, spiced apples, cranberries

*Veal:* bay leaf, curry, dill seed, ginger, marjoram, oregano, summer savory; currant jelly; broiled apricots or peaches

*Fish:* bay leaf, curry, dill, garlic, lemon juice, mushrooms, mustard, onion, paprika, pepper

*Eggs:* basil, chives, curry, mustard, parsley, green pepper, rosemary, diced tomato

## VEGETABLES

Add a dash of sugar while cooking vegetables to bring out flavor.

*Asparagus:* lemon juice, caraway; unsalted chopped nuts

*Green beans:* dill, lemon, marjoram, nutmeg, onion, rosemary; slivered almonds

*Broccoli:* lemon juice, oregano, tarragon

*Corn:* chives, parsley, green pepper, pimento, tomato

*Peas:* mint, mushroom, onion, parsley, green pepper

*Potatoes:* chives, mace, onion, parsley, green pepper

*Squash:* basil, ginger, mace, onion, oregano

*Sweet potatoes:* cinnamon, nutmeg; brown sugar

*Tomatoes:* basil, marjoram, oregano, parsley, sage

Homemade quick breads, biscuits, and muffins may be made by using low-sodium baking powder instead of regular baking powder. For each teaspoon of regular baking powder, it is necessary to use 1½ teaspoons low-sodium baking powder. The salt specified in the recipe should be omitted.

Homemade bread, waffles, and rolls may be made by using yeast and omitting the salt from the recipe. The yeast dough may be rolled out, spread with unsalted butter, and sprinkled with sugar and cinnamon for delicious cinnamon rolls.

The booklets prepared by the American Heart Association contain menu suggestions and helpful hints in the prepartion of food, as well as guides for eating out.

## REVIEW QUESTIONS AND PROBLEMS

1. What are the circumstances that lead to the formation of edema in patients who have had a heart attack?

2. What is the chief source of sodium in the diet?

3. How do sodium-restricted diets compare with the normal diet in the amounts of sodium contained in them?

4. Classify the following foods as (1) low in sodium; (2) naturally high in sodium; or (3) containing much added salt: oranges, shredded wheat, cornflakes, peaches, catsup, American cheese, skim milk, sardines, peanut butter, potato chips, sugar, fresh peas, canned apricots, canned tuna fish, roast beef, pickles.

5. For a patient with cardiac failure and edema, what factors would be important in dietary care in addition to sodium restriction?

6. How would you change a 500-mg-sodium diet to 250-mg-sodium? To 1000-mg-sodium?

7. List the foods that often cause discomfort and distention for cardiac patients.

8. How could you make each of the following foods more palatable for a sodium-restricted diet: sweet potatoes, frozen green beans, roast pork, unsalted bread?

9. A patient asks if he may use a salt substitute. What should you tell him?

10. Modify the 1800-kcal diet in Table 25–2 so that it is low in cholesterol and saturated fat, and increased in polyunsaturated fats. (See Chap. 24.)

## REFERENCES

American Heart Association. *Your Sodium-Restricted Diet: 500 mg, 1000 mg, Mild Restriction,* 1958; Fold-out charts: *Sodium-Restricted Diet, 500 mg,* 1965; *Sodium-Restricted Diet, 1000 mg,* 1966; *Sodium-Restricted Diet, Mild Restriction,* 1967.

Deutsch, P., and Deutsch, R.: "The Heart Attack You Didn't Know You Had," *Today's Health,* 47:42, July 1969.

Mason, M. A.: *Basic Medical-Surgical Nursing,* 3rd ed. New York: Macmillan Publishing Co., Inc., 1974, Chap. 9, pp. 137–41, 148–55, 161–65.

Searight, M. W.: "A Low-Sodium Potluck Luncheon," *Nurs. Outlook,* 16:30–32, August 1968.

Soffer, A.: "What You Should Know About Stroke," *Today's Health,* 46:40, August 1968.

# DISEASES OF THE KIDNEY

*Diets Controlled for Protein, Potassium, and Sodium*

## FUNCTIONS OF THE KIDNEY

There are about one million working units called *nephrons* in each kidney. Each nephron consists of a tuft of capillaries known as the *glomerulus* attached to a long winding *tubule* that empties into collecting tubules.

The glomerulus filters the blood that circulates through it. Water together with glucose, amino acids, urea, sodium chloride, and other small molecules filter into the tubules. Large molecules such as the blood proteins are held back in the circulation. Each glomerulus filters only a tiny drop of fluid in a day, but the volume of plasma filtered by the two million glomeruli amounts to about 180 liters in 24 hours. The amounts of glucose, sodium chloride, and other substances filtered are equally large; for example, the sodium chloride filtered is over 1 kilogram which is roughly 100 times the daily intake of salt!

The winding tubules bring about *selective reabsorption* so that the normal concentration of substances in the blood is maintained at all times. Normally, the urine volume ranges from 1000 to 2000 ml, which means that over 99 per cent of the filtered water has been returned to the circulation. Likewise, all of the glucose and vitamin C, and almost all of the amino acids, sodium, and other substances have been returned to the blood. For example, if you eat foods containing more salt than your body needs, the renal excretion of water and sodium will be increased. On the other hand, if you greatly reduce your salt intake or if the body sodium is depleted, the excretion in the urine will be very small. Several hormones such as the antidiuretic hormone and adrenal cortical hormones control the amounts of fluid and electrolytes that will be reabsorbed from the tubules.

Most of the wastes of metabolism are excreted by the kidney. Urea is the principal waste from the metabolism of protein, but uric acid, creatinine, and ammonia are also excreted. The kidney is an important regulator of acid-base balance. It secretes a more acid urine if there is increased production of metabolic acids, and it synthesizes ammonia which can neutralize acids so that there is less loss of base.

## NEPHRITIS

*Acute glomerulonephritis* (inflammation of the glomeruli) frequently follows a streptococcic infection of the respiratory tract or scarlet fever. It is often seen in young children. During the acute stage of the illness there is nausea, fever, vomiting, hematuria, oliguria, and hypertension. The appetite is usually very poor, and little is gained by forcing food when the gastrointestinal symptoms are present. The fluid intake is usually restricted, but the patient is likely to tolerate the fluid allowance as fruit juices, fruit ices, ginger ale, sweetened weak tea, and hard candy. Even these small amounts of carbohydrate help to reduce tissue breakdown. As soon as the acute symptoms subside the patient should be given a normal diet in which the protein intake is at, or slightly below, the recommended allowances for age and body size. See Table 4–1. Sodium restriction is not necessary except when edema is present. The amounts of food listed for the 40- to 60-gm protein diets in Table 26–2 (p. 262) are usually satisfactory. However, limitation of the potassium intake is not required.

*Chronic glomerulonephritis* may be present in a latent stage for years before symptoms are detected. When the kidney function is below 20 to 10 per cent of normal, the patient begins to complain of headache, fatigue, nocturia, and sometimes blurring of the vision. Hypertension, proteinuria, and hematuria may also be present.

Sufficient nutrients to meet body requirements are of utmost importance so that the sense of well-being can be maintained as long as possible. Anemia is relatively common and persistent, and a supplement of iron salts is usually prescribed.

If the blood urea is only moderately high, about 60 to 70 gm protein are included daily, with particular emphasis upon sources of high biologic value. If there is proteinuria, the daily protein intake should be increased by the amount lost in the urine.

Sodium restriction is not necessary except when there is edema, although some physicians routinely prescribe mild restriction. (See Chap. 25.) Because the kidneys are usually unable to concentrate urine, the fluid loss can be high, and must be compensated by an increased intake of fluid.

# Nutritional Care in Renal Failure

### CLINICAL FINDINGS

Renal failure indicates that the kidneys are no longer able to fulfill their functions adequately. Acute renal failure sometimes occurs from the trauma of surgery or accidents or from the ingestion of poisons. It is an emergency situation that often requires dialysis. Chronic renal failure is the final outcome of chronic glomerulonephritis or may be associated with poor circulation because of extensive atherosclerosis or cardiac failure.

In renal failure the patient has an elevated blood urea nitrogen (uremia), acidosis, anemia, and usually excretes little or no urine. These changes produce gastrointestinal upsets such as anorexia, nausea, vomiting, bad breath, and ulcerations of the mouth. These symptoms make it difficult for the patient to eat. Marked retention of potassium and severe edema interfere with heart action, thus further endangering the life of the patient.

### PLANNING NUTRIENT LEVELS

A carefully controlled diet is primary therapy whether the patient is being maintained as comfortably as possible or is a candidate for transplant or dialysis. The dietary control can make the difference between being able to hold a job and maintain reasonably normal activities or being miserable and dependent. The diet is complex and requires individual planning for each patient according to his symptoms, the laboratory tests, and his nutritional status. From time to time dietary adjustments must be made to coincide with changes in his condition.

The diet is controlled for protein, potassium, sodium, and fluid intake. The following factors are considered:

*Energy.* Any breakdown of body tissues releases both nitrogen and potassium to the circulation, causing dangerous increases in the blood levels. Therefore, it is essential to prevent this by giving sufficient calories (about 2000 to 3000 kcal) from carbohydrate and fat so that tissue catabolism is kept at a minimum.

*Protein.* Most frequently protein is restricted to 40 gm, but it may be as low as 20 gm or as high as 60 gm. In renal failure the excess of nitrogenous constituents in the blood can be used to synthesize the nonessential amino acids. The protein in the diet must supply the essential amino acids. Foods such as eggs, milk, and meat will furnish most of the protein in the diet.

*Potassium.* In severe renal failure the blood concentration of potassium is sometimes at dangerously high levels. This interferes with the normal rhythm of the heart. This can be minimized by giving a diet restricted in potassium; 40 mEq (1560 mg) is a level often prescribed.

*Sodium.* Restriction of sodium ranging from 500 mg to mild restriction is ordered if there is edema. Some patients are "salt losers." If they are placed on a sodium-restricted diet they will lose more sodium than they are ingesting, and they will become dehydrated.

*Minerals and vitamins.* The protein-restricted diets do not provide recommended daily allowances of calcium, iron, vitamin B complex, and vitamin D. Supplements of these nutrients should be prescribed.

*Fluid.* When there is oliguria the fluid intake is restricted to the daily volume in the urine plus about 500 to 700 ml which represents the approximate loss from the skin, lungs, and bowel. For example, a urinary excretion of 250 ml daily would permit a fluid intake of 750 ml. This includes all the water present in foods as well as that in beverages. A 100-gm portion of fruits and vegetables supplies 80 to 90 ml water, and 100 ml of milk is equal to 87 ml water. See Table A–1 for per cent of water in foods.

### FOOD LISTS AND MEAL PLANS

*Protein-free electrolyte-free diet.* In anuria a patient is sometimes given for a few days a mixture that contains no protein, but that supplies sufficient calories to prevent tissue breakdown. One such mixture is a butter-sugar "soup" prepared by cooking together 2 tablespoons flour, ¾ cup sugar, and 2 cups water. The mixture is flavored with vanilla, chilled, and served as six equal feedings. It provides 1800 kcal.

*Sources of protein.* Almost all of the protein in the restricted diets must come from milk, eggs, and meat. Cereals, bread, rice, macaroni, spaghetti, and noodles are usually depended upon as good sources of calories. However, 6 to 8 servings of these foods a day would account for 15 to 25 gm protein, which is not of high biologic value. Obviously not much of these foods could be used on diets restricted to 40 gm protein or less.

Special flours and breads have been developed by food processors that are protein-free and low in potassium and sodium.* Recipes for using these products have been developed by the manufacturers. The absence of protein in the flour means that breads will not have the texture qualities provided by gluten, and they are generally less acceptable to the patient. Jellies, unsalted butter and margarine, and honey improve the palatability as well as enhancing the caloric intake. The nurse must emphasize to the

---

* Dietetic Paygel-P, General Mills, Minneapolis, Minnesota.
  Cellu Wheat Starch and Cellu Low Protein Baking Mix, Chicago Dietetic Supply House, LaGrange, Illinois.

patient that it is important to consume all the food allowed on the diet; it is not sufficient to restrict protein only.

*Sources of potassium.* The normal intake of potassium varies from 3000 to 8000 mg, being at the higher levels when protein and calorie intakes are also high. One way to reduce the potassium intake is to reduce the intake of protein as in the diets restricted to 20 and 40 gm.

Vegetables and fruits are also good sources of potassium, but there is a wide variability from one food to another. Potassium salts are quite soluble in water. A potato that is boiled in a fairly large amount of water will contain less potassium than the same potato if it were baked. If the potato is cut into small pieces before cooking it will furnish less potassium than if it is boiled whole.

*Exchange lists.* Foods for these diets are grouped according to their contributions of protein, sodium, and potassium. See Table 26–1 for summary of values to be used in calculating diets.

Fruits have been grouped in two lists, one providing less than 0.5 gm protein per serving, and one containing 1.0 gm protein per serving. There are three lists for vegetables, furnishing 0.5, 1.0, and 2.0 gm protein respectively. In the protein-restricted diets outlined in Table 26–2 it is essential that the foods be used in the amounts and kinds listed.

Sometimes potassium restriction need not be severe. With more liberal allowances, a wider choice of low-protein foods is permitted. Note that each fruit and vegetable list includes a selection of foods that contains somewhat higher levels of potassium.

The daily allowance for protein is divided approximately evenly in the three meals so that there is maximum utilization. These patients cannot afford to cheat on their diets. To do so means that the body is overloaded with nitrogen, potassium, sodium, and fluid. On the other hand there is decided improvement of the appetite and sense of well-being when the patient consumes all the foods planned for his controlled diet. (See Fig. 26–1.)

TABLE 26–1   PROTEIN, SODIUM, AND POTASSIUM VALUES FOR FOOD LISTS

| Food List | Household Measure | Weight gm | Protein gm | Sodium * mg | Potassium mg |
|---|---|---|---|---|---|
| Milk, whole or nonfat | 1 cup | 240 | 8 | 120 | 335 |
| Milk, low sodium | 1 cup | 240 | 8 | 7 | 600 |
| Meat, poultry, fish, cooked | 1 ounce | 30 | 7 | 25 | 100 |
| Egg | 1 | 50 | 7 | 60 | 65 |
| Cheese, American, salted | 1 ounce | 30 | 7 | 210 | 25 |

* Except for cheese, regular bread, and salted butter, the values listed for sodium are those that apply when no salt is used in processing or preparation of the food. Also, certain high-sodium items in the meat and vegetable lists would be omitted if the diet is restricted in sodium.

TABLE 26–1 (Continued)

| Food List | Household Measure | Weight gm | Protein gm | Sodium * mg | Potassium mg |
|---|---|---|---|---|---|
| Cheese, cottage, salted | 1 ounce | 30 | 7 | 85 | 25 |
| Fruits, list 1 | ½ cup | 100 | less than 0.5 | 2 | 85 |
| Fruits, list 2 | ½ cup | 100 | 1 | 2 | 135 |
| Vegetables, list 1 | ½ cup | 100 | 0.5 | 9 | 110 |
| list 2 | ½ cup | 100 | 1 | 9 | 125 |
| list 3 | ½ cup | 100 | 2 | 9 | 160 |
| Bread, low sodium | 1 slice | 30 | 2 | 5 | 30 |
| Bread, regular | 1 slice | 30 | 2 | 160 | 30 |
| Bread, low-protein, low-electrolyte | 1 slice | 30 | 0.1 | 9 | 3 |
| Butter, unsalted | 1 teaspoon | 5 | tr | tr | tr |
| Butter, salted | 1 teaspoon | 5 | tr | 50 | tr |

## FOOD LISTS FOR CONTROLLED PROTEIN, SODIUM, AND POTASSIUM DIETS *

### Milk List

Buttermilk, unsalted
Evaporated milk, reconstituted
Low sodium milk
Nonfat dry milk, reconstituted
Skim milk
Whole milk

### Meat or Substitute List

Beef, chicken, duck, lamb, liver, pork, tongue (unsalted), turkey, veal
Cod, flatfish (flounder or sole), kingfish (whiting), haddock, perch, canned salmon and tuna (omit on sodium-restricted diet)
Clams, crab, lobster, scallops, shrimp (all omitted on sodium-restricted diet)
Egg
Cheese—Cheddar, cottage, American, Swiss (omit on sodium-restricted diet)

### Fruit, List 1

Apple, raw        1 small
Grapes, European    12

### Fruit, List 1 (Continued)

½ cup servings of: applesauce, pears, pineapple, diced watermelon
½ cup of juices: apple, grape, peach nectar, pear nectar, orange-apricot, pineapple-grapefruit, pineapple-orange

With liberal potassium allowance
  (145 mg potassium per serving)
½ cup of: apricot nectar, pineapple juice, canned fruit cocktail, purple plums

### Fruit, List 2

Pear, raw        1 small
Tangerine        1 small
½ cup servings of fresh or frozen blackberries, blueberries, boysenberries, canned cherries, figs; canned or fresh grapefruit; frozen red raspberries

With liberal potassium allowance
  (200 mg potassium per serving)
Orange        1 small
Peach, raw        1 small
Plums, fresh        2 medium

* Adapted from *Manual of Diets*, Departments of Dietetics, Hospital of St. Raphael, Veterans Administration Hospital, and Yale–New Haven Hospital, New Haven, Conn.

## Fruit, List 2 (Continued)

Strawberries, fresh ⅔ cup

½ cup servings of cantaloupe, honeydew, frozen melon balls, fresh or frozen rhubarb

½ cup of these juices: grapefruit, grapefruit-orange, orange, tomato

## Vegetable, List 1

½ cup servings of raw cabbage, cucumber, lettuce, onion, tomato

### With liberal potassium allowance

(165 mg potassium per serving)

Carrot, raw          1 small (+)†
Celery, raw          1 stalk (+)
Endive, raw          ½ cup

## Vegetables, List 2

½ cup servings of canned green or wax beans, carrots (+), spinach (+), fresh cooked cabbage, eggplant, mustard greens, onion, summer squash

### With liberal potassium allowance

(190 mg potassium per serving)

½ cup servings of canned beets (+), rutabagas, tomatoes; fresh cooked carrots (+), turnips (+); frozen summer squash, winter squash

## Vegetables, List 3

½ cup servings of canned asparagus; fresh or frozen green or wax beans, okra

### With liberal potassium allowance

(245 mg potassium per serving)

½ cup servings of fresh or frozen cauliflower; cooked dandelion greens (+); potato, boiled and peeled before cooking; mashed potato

## Bread and Substitutes

| | |
|---|---|
| Bread | 1 slice |
| Cereals, dry | 1 cup |
| Cornflakes, Puffed Rice, Puffed Wheat, shredded wheat | |
| Cereals, cooked | ½ cup |
| cornmeal, farina, oatmeal, rice, rolled wheat | |
| Crackers, soda | 3 squares |
| Flour | 2 tablespoons |
| Grits | 1 cup |
| Macaroni, noodles, or spaghetti | ¼ cup |
| Rice | ½ cup |

## Fats

Butter
Cream (1 ounce contains 35 mg potassium)
Fat or cooking oil
Margarine
Salad dressings: French or mayonnaise

### Miscellaneous

Cornstarch
Flavoring extracts
Ginger ale
Hard candies
Herbs (see suggestions page 252)
Honey
Jam or jelly
Jellybeans
Rice starch
Spices (see suggestions page 252)
Sugar, white, confectioners'
Syrup
Tapioca
Vinegar
Wheat starch

† All items marked (+) are omitted when sodium restriction is ordered.

TABLE 26–2  SUGGESTED DAILY MEAL PATTERN FOR CONTROLLED PROTEIN, SODIUM, AND POTASSIUM DIET *

| | | Protein | | |
|---|---|---|---|---|
| | Measure | 20 gm | 40 gm | 60 gm |
| Breakfast | | | | |
| Fruit, list 1 | 1 exchange | 1 | 1 | 1 |
| Egg | 1 | — | 1 | 1 |
| Cereal | 1 exchange | 1 | 1 | 1 |
| Low-protein bread | 1 slice | 2 | — | — |
| Bread, enriched | 1 slice | — | 1 | 1 |
| Milk | cup | ¼ | ¼ | ¼ |
| Lunch | | | | |
| Egg | 1 | 1 | — | — |
| Meat or equivalent | 1 ounce | — | 1 | 2 |
| Bread or substitute | 1 exchange | — | 1 | 2 |
| Low-protein bread | 1 slice | 2 | — | — |
| Vegetable, list 1 | 1 exchange | — | 1 | 1 |
| Milk | cup | — | ½ | ½ |
| Low-protein dessert | 1 serving | 1 | 1 | 1 |
| Fruit, list 1 | 1 exchange | 1 | 1 | 1 |
| Dinner | | | | |
| Meat or equivalent | 1 ounce | — | 1 | 2 |
| Bread or substitute | 1 exchange | 1 | 1 | 2 |
| Low-protein bread | 1 slice | 2 | — | — |
| Vegetable, list 1 | 1 exchange | 1 | — | — |
| Vegetable, list 2 | 1 exchange | — | 1 | 1 |
| Fruit, list 2 | 1 exchange | — | 1 | 2 |
| Milk | cup | ½ | — | — |
| Low-protein dessert | 1 serving | 1 | — | — |

* *Manual of Diets*, Department of Dietetics, Hospital of St. Raphael, Veterans Administration Hospital, Yale–New Haven Hospital, New Haven, Conn.

## Other Renal Disorders

### NEPHROTIC SYNDROME

The nephrotic syndrome is not a specific disease entity but a combination of symptoms that are often seen in certain stages of renal disease. These include severe edema, heavy albuminuria, very low serum proteins—especially albumin, high serum lipids, anemia, and oliguria.

The dietary management consists of a high-protein diet with ample

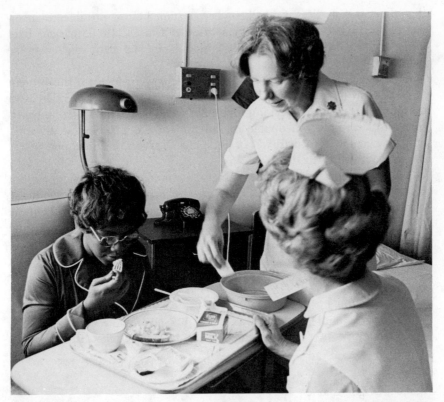

FIGURE 26–1 Patients with chronic renal failure often have poor appetites. They may need assistance as well as encouragement to consume sufficient food to meet caloric requirements. The nurse and dietitian must also explain the nature of the diet to the patient. (*Courtesy, Department of Nursing, Delaware County Community College, Media, Pennsylvania.*)

calorie intake. To correct the large losses of protein in the urine and to raise the level of blood albumin, young children need 3 to 4 gm protein per kg, and older persons require up to 125 gm protein per day. Because of the severity of edema, sodium is sometimes restricted to as low as 500 to 1000 mg per day. With such restriction it may be necessary to use low-sodium milk so that the protein intake is adequate. (See Chap. 25.)

The appetite is usually poor, and the nurse and parents of a child must use great patience and persuasion to encourage food intake. It is questionable whether severe sodium restriction is of value if it means that the patient will not eat.

*High-protein diet.* As in all therapeutic diets, the planning for high protein intake begins with the normal diet. The basic diet outlined on page 37 furnishes about 70 gm protein. To achieve a level of 125 gm protein means that concentrated sources of protein would be useful so that there is not excessive bulk to be consumed. It is possible to incorporate one or two additional eggs in the day's meals. If the patient likes meat, fish, or poultry the modest amounts in the basic diet may be increased by 2 or 3 ounces.

Additional milk is usually included. One way to increase the protein in the diet at low cost and with little increase in volume of the diet is to use nonfat dry milk. Depending upon the brand used, 4 to 5 tablespoons added to 8 oz milk will double the amount of protein. Nonfat dry milk may also be added to mashed potatoes, cream sauces, cream soups, baked custard, and other foods.

Many patients who require a high-protein diet have poor appetites. It is better to start with the patient's present food intake and to gradually increase the protein and calorie intake. The portions served should be of such size that the patient is able to eat all the foods offered. A bedtime snack is a good way to increase protein and calorie intakes. Two examples of such snacks are:

Sandwich
   2 slices bread
   2 teaspoons butter, mayonnaise
   1½ oz. roast beef
   1 oz cheese
Milk, 1 cup

Protein, 29 gm; calories, 585

High-protein milk shake (tall glass)
   1 cup milk
   4–5 tablespoons nonfat dry milk
   2 tablespoons chocolate syrup

Protein, 16 gm; calories, 345

Food allowances to provide 125 gm protein and approximately 2500 kcal:

   4 cups milk
1–3 eggs
7–9 ounces meat, poultry, fish, cheese
3–4 servings vegetables
      1 green leafy or deep yellow
      1 raw
      1 potato or substitute
   3 servings fruit, including 1 citrus fruit
6–7 servings cereals, breads
Butter, margarine, salad dressings
Sugar, jelly, jam
Desserts such as puddings, custard, ice cream

The following menu illustrates the kinds and amounts of foods used for a diet providing 125 gm protein and 2500 kcal:

*Breakfast*
Stewed prunes
Scrambled eggs, 2
Wheat flakes *with*
Milk, 1 cup
Sugar
Toast, enriched, 1 slice
Butter or margarine
Jelly
Coffee with cream, sugar

*Luncheon*
Cold sliced ham, bologna, cheese, 3 oz
Potato salad
Lettuce, sliced tomato
Mayonnaise
Roll
Butter or margarine
Fresh peach ice cream
Cookie
Milk, 1 cup
Tea, if desired

*Dinner*
Swiss steak, 4 oz
Parsley buttered noodles
French green beans with slivered almonds
Grapefruit avocado salad on water cress
French dressing
Dinner roll with butter or margarine
Floating Island
Milk, 1 cup
Tea or coffee, if desired

*Bedtime*
Egg salad sandwich
Milk, 1 cup

## URINARY CALCULI

Most kidney stones contain calcium as calcium carbonate, phosphate, or oxalate. There are also uric acid stones and cystine stones. Some stones dissolve in acid and some in alkali. Medications are usually prescribed to increase the acidity or alkalinity of the urine. Diet alone does not sufficiently change the pH of the urine, but modifications are sometimes prescribed so that the diet will not counteract the effectiveness of the medication.

A *calcium- and phosphorus-restricted diet* limits milk to 1½ cups or less, and eliminates cheese and all foods prepared with milk.

If an *acid-ash diet* is ordered the emphasis is upon meat, eggs, fish, poultry, cereals, and breads, macaroni and other pastas, rice, cranberry juice, prunes, and plums. The amounts of milk, vegetables, and fruits are included at levels suggested in the basic diet. (See p. 37.)

For oxalate and uric acid stones an *alkaline-ash diet* is sometimes ordered. This diet restricts the amount of eggs, meat, cereals, and breads, and emphasis is placed upon milk, fruits, and vegetables.

Butter, margarine, shortenings, oils, sugar, hard candies, gumdrops, honey, and pure starches are neutral and may be used on either acid-ash or alkaline-ash diets.

A diet restricted in oxalate is sometimes ordered, but its effectiveness is unknown. Such a diet would eliminate almonds, beets and beet greens, cashew nuts, chard, chocolate, cocoa, coffee, corn, currants, endive, figs, Concord grapes, okra, plums, potatoes, raspberries, rhubarb, spinach, sweet potatoes, tea, and tomatoes.

Uric acid stones are sometimes a complication of gout. (See p. 230.)

## REVIEW QUESTIONS AND PROBLEMS

1. What changes take place in the composition of urine of the normal individual in these situations: a diet containing many salty foods is eaten; a diet containing very little salt is eaten; the protein intake is about 100 gm or more each day?

2. What problems might arise for the patient with chronic renal failure in the three situations listed in question 1?

3. Why is it so important to emphasize liberal intakes of carbohydrate and fat by patients with renal failure?

4. An increase in fluid intake is usually recommended when a high-protein diet is ordered. Why?

5. What would be the total fluid intake from the following meal: 1 egg, 2 slices bread, ½ cup green beans, ½ cup applesauce, ½ cup milk? See Table A–1 (p. 306) for information on water contents of food.

6. A patient on a potassium-restricted diet is told not to use the juices from canned vegetables and fruits. Why?

7. A patient on a potassium-restricted diet is advised that he may include a small potato in his diet two or three times a week. What directions should be given for the preparation of the potato?

8. Using the 60 gm-protein diet plan in Table 26–2 and the food exchange lists, plan a menu for one day that is low in potassium and sodium.

9. In the sample menu for the high-protein diet on page 265 arrange the food items under these four headings: acid ash; alkaline ash; neutral; and high in oxalates.

10. Which foods would be emphasized for a patient with renal calculi that are more soluble in acid?

## REFERENCES

Anderson, C. F., et al.: "Nutritional Therapy for Adults with Renal Disease," JAMA, 223:68–75, 1973.

Bugg, R.: "Your Body's Silent Partners," Today's Health, 7:54, January 1969.

Cost, J. S.: "Diet in Chronic Renal Disease: A Focus on Calories," J. Am. Diet. Assoc., 64:186–87, 1974.

Downing, S. R.: "Nursing Support in Early Renal Failure," Am. J. Nurs., 69:1212–16, 1969.

Gillette, E.: "A Patient During Dialysis Treatment," *Nurs. Care*, 6:17, January 1973.

Mason, M. A.: *Basic Medical-Surgical Nursing*, 3rd ed. New York: Macmillan Publishing Co., Inc., 1974, Chap. 16, pp. 358–62, 373–74, 376–82.

Robinson, C. H.: *Normal and Therapeutic Nutrition*, 14th ed. New York: Macmillan Publishing Co., Inc., 1972, Chap. 44.

Robinson, L. G., and Paulbitski, A. H.: "Diet Therapy and Educational Program for Patients with Chronic Renal Failure," *J. Am. Diet. Assoc.*, 61:531–38, 1972.

Stein, P. G., and Winn, N. I.: "Diet Controlled in Sodium, Potassium, Protein, and Fluid: Use of Points for Dietary Calculation," *J. Am. Diet. Assoc.*, 61:538–41, 1972.

**27**  General Dietary Considerations | FIBER | FLAVOR | FLAVOR AND
DIGESTION | OTHER FACTORS IN FOOD TOLERANCE •
Peptic Ulcer | CLINICAL FINDINGS | TREATMENT | LIBERAL
DIET | BLAND FIBER-RESTRICTED DIET • Other Diseases of the
Gastrointestinal Tract | HIATAL HERNIA | DIVERTICULITIS |
CONSTIPATION

# DISEASES OF THE
# GASTROINTESTINAL TRACT

*Bland Fiber-Restricted Diet; High-Fiber Diet;*
*Very Low-Residue Diet*

The dietary modifications used for diseases of the gastrointestinal tract
are discussed in three chapters: peptic ulcer, hiatal hernia, diverticulitis,
and constipation in this chapter; diseases of malabsorption in Chapter 28;
and diseases of the liver, gallbladder, and pancreas in Chapter 29. Any
disease of the gastrointestinal tract leads to some changes in function.
The student should first review the normal digestive processes discussed
in Chapter 3.

## General Dietary Considerations

The maintenance of good nutrition is basic to all dietary modifications
for diseases of the gastrointestinal tract. For most patients the recommended dietary allowances will meet the needs. (See Table 4–1, p. 32.)
Some patients require additional calories, protein, minerals, and vitamins
because their symptoms have prevented them from eating an adequate
diet or because they have been afraid to eat a wide variety of foods. In
other patients, especially those with diseases of malabsorption, the large
losses from the bowel result in poor nutrition, and these losses must be
made up.

Two widely differing approaches are used in dietary modification
for some diseases, especially peptic ulcer and colitis. One of these is termed
"liberal" and the other is "traditional," or "conservative." The differing

points of view are concerned especially with the fiber and flavor characteristics of the diet.

## FIBER

The terms "fiber" and "residue" are not clearly differentiated. Fiber consists of the indigestible parts of foods. It includes cellulose, hemicellulose, lignins, gums, and related substances of plants, and the tough connective tissue from meats. Residue refers to the bulk remaining in the lower part of the gastrointestinal tract. It is derived from the indigestible fibers of the food, but may also be modified by the effect of the food on the growth of intestinal bacteria and their residues. For example, milk that contains no fiber may increase the residue in the feces.

Some foods contain much more fiber than others. Contrast the fibrous nature of cabbage, celery, and pineapple with the finer texture of spinach, lettuce, and banana; or the toughness of mature peas and Lima beans with the tenderness of the young seeds. The structural parts of the plant, skins, and seeds are indigestible. They lend bulk to the normal diet and encourage normal elimination.

The fiber content of the diet may be progressively reduced in the following ways:

1. Selecting only young tender vegetables.

2. Omitting those foods that have seeds, tough skins, or much structural fiber; for example, berries, celery, corn, cabbage, stalks of asparagus, mature beans, and peas.

3. Peeling fruits and vegetables, such as apples, pears, potatoes, stalks of broccoli.

4. Cooking foods to soften the fiber.

5. Pressing foods through a sieve (puréeing or straining).

6. Using refined cereals and white breads in place of whole-grain cereals and breads.

7. Omitting fruits and vegetables entirely; using only strained juices.

Strained vegetables and fruits are extremely unpopular with patients. They have lost appeal in appearance, texture, and in flavor, and are looked upon as baby foods. Undoubtedly, these foods are necessary when a very smooth diet is required, as for a patient with bleeding esophageal varices; they are also useful in the construction of tube feedings. However, physicians have questioned the need for these foods in many diets for gastrointestinal disorders. Thus the soft and bland diets to be described in this chapter are much more liberal than they were a number of years ago.

Meats on low-fiber diets must be tender. Steaks, chops, and roasts with little connective tissue may be broiled and roasted. The less tender cuts of meat become tender when cooked with moist heat at low temperature; for example, stews that are simmered rather than boiled and pot roasts cooked at low heat. Tender cuts of meat need not be ground except when the patient should not exert the effort to chew or when the patient has no teeth.

## FLAVOR

The flavors that are conveyed by foods are a composite of the taste qualities and the odors. Characteristic flavors are given to foods by various oils and water-soluble compounds. Fruits taste sweet or sour, depending upon the amounts of sugar or acid. Fruits also give off typical odors that add much to their enjoyment.

Vegetables are classed as strong- or mild-flavored, depending upon the amounts of sulfur compounds that are present. Such compounds enhance the flavor of properly cooked vegetables, but they are objectionable when vegetables are overcooked.

Meat extractives (purines) are nonprotein, nitrogen-containing compounds that are responsible for the flavor of meat. They give rich flavor to a gravy or soup.

The flavor of a food is modified by cooking procedures. The volatile substances that escape into the air lead to some loss and change of flavor. Would you expect cabbage to be stronger in flavor if cooked in an open or covered saucepan? Overcooking leads to loss of flavor, because some of the flavor compounds are dissolved out into the cooking water. On the other hand, some vegetables like cabbage develop strong flavors if overcooked.

The flavor of foods is enhanced by the addition of flavoring substances, including spices, herbs, salt, vinegar, sugar, and flavoring extracts. The effect of their use depends upon the choice of the condiment and the amount that may be used. Good cooks know that they must use a light hand in the use of herbs, for a little goes a long way. Chili con carne is normally classed as a highly flavored dish; yet it could range in seasoning from relatively mild to decidedly hot.

## FLAVOR AND DIGESTION

Certain categories of foods are considered by many to cause gastrointestinal discomfort. Included are strongly flavored vegetables—broccoli, Brussels sprouts, cabbage, cauliflower, cucumber, leeks, onions, radishes, turnips; melons; and dry beans and peas.

Other foods are thought to be chemically stimulating; that is, they presumably increase the flow of gastric juices. Among these are meat extractives—broth, gravies, all meat stock soups; certain spices and season-ings—catsup, chili, garlic, horseradish, meat sauces, mustard seed, pepper, pickles, excessive salt, tabasco sauce, vinegar, Worcestershire sauce; and coffee and tea.

Considerable difference of opinion exists concerning the effects of eating the foods just discussed. On the one hand, people of several cultures—Indians and Africans, for example—use highly seasoned foods all their lives and appear to suffer no ill effects. Contrariwise, you undoubtedly know someone who complains of indigestion with the merest suggestion of garlic, onion, cucumber, or other items in the diet.

Specialists in medicine and dietetics believe that bland diets need have fewer restrictions placed upon them. Many persons should be permitted the wider range of many food choices that so often appear on "avoid" lists. Omissions of food should be made without hesitation for those indi-viduals who have a definite intolerance for them.

## OTHER FACTORS IN FOOD TOLERANCE

Patients with gastrointestinal disturbances are often nervous, anxious, worried, and tense. Their emotions influence the digestion of foods. They have many dislikes and expressed intolerance to food. It is important to give every consideration to the planning of meals that are enjoyable to the patient. The patient must also see the need for including nutritionally important foods from all major food groups.

Rapid eating and failure to relax are frequently noted in these patients. They need to take adequate time for meals and to learn to eat slowly. They need, moreover, to learn to rest before and after meals and to look for diversions that are relaxing.

## Peptic Ulcer

### CLINICAL FINDINGS

A peptic ulcer is an erosion of the gastrointestinal mucosa. It may be found in the esophagus, stomach, and most often in the duodenum. Pain is caused by contact of the hydrochloric acid with the eroded surface. The pain is described as dull, gnawing, burning, or even piercing. The patient with a peptic ulcer is often anxious, tense, emotional, and one who strives for perfection in whatever he does. Usually there is increased secretion of gastric juice and increased motility. Many patients who have restricted their intake to relatively few foods have low blood proteins, anemia, and weight loss.

## TREATMENT

A number of drugs are available to reduce the secretion of acid and the motility. Antacids to be taken between meals are usually prescribed to neutralize the acid, thus permitting the ulcer to heal. When used over a long period of time antacids are likely to reduce the absorption of iron.

The objectives of dietary management are to maintain good nutrition; to supply the nutrients needed to heal the ulcer, protein and ascorbic acid being especially important; and to provide foods that give the patient satisfaction and comfort. The presence of foods in the stomach dilutes the acid and reduces pain; therefore, six or more meals are given instead of three large meals. Protein foods, including milk, eggs, meat, poultry, and fish, neutralize acid for relatively short periods of time.

### LIBERAL DIET

Those who recommend a liberal diet believe that healing of the ulcer is more rapid if a nutritionally adequate diet that is pleasing to the patient is used from the beginning of treatment. Most people do not enjoy ground or puréed foods. Patients who eat foods that include spices, flavorings, and strongly flavored vegetables do not have discomfort more frequently than those on the conservative diets. The fiber in fruits and vegetables does not irritate the ulcer, and healing is not slower when these foods are included. (See Fig. 27–1.)

The patient should eat three small meals with midmorning, mid-afternoon, and evening snacks. Preference for snacks should be given to protein-rich foods. Although all foods are permitted, the patient's individual tolerances must be respected. For example, one patient may not tolerate Brussels sprouts, so there is no point in suggesting that he eat them; another patient likes Brussels sprouts and eats them without discomfort, so he should not be denied them.

Tobacco, alcohol, and caffeine are strong stimulants to acid production and they should not be used. Sometimes coffee with milk and weak tea are permitted in limited amounts.

### BLAND FIBER-RESTRICTED DIET

The conventional approach to diet allows a limited selection of food at first and progressing through three or four stages to a normal diet. For some patients this approach is psychologically more satisfying. A moderately liberal progression is described below.

*Stage 1.* Milk at two-hourly intervals: 180 ml (6 oz). In addition at mealtimes 1 serving (3 to 4 oz) of any one of these foods: strained cream soup, eggs, cottage cheese, white potato, white toast or crackers, refined

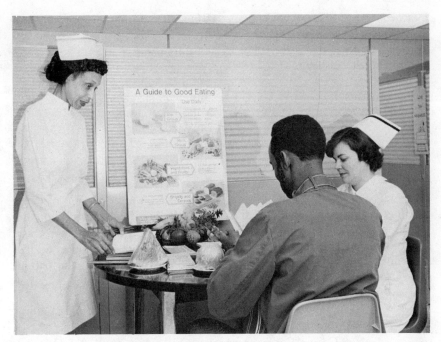

**FIGURE 27-1** A patient convalescing from peptic ulcer learns, to his surprise, that he will be able to enjoy most foods from a normal diet. Selecting a nutritionally adequate diet is important. The nurse will be able to reinforce the instruction from time to time. (*Courtesy, Dietetic Service, Veterans Administration Hospital, Coatesville, Pennsylvania.*)

cereals, plain cake or cookies, gelatin, and plain puddings. This stage is used for only a few days.

*Stage 2.* Milk is given on awakening, midmorning, midafternoon, and before bedtime: 240 ml (8 oz). At mealtime the total volume of food is about 350–450 gm (12–16 oz). All foods of stage 1 are used. In addition allow tender meat, poultry, fish, prepared any way except fried; fruit juices, banana, orange or grapefruit sections, canned fruits except berries; cooked or canned tender asparagus, wax or green beans, beets, spinach, sweet potato, winter squash. The following menu is typical of allowances for stage 2:

*On Awakening*
Milk—8 oz

*Breakfast*
Oatmeal
Milk, sugar
Egg—1

Enriched toast
Butter or margarine
Orange juice—½ cup

*Midmorning*
Milk—8 oz
Crackers—2

*Luncheon*

Cream of pea soup—½ cup
Crackers—2
Chicken-noodle casserole
White bread
Butter or margarine
Canned peaches
Milk

*Midafternoon*

Vanilla pudding
Milk

*Dinner*

Roast beef—3 oz
Mashed potato
Asparagus tips
Bread or roll
Butter or margarine
Vanilla ice cream
Milk

*Bedtime*

Milk shake
Plain sugar cookies

*Stage 3.* Six feedings a day are continued. The foods allowed on the soft diet, page 197, are used with two exceptions: broth, meat soups, and gravies are omitted; and coffee is limited to 1 cup per day and is diluted with milk. In addition to the foods included on the soft diet, the patient may also use raw apples, cherries, peaches, pears, and plums; and raw tomato, tender salad greens, and celery.

## Other Diseases of the Gastrointestinal Tract

### HIATAL HERNIA

Hiatal hernia is an abnormal gap in the diaphragm so that parts of the stomach and other organs slip into the chest cavity. It is found in about 10 per cent of all people, although most of them have no symptoms. Patients complain of heartburn because of the reflux of gastric juice into the esophagus. Those who are obese should lose weight, since excessive weight causes increased pressure, just as do tight garments. A normal diet is usually tolerated, although some patients omit certain foods to which they are intolerant. Small meals with midmorning and midafternoon snacks are better than three large meals. No food should be taken for several hours prior to bedtime. If the symptoms are severe the bland fiber-restricted diet, stages 2 and 3, described on page 273 should be tried.

### DIVERTICULITIS

A *diverticulum* is a tiny sac or pouch in the intestinal wall, most often in the colon. Diverticula become filled with food and bacteria, but produce no symptoms until they become infected and inflamed. Pain in diverticulitis is sometimes severe.

*Very low-residue diet.* During an acute attack of diverticulitis the diet should furnish as little residue as possible. The diet allows tender meats, poultry, fish, eggs, white bread, rice, macaroni, noodles, simple desserts, clear soups, tea, and coffee. It omits all fruits, fruit juices, vegetables, and usually milk. Such a diet is obviously lacking in calcium, iron, and vitamins, and should be used for only a few days. A typical menu is as follows:

| *Breakfast* | *Luncheon* | *Dinner* |
|---|---|---|
| Cream of wheat | Tomato bouillon | Small club steak |
| Milk for cereal | Crackers | Baked potato without skin; |
| Sugar | Roast chicken | butter |
| Soft-cooked egg | Buttered rice | Roll with butter |
| White toast | White bread or roll | Whipped raspberry gelatin |
| Butter | Butter or margarine | Plain sugar cookies |
| Coffee | White cake with icing | Tea with lemon and sugar |
| | Tea with lemon and sugar | |

Long, continued use of low-fiber diets are believed to contribute to the development of diverticuli in older persons. The swallowing of air together with the gases resulting from the overproduction of bacteria in the intestines leads to increased gas pressure. Diets that are low in fiber cause the colon to contract more tightly; this further increases the gas pressure. The walls of the colon then bulge out to form the diverticulum. Older people should be encouraged to eat a greater amount of whole-grain cereals and breads, fruits, and vegetables.

## CONSTIPATION

Atonic constipation occurs more frequently in elderly persons and those who are physically handicapped. They have little exercise and often confine their food selection to low-fiber foods. In addition they may drink little liquid, resort to the use of laxatives, and have irregular habits of elimination. Obviously these practices must be changed to correct the constipation. Unless the physician indicates otherwise, the patient should be encouraged to drink 1200 to 1500 ml fluid daily; to exercise as the condition warrants; and to develop regular habits of elimination.

*High-fiber diet.* The normal diet is increased in fiber content by including two or more servings of raw fruit and vegetable daily. A salad may be given at noon and evening meals. Raw fruit may be used in place of pudding or cake. Whole-grain breads and cereals with some bran are substituted for white breads and refined cereals. Prunes and prune juice have particular laxative properties.

## REVIEW QUESTIONS AND PROBLEMS

1. What are the sources of fiber in the diet? What is meant by residue?

2. What are some factors that explain the intolerances that people have to foods?

**3.** Take a survey of five people you know to find out what foods they do not tolerate. What reasons do they give for any intolerance they have?

**4.** What is the relationship of fiber and strongly flavored vegetables to the discomfort that patients with gastrointestinal diseases often describe?

**5.** What are the advantages of a liberal diet in the treatment of patients with peptic ulcer? When would a progressive regimen be better?

**6.** Write a menu for one day for a patient who carries his lunch to work and who is following a bland fiber-restricted diet, stage 3.

**7.** A high-fiber diet is recommended for reducing the incidence of diverticulitis. Explain why such a diet would be useful.

## REFERENCES

Donaldson, R. M.: "The Muddle of Diets for Gastrointestinal Disorders," *JAMA,* 225:1243, 1973.

Ingelfinger, F. J.: "Gastric Function," *Nutr. Today,* 6:2–11, September 1971.

Ingelfinger, F. J.: "Gastrointestinal Absorption," *Nutr. Today,* 2:2–10, 1967.

Joint Committee of the American Dietetic Association and the American Medical Association: "Diet as Related to Gastrointestinal Function," *J. Am. Diet. Assoc.,* 38:425, 1961; also, *JAMA,* 176:935–41, 1961.

Mason, M. S.: *Basic Medical-Surgical Nursing,* 3rd ed. New York: Macmillan Publishing Co., Inc., 1974, Chap. 12.

Painter, N. S., *et al.*: "High-Residue Diet for Diverticular Disease of the Colon (Questions and Answers)," *JAMA,* 221:1058, 1972.

Plumley, P.F., and Francis, B.: "Dietary Management of Diverticular Disease," *J. Am. Diet. Assoc.,* 63:527–30, 1973.

Ratcliff, J. D.: "America's Laxative Addicts," *Today's Health,* 40:52, November 1962.

Robinson, C. H., *Normal and Therapeutic Nutrition,* 14th ed. New York: Macmillan Publishing Co., Inc., 1972, Chap. 34.

# MALABSORPTION DISORDERS

*Lactose-Free Diet; Gluten-Restricted Diet*

Malabsorption is a general term that describes incomplete absorption of one or more nutrients. There are many causes. In diseases characterized by diarrhea the nutrients pass through the gastrointestinal tract too rapidly to be absorbed. In some conditions a specific function is diminished or absent; for example, failure to produce pancreatic or intestinal enzymes, or a diminished area of intestinal surfaces for absorption. The malabsorption resulting from pancreatic disease is discussed in Chapter 29.

### DIARRHEA

Diarrhea is the frequent passage of liquid to semisolid stools. It is a symptom in numerous functional and organic disorders. In acute diarrhea, such as that from a staphylococcal infection, a clear-fluid diet (p. 195) is given for 12 to 24 hours, and then progressed to a soft fiber-restricted diet (p. 197) and a regular diet.

Diarrheas that are of prolonged duration lead to serious losses of fluids, electrolytes, proteins, fats, carbohydrates, and vitamins. These losses must be replaced by high-protein high-calorie diets that are often supplemented with minerals and vitamins. Additional dietary modifications depend upon the nature of the disorder; for example, the gluten restriction in sprue, and the lactose omission in lactase deficiency.

## ULCERATIVE COLITIS

This is an inflammation of the colon, occurring more frequently in young adults. The causes are unknown. Many of the patients are nervous, worried, and emotionally unstable. Any upsets aggravate the condition. In severe colitis there is much loss of water, electrolytes, and protein in the numerous stools. Weight loss, dehydration, anemia, and general weakness are outstanding.

*Dietary management.*    Because of the considerable protein losses the diet should supply 100 to 150 gm protein. About 2500 to 3000 kcal are needed. In severe illness the very low-residue diet (p. 274) is used first, and then progressed to a soft fiber-restricted diet. Supplements of vitamins and minerals, especially iron, are required. Some patients do not tolerate milk and require calcium supplements as well.

The nurse and dietitian must convince the patient by frequent visits, especially at mealtime, that they are sincerely interested in his welfare and that the foods served to him are alright for him to eat. They must be prepared to listen patiently to many complaints and to reassure constantly. The patient may be helped to select his own diet from a list of appropriate foods. (See Fig. 28–1.)

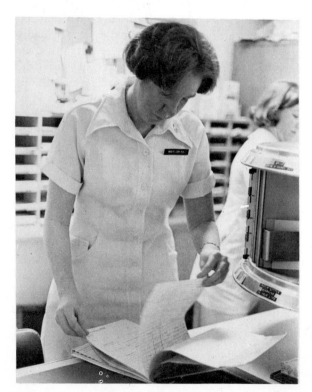

FIGURE 28–1  A nurse reviews the patient's chart and makes notations regarding the patient's acceptance of his diet. (*Courtesy, Department of Nursing, Delaware County Community College, Media, Pennsylvania.*)

## LACTOSE INTOLERANCE

*Congenital lactase deficiency.* A small percentage of infants are born with a lack of lactase and therefore they are unable to digest the lactose in milk. The infants become severely ill within a few days of birth. They must be given a formula that is free of all sources of lactose, such as meat-base, soybean, or amino acid hydrolysate.*

*Acquired lactase deficiency.* Many individuals have adequate levels of lactase during infancy but lose some of the ability to digest lactose in later years. The deficiency occurs frequently in Oriental and African populations and in the Middle East. It occurs in only a small per cent of Caucasians. School children who are affected complain of abdominal bloating, flatulence, cramps, and diarrhea when they drink too much milk.

Nurses need to be alert to the complaints of patients and the possibility of lactose intolerance when relatively large amounts of milk are consumed; for example, in diets for peptic ulcer and in tube feedings. The deficiency is often observed in sprue, ulcerative colitis, cystic fibrosis, and kwashiorkor.

*Dietary management.* When there is a complete absence of lactase, the diet must be carefully planned to eliminate all sources of lactose. These include:

Milk in all forms: fresh whole or skim; buttermilk; dry evaporated; malted; yogurt

Beverages containing milk or milk powder: Cocomalt, cocoa, chocolate, Ovaltine

Breads and rolls made with milk; sweet rolls; bread mixes; griddle cakes; waffles; zwieback

Cereals: Cream of Rice, Instant Cream of Wheat, Special K, Total

Desserts: cakes, cookies, custard, ice cream, pies with cream fillings such as chocolate, coconut, cream, custard, pumpkin; puddings made with milk, sherberts

Fats: butter, cream, margarine

Meat: frankfurters and luncheon meats, unless 100 per cent meat

Sauces: cream, or containing butter, margarine

Soups: cream

Sweets: caramel or chocolate candy

Vegetables: seasoned with butter or margarine; with cream sauces; mashed potatoes

Most children and adults with lactase deficiency can tolerate small amounts of lactose, and the stringent omissions listed above can be relaxed according to the individual's tolerance. For example, the tiny amounts

* Mul-Soy ®, Borden Company, New York: MBF (Meat-Base formula), Gerber Products, Fremont, Michigan; Nutramigen ® and Sobee ®, Mead Johnson & Co., Evansville, Indiana.

of lactose in butter or margarine may have no adverse effect, and these table spreads can be used. Others learn that they can take small amounts of milk at a meal; for example, ½ to 1 cup of milk may produce no symptoms while any excess cannot be ingested at one time. When milk must be omitted entirely there must be supplementation with calcium.

### NONTROPICAL SPRUE

*Celiac disease* in children and *nontropical sprue* in adults are the same condition. The disease is also known as *gluten-induced enteropathy*. When gluten is ingested changes occur in the epithelial cells of the jejunum, and absorption of sugars, fats, and amino acids is greatly reduced. The stools are bulky, foamy, and foul; they have a high percentage of fat (steatorrhea) and there are serious losses of all nutrients. Many signs of malnutrition are present in the untreated patient: weight loss, muscle wasting, protruding abdomen, sore mouth, bone pain, increased fractures, peripheral neuritis, and prolonged bleeding time.

*Dietary management.* The elimination of all sources of gluten in the diet brings about remarkable improvement. This means that all products containing wheat, rye, oats, or barley must be omitted from the diet. The diet must be continued indefinitely. Even small amounts of wheat as that used for thickening gravy produces harmful symptoms. The patient requires much counseling regarding the foods that he may have, how to prepare them, how to interpret labels, and so on. The characteristics of a gluten-restricted diet are given below.

## Gluten-Restricted Diet

The diet excludes all sources of wheat, rye, oats, and barley. Read labels carefully.

Aqueous multivitamins are usually prescribed in addition to the diet.

The diet may be progressed gradually; that is, small amounts of unsaturated fats may be used at first, adding harder fats later. Fiber may be reduced initially by using only cooked fruits and vegetables. Strongly flavored vegetables may be poorly tolerated at first.

INCLUDE THESE FOODS, OR THEIR NUTRITIVE EQUIVALENTS, DAILY:
    4 cups milk
6–8 ounces (cooked weight) lean meat, fish, or poultry
    1 egg
    4 vegetables including:
        1 dark green or deep yellow
        1 potato

2 other vegetables
Other to be served raw, if tolerated
3 fruits including:
1–2 servings citrus fruit or other good source ascorbic acid
1–2 other fruits
4 servings bread and cereals: corn, rice, soybean
NO WHEAT, RYE, OATS, BARLEY
2 tablespoons fat
Additional calories are provided by using more of the foods listed, desserts, soups, sweets

## FOODS ALLOWED

*Beverages*—carbonated, cocoa, coffee, fruit juices, milk, tea

*Breads*—cornbread, muffins, and pone with no wheat flour; breads made with cornmeal, cornstarch, potato, rice, soybean, wheat starch flour

*Cereals*—cooked cornmeal, Cream of Rice, hominy or grits, rice; ready to eat: corn or rice cereals such as cornflakes, rice flakes, Puffed Rice
*Cheese*—cottage; later, cream cheese
*Desserts*—custard, fruit ice, fruit whips, plain or fruit ice cream (homemade), plain or fruit gelatin, meringues; homemade puddings—cornstarch, rice, tapioca; rennet desserts; sherbet; cakes and cookies made with allowed flours
*Eggs*—as desired
*Fats*—oil: corn, cottonseed, olive, sesame, soybean; French dressing, pure mayonnaise, salad dressing with cornstarch thickening
Later addition: butter, cream, margarine, peanut oil, vegetable shortening
*Flour*—cornmeal, potato, rice, soybean

*Fruits*—all cooked, canned, and juices; fresh and frozen as tolerated, avoiding skin and seeds initially

## FOODS TO AVOID

*Beverages*—ale, beer, instant coffee containing cereal, malted milk, Postum, products containing cereal
*Breads*—all containing any wheat, rye, oats, or barley; bread crumbs, muffins, pancakes, rolls, rusks, waffles, zwieback; all commercial yeast and quick bread mixes; all crackers, pretzels, Ry-Krisp
*Cereals*—cooked or ready-to-eat breakfast cereals containing wheat, oats; barley, macaroni, noodles, pasta, spaghetti, wheat germ

*Desserts*—cake, cookies, doughnuts, pastries, pie; bisques, commercial ice cream, ice cream cones; prepared mixes containing wheat, rye, oats, or barley; puddings thickened with wheat flour

*Fats*—bacon, lard, suet, salad dressing with flour thickening

*Flour*—barley, oat, rye, wheat—bread, cake, entire wheat, graham, self-rising, whole wheat, wheat germ
*Fruits*—prunes, plums, and their juices; those with skins and seeds at first

Meat—all lean meats, poultry, fish: baked, broiled, roasted, stewed

Meat—breaded, creamed, croquettes, luncheon meats unless pure meat, meat loaf, stuffings with bread, scrapple, thickened stew

Fat meats such as corned beef, duck, frankfurters, goose, ham, luncheon meats, pork, sausage

Fatty fish such as herring, mackerel, sardines, swordfish, or canned in heavy oil

Milk—all kinds

Soups—broth, bouillon, cream if thickened with cornstarch, vegetable

Soups—thickened with flour; contain barley, noodles, etc.

Sweets—candy, honey, jam, jelly, marmalade, marshmallows, molasses, syrup, sugar

Sweets—candies with high fat content, nuts; candies containing wheat products

Vegetables—cooked or canned: buttered; fresh as tolerated

Vegetables—creamed if thickened with wheat, oat, rye, or barley products. Strongly flavored if they produce discomfort: baked beans, broccoli, Brussels sprouts, cabbage, cauliflower, corn, cucumber, lentils, onions, peppers, radishes, turnips

Miscellaneous—gravy and sauces thickened with cornstarch; olives, peanut butter, pickles, popcorn, potato chips

Miscellaneous—gravies and sauces thickened with flours not permitted

## TYPICAL MENU FOR GLUTEN-RESTRICTED DIET

### Breakfast

Tomato juice
Rice Krispies with milk, sugar
Poached eggs—2
Corn sticks (cornmeal; no wheat flour)
Butter, jelly
Coffee with cream, sugar

### Luncheon

Baked breast of chicken (egg-cornflake crust)
Savory rice
Buttered spinach

Celery and carrot sticks
Vanilla tapioca pudding with sliced orange sections
Milk

### Dinner

Pot roast of beef *with*
Gravy (thickened with cornstarch)
Parsley potato
Mashed winter squash
Tossed green salad
French dressing
Coffee ice cream
Coffee or tea

*Bedtime*

Strawberry milk shake

## REVIEW QUESTIONS AND PROBLEMS

1. What symptoms would lead you to suspect that an individual may have an intolerance to lactose? What causes this intolerance?

2. What substitutes are used in formulas for infants who have lactase deficiency?

3. Modify the following dinner menu so that it is suitable for (a) a young adult who needs a lactose-free diet; (b) a young woman with ulcerative colitis who needs a high-protein very low-residue diet; (c) a man with sprue for whom a gluten-restricted diet has been ordered.

Cream of tomato soup with crackers
Roast chicken with stuffing, gravy
Mashed potatoes
Creamed spinach
Dinner roll
Butter
Mixed vegetable salad with blue cheese dressing
Angel food cake with sliced peaches
Coffee; cream; sugar

## REFERENCES

Bayless, T. M.: "Disaccharidase Deficiency," *J. Am. Diet. Assoc.*, 60:478–82, 1972.

Commentary: "Lactose, Milk Intolerance, and Feeding Programs," *J. Am. Diet. Assoc.*, 61:241–42, 1972.

DeRisi, L. L.: "Starving in the Midst of Plenty; Adult Celiac Disease," *Am. J. Nurs.*, 70:1048–53, 1970.

"How to Eat Well on a Gluten-Free Diet," *Today's Health*, 43:38, October 1965.

Kowlessar, O. D.: "Dietary Gluten Sensitivity Updated," *J. Am. Diet. Assoc.*, 60:475–77, 1972.

Rosensweig, N. S.: "Dietary Sugars and Intestinal Enzymes," *J. Am. Diet. Assoc.*, 60:483–86, 1972.

# DISEASES OF THE LIVER,
# GALLBLADDER, AND PANCREAS

The diets required for diseases of the liver, gallbladder, and pancreas are further applications of diets described in preceding chapters, namely the fat-restricted diet (Chap. 24), the sodium-restricted diet (Chap. 25), and the high- and low-protein diets (Chap. 26).

## FUNCTIONS OF THE LIVER

The liver is probably the most complex organ in the body with numerous functions that are listed only briefly here. It synthesizes plasma proteins, hemoglobin, prothrombin, heparin, glycogen, lipoproteins, phospholipids, cholesterol, and numerous other substances. It stores glycogen, iron, copper, and vitamins A and D. It participates in the metabolism of nutrients by the removal of the amino group from amino acids, the synthesis of urea, the formation of bile for the normal digestion of fats, the oxidation of fatty acids, and the conversion of carotene to vitamin A. It detoxifies poisons that would otherwise be harmful to the body. With such a variety of functions it is evident that any disease can seriously interfere with nutritional status and health.

## HEPATITIS

Hepatitis is an inflammation of the liver. One cause is viral infection transmitted by contaminated food or water or from transfusion of blood products that contain the virus. Hepatitis is also caused by drugs to which

284

a person is sensitive or by toxic agents such as carbon tetrachloride. Among the symptoms that interfere with food intake are anorexia, nausea, vomiting, fever, and abdominal discomfort. Weight loss is often great.

*Dietary management.* A nutritionally adequate diet is an important aspect of therapy, since poor nutritional status can result in permanent damage to the liver. Because of nausea and vomiting in the early stages it may be necessary to resort to parenteral fluids or to tube feedings.

The appetite usually remains poor, so that the nurse and dietitian must be sure that the diet is attractive and appealing to the taste, and must use a good deal of persuasion to get the patient to eat. Each meal should include only the amounts of food that the patient can be expected to eat; six small meals may be better than three overly large meals. The diet is based upon the following modifications:

1. From 2500 to 4000 kcal, depending upon extent of fever and weight loss. See Chapter 21 for high-calorie diet.

2. High protein: 100 to 150 gm. Include 4 to 5 cups of milk daily if it is tolerated, and 6 to 9 ounces meat, fish, or poultry.

3. Fat: normal intake; fats are useful for supplying additional calories. Fats should be easily digestible, omitting fried foods. If there is obstruction of the biliary tract, a low-fat diet is used.

4. Liberal carbohydrate as a source of calories and to provide for continuous glycogen storage—a protection against liver damage.

5. Consistency adjusted according to gastrointestinal symptoms: may progress from full-fluid to soft fiber-restricted to normal. (See Fig. 29–1.)

### CIRRHOSIS

This is a chronic disease with degenerative changes, fatty infiltration, and fibrosis. It is sometimes the outcome of inadequately treated hepatitis, and more often is associated with chronic alcoholism.

*Dietary management.* The normal diet is satisfactory for many patients and should be used as long as the clinical findings permit. When a patient is in poor nutritional status, the recommendations given above for hepatitis are appropriate. However, patients with severe cirrhosis should always be watched carefully if their protein intakes are high because hepatic coma (discussed in the section that follows) can be a serious complication.

Two symptoms pose particular problems for patients with cirrhosis. *Ascites* is the abnormal accumulation of fluid in the abdomen. When it is present a 250 mg-sodium diet is often ordered. (See pp. 248–53.) The serum proteins are usually low in these patients, a finding that supports the need for additional protein in the diet. At a 250 mg-sodium restriction, the protein intake can be raised above normal levels only by the inclusion of 1 quart low-sodium milk each day.

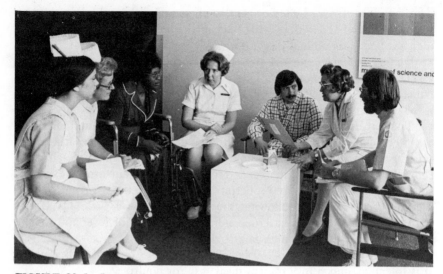

FIGURE 29–1 In a clinical conference the patient's nutritional needs are discussed. The patient should have an opportunity to present his problems and to participate in the planning of his diet. (*Courtesy, Department of Nursing, Delaware County Community College, Media, Pennsylvania.*)

*Esophageal varices* are easily irritated by the swallowing of coarse, fibrous foods or a large bolus of food, thus initiating hemorrhage. The diet must be smooth in texture. The soft fiber-restricted diet described on pages 197–99 may require further restriction by grinding meats and purée-ing fruits and vegetables.

### HEPATIC COMA

This is a complication of severe liver disease caused by a high blood level of ammonia. It is especially likely to occur following gastrointestinal hemorrhage, surgery, or the use of a high-protein diet in severe liver disease. The ammonia that enters the general circulation from the intestinal tract is toxic to the central nervous system so that the typical symptoms are drowsiness, irritability, restlessness, poor coordination of the arms and legs, fecal odor to the breath, and eventually loss of consciousness.

*Dietary management.* The principal treatment is to reduce the protein metabolism to a minimum. This is accomplished by:

1. Sufficient calories from carbohydrate and fat to prevent tissue breakdown; about 1500 to 2000 kcal.

2. Protein-free to low-protein diet—about 20 to 30 gm protein—for a few days. See low-protein diet, page 262.

With improvement the diet is cautiously increased by 10 gm of protein every few days until a normal diet is again achieved. Many patients use a 40- to 50 gm-protein diet for long periods of time.

## DISEASES OF THE GALLBLADDER

*Function.* The gallbladder concentrates the bile and stores it. Upon entering the duodenum, fat stimulates the secretion of a hormone, *chole-cystokinin.* This hormone is carried by the blood stream to the gallbladder and forces contraction, so that the bile is released into the common duct and then into the duodenum. Bile emulsifies fats so that they can be hydrolyzed by the fat-splitting enzymes, the lipases. If there is any interference with the flow of bile, fat digestion is impaired.

Inflammation of the gallbladder is known as *cholecystitis,* and formation of gallstones is *cholelithiasis.* Stones are often present without symptoms. If the gallbladder is inflamed or if there are stones blocking the flow of bile, there is pain when the gallbladder contracts.

*Dietary modification.* The aim of diet therapy is to reduce the discomfort by minimizing the contraction of the gallbladder. In acute cholecystitis no food is given for the first 12 to 24 hours. A clear-fluid diet (p. 195) is followed by a soft very low-fat diet, allowing only 20 to 30 gm fat per day. This allows skim milk, 5 to 6 ounces of very lean meat, fish, or poultry, not over 3 eggs per week, and customary amounts of breads, cereals, fruits, and vegetables. This food allowance is low in cholesterol, but it is not known whether cholesterol restriction reduces the formation of stones or not.

Once the acute attack subsides, the patient is progressed gradually to a diet that includes 50 to 60 gm fat daily. Such an allowance permits the use of whole milk (2 cups) and 2 to 3 teaspoons butter or margarine in addition to foods allowed on the very low-fat diet. Obesity is frequent in patients with gallbladder disease, and a low-calorie low-fat diet should be used. (See fat-restricted diet, p. 242.)

Many patients with gallbladder disease complain of abdominal discomfort when they eat certain foods such as eggs, legumes, melons, berries, and strongly flavored vegetables. Although these foods need not be omitted for all patients, the individual tolerances should be respected.

## PANCREATITIS

Disease of the pancreas interferes with the normal production of pancreatic enzymes, and therefore the digestion of fats, protein, and starches is reduced. Undigested fat, starch, and protein are present in the stools in increased amounts. Fat-soluble vitamins are poorly absorbed. Such losses if not corrected lead to general malnutrition.

Acute pancreatitis is often accompanied by severe pain, distention, nausea, vomiting, and constipation. Nothing is given by mouth initially, but fluids and electrolytes are replaced parenterally. Then the diet is progressed from clear fluids to a soft diet.

Chronic pancreatitis is often caused by alcoholism. A disorder of lipid metabolism is also associated with pancreatitis and abdominal pain. (See Type 1 and 5 hyperlipoproteinemias, Chapter 24.) The pain is often severe with the ingestion of fat or alcohol. Pancreatic extract may be used to aid digestion. The maintenance diet is very low in fat—20 to 30 gm per day, and high in protein and carbohydrate to supply calories. (See pp. 236–37 for fat-restricted diet, types 1 and 5.)

## CYSTIC FIBROSIS

This is an inherited disease that affects the exocrine glands (glands that excrete to the outside of the body). There is excessive secretion of thick mucus which often blocks the ducts of the liver, pancreas, and lungs. Large amounts of sodium chloride are excreted in the perspiration.

If the pancreatic ducts are blocked, the pancreatic enzymes cannot reach the duodenum, and malabsorption is often severe. The child appears haggard, shows signs of tissue wasting, has a large protruding abdomen, and excretes large, foul stools with much fat, starch, and protein.

*Dietary management.* In pancreatic dysfunction pancreatic extract is given before each meal to aid digestion. A high-calorie high-protein diet is essential. If fats cannot be tolerated medium-chain triglycerides (MCT) are useful to increase the caloric intake. MCT is an oil available in a pharmacy that can be used for food preparation. Because the oil is made up of short-chain fatty acids, it is more readily absorbed.* Supplements of the B-complex vitamins, ascorbic acid, and water-soluble preparations of vitamins A and D are usually required. Patients find it difficult to eat if their breathing is affected. They must eat slowly and should be given small meals at frequent intervals.

## REVIEW QUESTIONS AND PROBLEMS

1. Prepare a table that summarizes the dietary changes made for each of these conditions: hepatitis; hepatic coma; esophageal varices; ascites; cholecystitis; cystic fibrosis. Use these headings in your table: calories; protein; fat; carbohydrate; sodium; texture.

2. Plan a menu for a young man who has hepatitis. Include at least 100 gm protein and 3000 kcal.

---

* Mead Johnson and Company, Evansville, Indiana.

3. Modify the menu you have planned in question 2 so that it will provide no more than 250 mg sodium. What reasons can you give for restricting sodium?

4. What symptoms would suggest to you that a patient may have impending hepatic coma? Plan a 20 gm protein 1500 kcal diet for such a patient.

## REFERENCES

Bielski, M. T., and Molander, D. W.: "Laennec's Cirrhosis," *Am. J. Nurs.*, 65:82–86, 1965.

Bolt, R. J.: "Medical Treatment of Cholecystitis," *Mod. Treat.*, 5:514–27, 1968.

Carper, J.: "Cirrhosis: A Growing Threat to Life," *Today's Health*, 48:26–27, February 1970.

Davidson, C. S.: "Dietary Treatment of Hepatic Diseases," *J. Am. Diet. Assoc.*, 62:515–19, 1973.

Illingworth, C.: "Gallstones," *Nurs. Times*, 66:167–68, 1970.

Mason, M. A.: *Basic Medical-Surgical Nursing*, 3rd ed. New York: Macmillan Publishing Co., Inc., 1974, Chap. 13.

Paton, A.: "Hepatic Coma," *Nurs. Times*, 65:1351–52, 1969.

Robinson, C. H.: *Normal and Therapeutic Nutrition*, 14th ed. New York: Macmillan Publishing Co., Inc., 1972, Chap. 37.

# FOOD ALLERGIES AND SKIN DISORDERS

## NATURE OF ALLERGIES

A homemaker ate a piece of chocolate cake and a few hours later developed a migraine-type headache. A 10-year-old boy began to wheeze while eating in a restaurant; his fork had a tiny trace of egg on it. A girl ordered a seafood casserole in a restaurant and almost immediately after tasting it began to tremble, perspire, and later had severe vomiting and diarrhea. A newborn baby developed severe eczema within a few days after starting his milk formula. All of these individuals were allergic to some food. About one in every 10 persons, or roughly 22 million Americans has an allergy to some substance. Less than one third of these are caused by foods.

An *allergy* is a sensitivity or abnormal reaction to a substance that is harmless to the normal individual. An *allergen* is the substance that sets off the reaction. In most instances the allergen is protein in nature, but nonprotein substances such as aspirin can also cause reactions.

Allergies are initiated in four ways: (1) by contact with foods, drugs, aerosol sprays, pesticides, poison ivy, hair, molds; (2) by ingestion of foods, drugs; (3) by inhalation of pollens, dust, cosmetics, sprays, molds, perfumes; (4) by injection of vaccines, serums, hormones, insect bites.

*Food allergens.* The most frequent food allergens are milk, wheat, eggs, fish, shellfish, citrus fruits, strawberries, tomatoes, and chocolate. Milk is the most frequent allergen in infants. Other foods to which people are sometimes sensitive are pork, nuts, peanut butter, corn, onion, garlic, cabbage, and potatoes. Foods that belong to the same botanic class are likely to produce reactions; for example, oranges, grapefruits, and lemons, or cabbage, cauliflower, and broccoli.

### SYMPTOMS

The tendency to allergy is inherited, but the individual does not inherit the allergy to the same substances, nor does he have the same symptoms as his parents. Any kind of physical or emotional stress—anger, fear, fatigue, illness, family or school problems—often provokes the allergic reaction or makes it more severe.

An allergen may produce only one symptom such as a skin rash or headache, or a combination of symptoms such as itching, diarrhea, and asthma. The response is almost immediate in those who are severely allergic, but is delayed for hours or even days in persons who are mildly allergic.

The skin, the eyes, the respiratory system, or the gastrointestinal tract may be affected. Changes observed in the skin includes hives, eczema, fever blisters, itching, and edema. The eyes could be red, swollen, itchy, or burning. If the mucous membranes of the gastrointestinal tract are affected, symptoms such as bad breath, nausea, vomiting, stomatitis, abdominal distention, cramps, diarrhea, or constipation might be present. Even attacks of peptic ulcer, colitis, and gallbladder disease have on occasion been attributed to allergy. The changes in the respiratory tract range from a runny nose, to sinusitis, to severe bronchial asthma.

### DIAGNOSIS

*Diet history.* If food allergy is suspected, a comprehensive dietary history is essential. The patient should keep a complete food diary for a period of time as well as a record of the occurrence of symptoms. Sometimes the correlation of the dietary records and the symptoms establishes the cause of the allergy. More often these records help to determine which skin tests and elimination diets should be used.

*Skin tests.* The suspected substances are rubbed into scratches made on the back or arm (scratch test), or are injected underneath the skin (intradermal test), or are placed in contact with the skin and covered with a patch (patch test). After a period of time redness and swelling at the point of contact with the skin suggest the possibility of allergy. Skin tests, however, can give false-positive as well as negative results. They must be interpreted together with other information obtained in the medical history.

*Restrictive or elimination diets.* Based upon the dietary history, food diary, and/or skin tests, a diet that eliminates all foods likely to produce allergy is tried. One of the widely used systems of elimination diets is that developed by Dr. Albert Rowe. Three of the diets do not contain milk, wheat, or eggs, while the fourth diet consists only of milk, sugar, and tapioca. The patient is tested on one of the diets for one to three weeks, unless there is a severe reaction to the diet. If the diet produces no reaction, the other diets are similarly tested. If a reaction occurs on a diet, one or more food items on that diet or a nonfood source could be responsible. If no reactions occur, the diet serves as a starting point for building a permanent diet.

### TREATMENT

When the foods that cause the reaction are known, the simplest treatment is to completely avoid all sources of these foods. This is no problem when there is allergy to a single food such as chocolate or strawberries, but it is often difficult to avoid milk, wheat, and eggs that are present in so many food products.

Some infants who are allergic to pasteurized cow's milk can tolerate boiled milk, evaporated milk, goat's milk, or the commercial milk formulas. When all forms of milk produce reactions, a meat-base formula, soybean formula, or synthetic formula is substituted. In some children milk allergy disappears by 5 years of age.

*Building on the elimination diet.* Let us suppose that a patient remained symptom-free on a given elimination diet. Then, all foods on that diet become the starting point for building the diet. Cautiously, *one food at a time* is added to the diet, and the patient's reactions are observed for a few days. If the added food provokes no reaction, it is added to the list of foods allowed, and another food is tested in the same way.

*Hyposensitization.* When an important food such as milk or wheat is producing symptoms, hyposensitization (also known as desensitization) is practical. It consists in giving the patient orally or by injection minute amounts of the offending substance. For example, a drop of milk might be diluted in a pint of water, and a few drops of this dilution fed once a day. If there is no reaction after a few days, the patient is given a slightly greater amount of the dilution. If reactions do occur, it is necessary to move back to an amount that does not produce symptoms. Because additions must be made so gradually, the hyposensitization requires weeks, months, or even a year.

### PATIENT COUNSELING

Many foods contain minute amounts of substances to which some people react. Therefore, detailed lists of foods that are likely to contain these allergens must be given to the patient. The foods that contain milk have been listed for the lactose-free diet, page 279. Foods to avoid for egg-free and wheat-free diets are listed below.

DIET WITHOUT EGGS—
FOODS TO AVOID

Eggs in any form

*Beverages*—Cocomalt, eggnog, malted beverages, Ovaltine, root beer

*Breads and rolls* containing eggs—crust glazed with egg, French toast, sweet rolls, griddle cakes, muffins, waffles, pretzels, zwieback

*Desserts*—cake, cookies, custard, doughnuts, ice cream, meringue, cream-filled pies—coconut, cream, custard, lemon, pumpkin, puddings

*Meats*—meat loaf; breaded meats dipped in egg

*Noodles*

*Salad dressings*—mayonnaise, cooked dressing

*Sauces*—Hollandaise

*Soups*—broth, consommé

*Sweets*—many cake icings, candies: cream, chocolate, fondant, marshmallow, nougat

DIET WITHOUT WHEAT—
FOODS TO AVOID

*Beverages*—Cocomalt, malted milk, instant coffee unless 100 per cent coffee, coffee substitutes; beer, gin, whiskey

*Breads, crackers, and rolls*—all breads including rye, oatmeal, and corn; hot breads and muffins; baking-powder biscuits; gluten bread; matzoth, pretzels, zwieback; crackers; griddle cakes, waffles

Note: bread, crackers, or wafers made of 100 per cent rye, corn, rice, soy, or potato flours may be used.

*Cereals*

| | |
|---|---|
| All-bran | Muffets |
| Beemax | New oats |
| Bran flakes | Pablum |
| Cheerios | Pep |
| Crackels | Pettijohn's |
| Cream of | Puffed Wheat |
| Wheat | Ralston cereals |
| Farina | Shredded Wheat |
| Grape-Nuts | Special K |
| Grape-Nuts | Total |
| flakes | Wheatena |
| Kix | Wheat flakes |
| Krumbles | Wheat germ |
| Maltex | Wheaties |
| Mello-wheat | Wheatsworth |
| | Wheat Chex |

*Desserts*—cake or cookies, homemade, from mixes, or bakery; doughnuts, ice cream, ice-cream cones, pies, puddings

*Flour*—white, whole wheat, graham

*Gravies and sauces* thickened with flour

*Meats*—prepared with flour, bread, or cracker crumbs such as croquettes and meat loaf; stews thickened with flour or made with dumplings; frankfurters, luncheon meats, or sausage in which wheat has been used as a filler; canned meat dishes such as stews, chili

*Pastas*—macaroni, noodles, spaghetti, vermicelli, and so on

*Salad dressings*—thickened with flour

*Soups*—commercially canned

Reading labels on food packages and cans and interpreting the information is absolutely essential. The patient must also have detailed lists of foods to use, and a suggested meal plan that fits in with the family's food patterns and that assures a nutritionally adequate diet. An allergy to milk means that another source of calcium, usually a calcium supplement, and riboflavin must be supplied. Allergy to citrus fruits means that other foods that are good sources of ascorbic acid must be emphasized.

Patients who have severe asthma must avoid large meals because gastrointestinal distention increases the likelihood of attack. The patient is advised to eat his meals slowly. Midmorning and midafternoon feedings help to assure adequate food intake, but a late evening meal is not advisable. Any kind of stress at mealtimes must be avoided.

### SKIN DISEASES

*Nutritional deficiencies.* Deficiencies of nutrients result in a variety of skin disorders. Usually these are associated with other symptoms. Eczema is a frequent disorder in infants that may be traced to lack of linoleic acid or vitamin $B_6$ or an imbalance of isoleucine and leucine in maple syrup urine disease. Other nutrient deficiencies are manifested as *keratinization* in vitamin A deficiency, *cheilosis* in riboflavin deficiency, and *symmetrical dermatitis* in niacin lack. (See Chaps. 11 and 12.)

*Acne vulgaris.* This is a chronic inflammation of the sebaceous glands accompanied by pimples and blackheads. It is especially trying during the adolescent period.

The treatment has been described as "confusing, contradictory, and controversial." Chocolate, candies, sweets, fried foods, rich desserts are often blamed for the condition, but research has shown that they apparently have little effect. Although there is no harm in the restriction of these foods, it is probably futile to expect improvement in the skin condition if they are omitted. The most positive approach that can be taken is to emphasize the need for a nutritionally adequate diet and to stress principles of hygiene such as skin cleanliness, exercise, elimination, and regular hours of rest.

### REVIEW QUESTIONS AND PROBLEMS

1. Define: allergy, allergen, elimination diet, hyposensitization.
2. What is the role of heredity in allergy?
3. List six foods that frequently produce allergy.
4. Plan a menu for a day for a young man who is allergic to wheat; for a 10-year-old boy who is allergic to eggs.
5. Prepare a list of good sources of ascorbic acid for a patient who is allergic to citrus fruits.
6. What nutritional problems should you anticipate for a person who is allergic to milk? How would you avoid these problems?

### REFERENCES

*Allergy Recipes.* Chicago, Ill.: The American Dietetic Association, 1969.
*Baking for People with Food Allergies.* Home and Garden Bulletin No. 147. Washington, D.C.: U.S. Department of Agriculture, 1968.

Feeney, M. C.: "Nutritional and Dietary Management of Food Allergy in Children," *Am. J. Clin. Nutr.*, 22:103–11, 1969.

Fulton, J. E., Jr., *et al.*: "Effect of Chocolate on Acne Vulgaris," *JAMA*, 210:2071–74, 1969.

Robinson, C. H.: *Normal and Therapeutic Nutrition*, 14th ed. New York: Macmillan Publishing Co., Inc., 1972, Chap. 46.

Smith, L.: "What Parents Can Do About Food Allergies," *Today's Health*, 47:55, July 1969.

Wood, M. N.: "Eating Well on a Wheat-Free Diet," *Today's Health*, 48:60, February 1970.

# NUTRITION IN SURGICAL CONDITIONS

*Tube Feedings; High-Protein, High-Fat Diet.*
*(for Dumping Syndrome)*

## Dietary Planning for Surgical Conditions

### NUTRITIONAL CONSIDERATIONS

Surgery or injury brings about important losses of nutrients through
losses of blood, plasma, or pus from the wound surface, hemorrhage, vomiting, and fever. These losses in turn lead to weight loss, poor wound healing,
edema or dehydration, anemia, and decubitus ulcers. The concentration of
serum proteins and hemoglobin may be reduced and the electrolyte balance
altered. Patients who come to surgery in poor nutritional status are at
greater risk. The increased needs, however, come at a time when food intake
is at a minimum.

*Protein.* Satisfactory protein nutrition is essential for normal wound
healing, and to protect the liver against possible injury from anesthesia.
When protein nutrition is poor, the wound heals slowly, is more likely
to become infected and edematous, and may break open. The breakdown
of protein tissues increases for several days following surgery. This is further
increased by immobilization. For well-nourished individuals no increase
in protein intake is necessary. When there has been malabsorption, or
following severe injury, the protein need may be well over 100 gm daily.

*Energy.* If the caloric intake is inadequate, protein will be used for
energy rather than for wound repair and tissue building. Even very small
amounts of glucose as in a parenteral feeding can have some protein-
sparing effect. The caloric requirements are very high when there is fever
or in patients with severe burns.

Obesity is a hazard to surgery. Whenever possible, the obese patient should lose some weight before surgery is attempted.

*Fluid-electrolyte balance.* Each day a significant amount of fluid is lost from the body (see p. 88). Ordinarily this is replaced not only by beverages but also by the food intake. In surgical procedures the losses are further increased through exudates, hemorrhage, and vomiting. The intake is usually decreased because of inability to eat.

Fluid and electrolyte imbalances must be corrected prior to surgery because of the great risks that accompany dehydration and acidosis. Fluids are given orally and parenterally as indicated. Subsequent to surgery parenteral fluids are given until the patient can take satisfactory amounts of fluids and food by mouth. The nurse should note the total intake and excretion of fluid.

*Vitamins.* Ascorbic acid is especially important for wound healing, and is sometimes prescribed in increased amounts prior to and following surgery. Vitamin K is of concern to the surgeon. Failure to synthesize vitamin K in the intestine may occur when antibiotics are given, or the liver may be unable to convert vitamin K to prothrombin. Either deficiency increases the likelihood of abnormal bleeding.

## PREOPERATIVE DIET

Sometimes it is possible to improve the state of nutrition prior to surgery. A high-protein high-calorie diet for the poorly nourished individual is of value for even a week or two before surgery (see pp. 214 and 263). Patients with metabolic diseases such as diabetes mellitus must be in metabolic balance before surgery is attempted.

In acute abdominal conditions such as appendicitis and cholecystitis no food is allowed by mouth until vomiting, pain, and distention have disappeared because of the danger of peritonitis. Most patients prior to surgery continue to ingest the diet they have been receiving, whether this be a normal diet or one modified for a particular condition. Prior to surgery on the gastrointestinal tract a very low-residue diet is often ordered for several days in order to reduce intestinal residue to a minimum (see p. 274).

Usually no food is allowed after the evening meal on the day before surgery. However, if surgery is planned for late afternoon or if a local anesthetic is to be used, a light breakfast is sometimes ordered. Fluids are generally permitted until midnight preceding the day of operation.

## POSTOPERATIVE DIET

The dietary progression depends upon the nature of the surgery. Food and fluids cannot be given orally until peristalsis has returned. Parenteral fluids maintain fluid and electrolyte balances.

When gastric secretions have begun and peristalsis resumes, clear fluids are given with the initial amounts being 30 to 60 ml. Warm fluids such as tea and broth are better than cold fluids. Patients respond better to solid foods than to liquid foods, and a very low-residue diet given in small amounts is usually the first order. Foods that are high in protein and fat are less distending than those high in carbohydrate. The patient should eat slowly and in small amounts to reduce the amount of air that is swallowed. The diet progresses to a soft fiber-restricted diet and then a regular diet, usually within a few days of surgery.

## PARENTERAL NUTRITION

Parenteral fluids may consist of physiologic saline or with additions of 5 per cent glucose, amino acids, electrolytes, vitamins, and medications. They are not nutritionally adequate, but they maintain fluid and electrolyte balance during the immediate postoperative period. One liter of 5 per cent glucose contains 50 gm glucose or 200 kcal. Even 400 kcal in a day can be beneficial in reducing tissue breakdown.

*Total parenteral nutrition (hyperalimentation).* A number of situations arise in which oral or tube feedings cannot be used for several weeks; for example, prolonged coma, severe uncontrolled malabsorption, extensive burns, and gastrointestinal fistulas. By techniques developed within the last decade a nutritionally adequate hypertonic solution consisting of glucose, protein hydrolysates, minerals, and vitamins can be given by means of an indwelling catheter into the superior vena cava. The high rate of blood flow brings about rapid dilution of the solution, and full nutritional requirements can be met indefinitely.

## TUBE FEEDINGS

A tube feeding is a nutritionally adequate allowance of liquefied foods that can be administered through a tube in the stomach or duodenum. A tube feeding is used in paralysis or obstruction of the esophagus, in anorexia nervosa, following mouth or gastric surgery, in severe burns, for unconscious patients, or in any situation where the patient is unable to chew or swallow.

A wide choice of these types of tube feedings is available: (1) blenderized feedings; (2) milk-base formulas; and (3) commercial preparations. Blenderized feedings include foods from a normal diet that are liquefied in a blender at high speed. These are generally preferred because diarrhea is a less frequent complication. To prepare a blenderized feeding the foods of a normal diet are placed in a blender with sufficient milk and other liquid to allow them to be blended. Homogenized milk must be used because plain milk would be churned into butter. The liquid mixture is strained several times through a fine-mesh sieve to remove all fiber. These feedings are usually given with a food pump.

Of the many formulas in use, two examples are shown in Table 31–1. The blenderized feeding includes strained baby foods, thereby reducing the amount of fiber and the need for repeated straining.

TABLE 31–1  TWO FORMULAS FOR TUBE FEEDING

| Blenderized Feeding* | | | Milk-Base Formula | |
|---|---|---|---|---|
| Strained liver | 150 | gm | Water (3 cups) | 720 gm |
| Egg | 50 | gm | Nonfat dry milk | 150 gm |
| Applesauce | 50 | gm | Pasteurized egg powder | 30 gm |
| Carrots, strained | 50 | gm | Sugar (¼ cup) | 50 gm |
| Orange juice, frozen, | | | Molasses (¼ cup) | 60 gm |
| reconstituted | 100 | gm | Brewer's yeast | 15 gm |
| Nonfat dry milk | 175 | gm | | |
| Sugar | 15 | gm | | |
| Brewer's yeast | 2.5 | gm | Total volume | 1000 ml |
| Water to make | 1000 | ml | Add supplement of vitamin | |
| | | | A to one feeding daily | |
| | | | Give 8 oz strained orange | |
| | | | juice in separate feeding | |
| Protein | 90 | gm | Protein | 72 gm |
| Calories | 1000 | | Calories | 1100 |

* Stumpf, G.L.: *Diet Manual—University of Michigan Hospital*, Ann Arbor, Mich.: The George Wahr Publishing Company, 1963, p. 41.

The normal daily intake of the formulas is about 2000 ml. The protein level may be reduced by decreasing the amount of nonfat dry milk. The calorie level may be adjusted by using light cream for part of the fluid.

The nurse should observe the patient carefully for the first few days after initiating a tube feeding, and be aware of complaints such as a feeling of fullness, gas, regurgitation, cramping, and diarrhea. Most if not all of these can be avoided by taking certain precautions. Initially tube feedings should be given at half to two-thirds strength, and in small volumes such as 30 to 60 ml. When it is evident that the patient tolerates the feeding, the concentration and the volume can be gradually increased until the desired calorie level is reached.

Some tube feedings are not well tolerated because they contain excess sugars, amino acids, and electrolytes that draw fluid from the blood circulation into the intestine. The patient complains of weakness and distention. When the protein intake needs to be high it is important that adequate fluids be supplied so that the nitrogenous wastes can be efficiently excreted by the kidney. Some patients do not tolerate lactose (see p. 279) and require feedings that do not contain milk.

Tube feedings are an excellent medium for bacterial growth. Feedings should be kept under constant refrigeration once they have been prepared or when a proprietary product has been opened. Any formula remaining at the end of a 24-hour period should be discarded. The tubes must be thoroughly flushed out.

## Diet for Special Surgical Procedures

### POSTGASTRECTOMY REGIMENS

Following gastrectomy a number of problems arise. In the absence of the gastric juices the entire digestion of protein must occur in the small intestine. Fat is less well utilized because of inadequate mixing of food with digestive juices. In the absence of gastric juice, iron is less well absorbed and iron-deficiency anemia occurs more often. Since the intrinsic factor is no longer produced from the stomach, the absorption of vitamin $B_{12}$ does not occur. Several years later the patient will have pernicious anemia unless vitamin $B_{12}$ is given by injection.

Immediately following gastrectomy, 30 to 60 ml of clear fluids are given hourly. By the third day a full-fluid or very low-residue diet is usually allowed. The foods are introduced gradually, however, keeping meals very small and at frequent intervals. Eggs, custards, cereals, milk, cream soups, and fruit purées are introduced first; then cottage cheese, tender chicken, and puréed vegetables are added. The emphasis is upon foods high in protein and fat and low in carbohydrate. Fluids are better tolerated if they are taken between meals.

*Dumping syndrome.* Certain patients who have had a gastrectomy complain of nausea, weakness, sweating, and dizziness shortly after meals. Vomiting, diarrhea, and weight loss are common.

The condition is caused by rapid entry of the food material directly into the intestinal tract. The large amount of carbohydrate draws water from the blood circulation into the small intestine and thus reduces the circulating blood volume. The sugars are rapidly absorbed into the blood. This causes too much insulin to be produced, and in a short time the blood sugar drops to very low levels. Thus the patient has the symptoms of insulin shock and also the symptoms that accompany reduction of the circulating blood volume.

The diet used for this condition is summarized below.

1. Give small meals every two hours consisting of meat, fish, poultry, eggs, or cheese with butter, margarine, or bacon.

2. As improvement occurs, add one to two small servings of one of

these: bread, crackers, cereals, vegetables, and finally unsweetened fruits. Gradually increase the amounts and variety of these foods until the diet approaches a normal pattern.

3. Omit fluids at mealtime; they may be taken after at least 45 minutes have elapsed.

4. Omit very cold foods.

5. Avoid sugar, jelly, jam, syrup, candy, soft drinks, sweetened fruit, gravies, sauces, cakes, cookies, pastries, ice cream, and other sweetened foods.

6. Relax and rest before and after meals.

### TYPICAL MENU FOR INITIAL STAGE

| *Breakfast, Noon, or Evening* | *Midmorning, Midafternoon, Bedtime* |
|---|---|
| 2 beef patties, or roast meat, chicken, fish, steaks, chops, or 2 to 3 eggs | 3 oz meat, fish, poultry |
| 2 to 3 pats butter or margarine | 2 to 3 pats butter or margarine |

### TYPICAL MENU FOR FIRST PROGRESSION

| *Breakfast* | *Midmorning, Midafternoon, Bedtime* |
|---|---|
| 2 scrambled eggs | 2 oz meat, fish, poultry |
| 2 strips bacon | 2 pats butter |
| ½ piece toast with butter | 2 thin slices bread for sandwich |

*Luncheon or Dinner*

4 oz meat, poultry, or fish
1 small serving green or yellow vegetable
½ slice bread with butter or margarine

### INTESTINAL SURGERY

Patients who have had an ileostomy or colostomy require a great deal of emotional support and continued assurance that the foods given to them can be safely eaten. The nurse also observes carefully the tolerance the patient has to the foods that are offered.

Following removal of a section of the ileum (ileectomy) a permanent opening in the abdominal wall (ileostomy) is provided through which digestive wastes are eliminated. The waste material is fluid and continuous and the losses of fluid, sodium, potassium, and nutrients are considerable. Fat absorption is poor and vitamin $B_{12}$ absorption is reduced or absent.

Clear fluids are given following surgery and then a very low-residue diet is introduced. Gradually foods containing a little fiber are added one by one to the low-residue diet, testing each food thoroughly for tolerance before adding a second. Weight loss is common and a high-protein high-calorie diet modified in fiber content is needed. Periodic injections of vitamin $B_{12}$ will be required to prevent pernicious anemia later in life.

A colostomy consists in attaching the proximal end of the resected colon to the opening in the abdominal wall. There is some ability to absorb water so that feces are more formed than in the ileostomy, and some bowel regularity can be established. Initially these patients are given a clear fluid and then a very low-residue diet. Most of them are eventually able to eat an essentially normal diet.

*Short bowel syndrome.* Massive resection of the intestine seriously reduces the amount of nutrient that can be absorbed. In this syndrome the section of bowel remaining is generally less than 2.46 m (8 ft ). Food materials move so rapidly through the remaining bowel that there is insufficient time for digestion and absorption of nutrients. If the jejunum has been removed some absorption can take place from the ileum. The jejunum, on the other hand, has only a small capacity to absorb water and electrolytes and cannot make up for a missing ileum.

Among the life-threatening problems following massive resection are severe changes in fluid and electrolyte balance, diarrhea, steatorrhea, extensive weight loss, and severe malnutrition. Diets containing up to 175 gm protein and 5000 kcal may be needed to prevent further weight loss. Medium chain triglycerides have been of some value in reducing the diarrhea and thus improving the electrolyte balance and nutritional status.

Recently it was found that diets developed for excursions into space were useful for patients with the short bowel syndrome. A number of commerial preparations are now available. They are called *elemental diets* or *chemically defined synthetic diets.* They consist of amino acids, simple carbohydrates, fats, and all the mineral and vitamin needs. They are taken as a flavored beverage several times a day or may be used as tube feedings. They require little if any digestive action, are readily absorbed from the upper intestine, and are practically residue-free. Their use substantially decreases the diarrhea and improves the nutritional status.

## BURNS

Fluid, electrolyte, and protein losses are tremendous from the burned surfaces. Edema at the burn site, failure to obtain satisfactory skin growth, atony of the gastrointestinal tract, vomiting, and diarrhea are frequently encountered. The excretion of large amounts of nitrogen, potassium, and other wastes places a tremendous load upon the kidneys. Large intakes of fluid are required to hold these wastes in solution and to replace body fluids.

Intravenous feedings including total parenteral nutrition are used until the patient is able to take oral feedings. When peristalsis is adequate tube feedings may be used instead of, or in addition to, oral feedings. A diet supplying 3000 to 5000 kcal and 150 gm or more of protein is usually needed (see pp. 214 and 263). Up to 1.0 gm ascorbic acid is often prescribed, as are also supplements of the B-complex vitamins.

## REVIEW QUESTIONS AND PROBLEMS

1. What is meant by blenderized tube feeding; elemental diet; milk-base formula?

2. What nutrients are especially important to promote wound healing?

3. Why is vitamin K of special importance in surgery?

4. Patients following surgery often complain of gastric fullness and cramping. What are some reasons for these symptoms? What dietary procedures may reduce them?

5. List several precautions that should be observed in using a tube feeding.

6. Why are injections of vitamin $B_{12}$ essential for patients who have had a gastrectomy? for those who have had massive intestinal resection?

7. When does the dumping syndrome occur? What are the symptoms? What are the important characteristics of the diet?

8. What is meant by the short bowel syndrome? What plans must be made for nutritional care?

9. Study the charts of four patients who have had surgery. Prepare a summary that shows the nature of the surgery, the postoperative orders for parenteral fluids, vitamin and mineral supplements, and diet. Indicate the postoperative days when each order was initiated.

## REFERENCES

Campbell, E. B.: "Nursing Problems Associated with Prolonged Recovery Following Trauma," *Nurs. Clin. North Am.*, 5:551–62, 1970.

Gormican, A., and Liddy, E.: "Nasogastric Tube Feedings: Practical Considerations in Prescription and Evaluation," *Postgrad. Med.*, 53:71–76, June 1973.

Grant, J. A., *et al.*: "Parenteral Hyperalimentation," *Am. J. Nurs.*, 69:2392–95, 1969.

Heidelbaugh, N. D., *et al.*: "Clinical Nutrition Applications of Space Food Technology," *J. Am. Diet. Assoc.*, 62:383–89, 1973.

McCarter, D.: "Nourishing the Solute-Sensitive Patient," *Am. J. Nurs.*, 73:1935–36, 1973.

Mason, M. A.: *Basic Medical-Surgical Nursing*, 3rd ed. New York: Macmillan Publishing Co., Inc., 1974, Chap. 5.

Robinson, C. H.: *Normal and Therapeutic Nutrition*, 14th ed. New York: Macmillan Publishing Co., Inc., 1972, Chap. 38.

White, D. R.: "I Have an Ileostomy," *Am. J. Nurs.*, 61:51, May 1961.

# APPENDIXES

## Table A–1. Nutritive Values of the Edible Part of Foods*

*[Dashes in the columns for nutrients show that no suitable value could be found although there is reason to believe that a measurable amount of the nutrient may be present]*

| Food, Approximate Measure, and Weight (in grams) | | gm | Water per cent | Food Energy calories | Pro-tein gm | Fat gm | Satu-rated (total) gm | Oleic gm | Lin-oleic gm | Carbo-hy-drate gm | Cal-cium mg | Iron mg | Vita-min A Value I.U. | Thia-mine mg | Ribo-flavin mg | Niacin mg | Ascor-bic Acid mg |
|---|---|---|---|---|---|---|---|---|---|---|---|---|---|---|---|---|---|
| | | | | | | | | **Fatty Acids** — Unsaturated | | | | | | | | | |

### Milk, Cheese, Cream, Imitation Cream; Related Products

| Food, Approximate Measure, and Weight | Measure | gm | Water % | Food Energy cal | Protein gm | Fat gm | Saturated (total) gm | Oleic gm | Linoleic gm | Carbohydrate gm | Calcium mg | Iron mg | Vit A Value I.U. | Thiamine mg | Riboflavin mg | Niacin mg | Ascorbic Acid mg |
|---|---|---|---|---|---|---|---|---|---|---|---|---|---|---|---|---|---|
| **Milk:** | | | | | | | | | | | | | | | | | |
| Fluid: | | | | | | | | | | | | | | | | | |
| 1 Whole, 3.5% fat | 1 cup | 244 | 87 | 160 | 9 | 9 | 5 | 3 | Trace | 12 | 288 | 0.1 | 350 | 0.07 | 0.41 | 0.2 | 2 |
| 2 Nonfat (skim) | 1 cup | 245 | 90 | 90 | 9 | Trace | — | — | — | 12 | 296 | 0.1 | 10 | 0.09 | 0.44 | 0.2 | 2 |
| 3 Partly skimmed, 2% nonfat milk solids added | 1 cup | 246 | 87 | 145 | 10 | 5 | 3 | 2 | Trace | 15 | 352 | 0.1 | 200 | 0.10 | 0.52 | 0.2 | 2 |
| Canned, concentrated, undiluted: | | | | | | | | | | | | | | | | | |
| 4 Evaporated, unsweetened | 1 cup | 252 | 74 | 345 | 18 | 20 | 11 | 7 | 1 | 24 | 635 | 0.3 | 810 | 0.10 | 0.86 | 0.5 | 3 |
| 5 Condensed, sweetened | 1 cup | 306 | 27 | 980 | 25 | 27 | 15 | 9 | 1 | 166 | 802 | 0.3 | 1,100 | 0.24 | 1.16 | 0.6 | 3 |
| Dry, nonfat instant: | | | | | | | | | | | | | | | | | |
| 6 Low-density (1 1/3 cups needed for reconstitution to 1 qt) | 1 cup | 68 | 4 | 245 | 24 | Trace | — | — | — | 35 | 879 | 0.4 | 120 | 0.24 | 1.21 | 0.6 | 5 |
| 7 High-density (7/8 cup needed for reconstitution to 1 qt) | 1 cup | 104 | 4 | 375 | 37 | 1 | — | — | — | 54 | 1,345 | 0.6 | 130 | 0.36 | 1.85 | 0.9 | 7 |
| **Buttermilk:** | | | | | | | | | | | | | | | | | |
| 8 Fluid, cultured, made from skim milk | 1 cup | 245 | 90 | 90 | 9 | Trace | — | — | — | 12 | 296 | 0.1 | 10 | 0.10 | 0.44 | 0.2 | 2 |
| 9 Dried, packaged | 1 cup | 120 | 3 | 465 | 41 | 6 | 3 | 2 | Trace | 60 | 1,498 | 0.7 | 260 | 0.31 | 2.06 | 1.1 | — |
| **Cheese:** | | | | | | | | | | | | | | | | | |
| Natural: | | | | | | | | | | | | | | | | | |
| Blue or Roquefort type: | | | | | | | | | | | | | | | | | |
| 10 Ounce | 1 oz | 28 | 40 | 105 | 6 | 9 | 5 | 3 | Trace | 1 | 89 | 0.1 | 350 | 0.01 | 0.17 | 0.3 | 0 |
| 11 Cubic inch | 1 cu. in. | 17 | 40 | 65 | 4 | 5 | 3 | 2 | Trace | Trace | 54 | 0.1 | 210 | 0.01 | 0.11 | 0.2 | 0 |
| 12 Camembert, packaged in 4-oz pkg. with 3 wedges per pkg. | 1 wedge | 38 | 52 | 115 | 7 | 9 | 5 | 3 | Trace | 1 | 40 | 0.2 | 380 | 0.02 | 0.29 | 0.3 | 0 |
| Cheddar: | | | | | | | | | | | | | | | | | |
| 13 Ounce | 1 oz | 28 | 37 | 115 | 7 | 9 | 5 | 3 | Trace | 1 | 213 | 0.3 | 370 | 0.01 | 0.13 | Trace | 0 |
| 14 Cubic inch | 1 cu in | 17 | 37 | 70 | 4 | 6 | 3 | 2 | Trace | Trace | 129 | 0.2 | 230 | 0.01 | 0.08 | Trace | 0 |
| Cottage, large or small curd: | | | | | | | | | | | | | | | | | |
| Creamed: | | | | | | | | | | | | | | | | | |
| 15 Package of 12 oz, net wt. | 1 pkg | 340 | 78 | 360 | 46 | 14 | 8 | 5 | Trace | 10 | 320 | 1.0 | 580 | 0.10 | 0.85 | 0.3 | 0 |
| 16 Cup, curd pressed down | 1 cup | 245 | 78 | 260 | 33 | 10 | 6 | 3 | Trace | 7 | 230 | 0.7 | 420 | 0.07 | 0.61 | 0.2 | 0 |
| Uncreamed: | | | | | | | | | | | | | | | | | |
| 17 Package of 12 oz net wt. | 1 pkg | 340 | 79 | 290 | 58 | 1 | 1 | Trace | Trace | 9 | 306 | 1.4 | 30 | 0.10 | 0.95 | 0.3 | 0 |
| 18 Cup, curd pressed down | 1 cup | 200 | 79 | 170 | 34 | 1 | Trace | Trace | Trace | 5 | 180 | 0.8 | 20 | 0.06 | 0.56 | 0.2 | 0 |

| No. | Food | Measure | Grams | Water (%) | Food energy (cal.) | Protein (g) | Fat (g) | Saturated (g) | Oleic (g) | Linoleic (g) | Carbohydrate (g) | Calcium (mg) | Iron (mg) | Vitamin A (I.U.) | Thiamin (mg) | Riboflavin (mg) | Niacin (mg) | Ascorbic acid (mg) |
|---|---|---|---|---|---|---|---|---|---|---|---|---|---|---|---|---|---|---|
| | **Cream:** | | | | | | | | | | | | | | | | | |
| 19 | Package of 8 oz, net wt. | 1 pkg | 227 | 51 | 850 | 18 | 86 | 48 | 28 | 3 | 5 | 141 | 0.5 | 3,500 | 0.05 | 0.54 | 0.2 | 0 |
| 20 | Package of 3 oz, net wt. | 1 pkg | 85 | 51 | 320 | 7 | 32 | 18 | 11 | 1 | 2 | 53 | 0.2 | 1,310 | 0.02 | 0.20 | 0.1 | 0 |
| 21 | Cubic inch | 1 cu in | 16 | 51 | 60 | 1 | 6 | 3 | 2 | Trace | Trace | 10 | Trace | 250 | Trace | 0.04 | Trace | 0 |
| | **Parmesan, grated:** | | | | | | | | | | | | | | | | | |
| 22 | Cup, pressed down | 1 cup | 140 | 17 | 655 | 60 | 43 | 24 | 14 | 1 | 5 | 1,893 | 0.7 | 1,760 | 0.03 | 1.22 | 0.3 | 0 |
| 23 | Tablespoon | 1 tbsp | 5 | 17 | 25 | 2 | 2 | 1 | Trace | Trace | Trace | 68 | Trace | 60 | Trace | 0.04 | Trace | 0 |
| 24 | Ounce | 1 oz | 28 | 17 | 130 | 12 | 9 | 5 | 3 | Trace | 1 | 383 | 0.1 | 360 | 0.01 | 0.25 | 0.1 | 0 |
| | **Swiss:** | | | | | | | | | | | | | | | | | |
| 25 | Ounce | 1 oz | 28 | 39 | 105 | 8 | 8 | 4 | 3 | Trace | 1 | 262 | 0.3 | 320 | Trace | 0.11 | Trace | 0 |
| 26 | Cubic inch | 1 cu in | 15 | 39 | 55 | 4 | 4 | 2 | 1 | Trace | Trace | 139 | 0.1 | 170 | Trace | 0.06 | Trace | 0 |
| | **Pasteurized processed cheese:** | | | | | | | | | | | | | | | | | |
| | American: | | | | | | | | | | | | | | | | | |
| 27 | Ounce | 1 oz | 28 | 40 | 105 | 7 | 9 | 5 | 3 | Trace | 1 | 198 | 0.3 | 350 | 0.01 | 0.12 | Trace | 0 |
| 28 | Cubic inch | 1 cu in | 18 | 40 | 65 | 4 | 5 | 3 | 2 | Trace | Trace | 122 | 0.2 | 210 | Trace | 0.07 | Trace | 0 |
| | Swiss: | | | | | | | | | | | | | | | | | |
| 29 | Ounce | 1 oz | 28 | 40 | 100 | 8 | 8 | 4 | 3 | Trace | 1 | 251 | 0.3 | 310 | Trace | 0.11 | Trace | 0 |
| 30 | Cubic inch | 1 cu in | 18 | 40 | 65 | 5 | 5 | 3 | 2 | Trace | 1 | 159 | 0.2 | 200 | Trace | 0.07 | Trace | 0 |
| | **Pasteurized process cheese food, American:** | | | | | | | | | | | | | | | | | |
| 31 | Tablespoon | 1 tbsp | 14 | 43 | 45 | 3 | 3 | 2 | 1 | Trace | 1 | 80 | 0.1 | 140 | Trace | 0.08 | Trace | 0 |
| 32 | Cubic inch | 1 cu in | 18 | 43 | 60 | 4 | 4 | 2 | 1 | Trace | 1 | 100 | 0.1 | 170 | Trace | 0.10 | Trace | 0 |
| 33 | Pasteurized process cheese spread, American | 1 oz | 28 | 49 | 80 | 5 | 6 | 3 | 2 | Trace | 2 | 160 | 0.2 | 250 | Trace | 0.15 | Trace | 0 |
| | **Cream:** | | | | | | | | | | | | | | | | | |
| 34 | Half-and-half (cream and milk) | 1 cup | 242 | 80 | 325 | 8 | 28 | 15 | 9 | 1 | 11 | 261 | 0.1 | 1,160 | 0.07 | 0.39 | 0.1 | 2 |
| 35 | | 1 tbsp | 15 | 80 | 20 | 1 | 2 | 1 | Trace | Trace | 1 | 16 | Trace | 70 | Trace | 0.02 | Trace | Trace |
| 36 | Light, coffee or table | 1 cup | 240 | 72 | 505 | 7 | 49 | 27 | 16 | 1 | 10 | 245 | 0.1 | 2,020 | 0.07 | 0.36 | 0.1 | 2 |
| 37 | | 1 tbsp | 15 | 72 | 30 | 1 | 3 | 2 | 1 | Trace | 1 | 15 | Trace | 130 | Trace | 0.02 | Trace | Trace |
| 38 | Sour | 1 cup | 230 | 72 | 485 | 7 | 47 | 26 | 16 | 1 | 10 | 235 | 0.1 | 1,930 | 0.07 | 0.35 | 0.1 | 2 |
| 39 | | 1 tbsp | 12 | 72 | 25 | Trace | 2 | 1 | 1 | Trace | 1 | 12 | Trace | 100 | Trace | 0.02 | Trace | Trace |
| 40 | Whipped topping (pressurized) | 1 cup | 60 | 62 | 155 | 2 | 14 | 8 | 5 | Trace | 8 | 67 | Trace | 570 | Trace | 0.04 | Trace | 0 |
| 41 | | 1 tbsp | 3 | 62 | 10 | Trace | 1 | 1 | Trace | Trace | Trace | 3 | Trace | 30 | Trace | Trace | Trace | 0 |
| | Whipping, unwhipped (volume about double when whipped): | | | | | | | | | | | | | | | | | |
| 42 | Light | 1 cup | 239 | 62 | 715 | 6 | 75 | 41 | 25 | 2 | 9 | 203 | 0.1 | 3,060 | 0.05 | 0.29 | 0.1 | 2 |
| 43 | | 1 tbsp | 15 | 62 | 45 | Trace | 5 | 3 | 2 | Trace | 1 | 13 | Trace | 190 | Trace | 0.02 | Trace | Trace |
| 44 | Heavy | 1 cup | 238 | 57 | 840 | 5 | 90 | 50 | 30 | 3 | 7 | 179 | 0.1 | 3,670 | 0.05 | 0.26 | 0.1 | 2 |
| 45 | | 1 tbsp | 15 | 57 | 55 | Trace | 6 | 3 | 2 | Trace | 1 | 11 | Trace | 230 | Trace | 0.02 | Trace | Trace |
| | **Imitation cream products (made with vegetable fat):** | | | | | | | | | | | | | | | | | |
| | Creamers: | | | | | | | | | | | | | | | | | |
| 46 | Powdered | 1 cup | 94 | 2 | 505 | 4 | 33 | 31 | Trace | Trace | 52 | 21 | 0.6 | 200[2] | — | — | Trace | — |
| 47 | | 1 tsp | 2 | 2 | 10 | Trace | Trace | Trace | 0 | 0 | 1 | 1 | Trace | Trace[2] | — | — | Trace | — |
| 48 | Liquid (frozen) | 1 cup | 245 | 77 | 345 | 3 | 27 | 25 | Trace | Trace | 25 | 29 | — | 2,100[2] | — | — | — | — |
| 49 | | 1 tbsp | 15 | 77 | 20 | Trace | 1 | 1 | Trace | Trace | 2 | 2 | — | 210[2] | — | — | — | — |
| 50 | Sour dressing (imitation sour cream) made with nonfat dry milk | 1 cup | 235 | 72 | 440 | 8 | 38 | 35 | Trace | 1 | 17 | 277 | 0.1 | 10 | 0.07 | 0.38 | 0.2 | 1 |
| 51 | | 1 tbsp | 12 | 72 | 20 | Trace | 2 | 2 | Trace | Trace | 1 | 14 | Trace | Trace | Trace | 0.02 | Trace | Trace |
| | Whipped topping: | | | | | | | | | | | | | | | | | |
| 52 | Pressurized | 1 cup | 70 | 61 | 190 | 1 | 17 | 15 | 1 | Trace | 9 | 5 | — | 340[2] | — | 0 | — | — |
| 53 | | 1 tbsp | 4 | 61 | 10 | Trace | 1 | 1 | Trace | 0 | Trace | Trace | — | 20[2] | — | 0 | — | — |

*Nutritive Value of Foods, Home and Garden Bulletin No. 72. U.S. Department of Agriculture, Washington, D.C., 1970.

[1]Value applies to unfortified product; value for fortified low-density product would be 1500 I.U. and the fortified high-density product would be 2290 I.U.

[2]Contributed largely from beta-carotene used for coloring.

# Table A-1. (Cont.)

| | Food, Approximate Measure, and Weight (in grams) | | gm | Water per cent | Food Energy calories | Protein gm | Fat gm | Fatty Acids Saturated (total) gm | Unsaturated Oleic gm | Unsaturated Linoleic gm | Carbohydrate gm | Calcium mg | Iron mg | Vitamin A Value I.U. | Thiamine mg | Riboflavin mg | Niacin mg | Ascorbic Acid mg |
|---|---|---|---|---|---|---|---|---|---|---|---|---|---|---|---|---|---|---|
| | Whipped topping (cont.) | | | | | | | | | | | | | | | | | |
| 54 | Frozen | 1 cup | 75 | 52 | 230 | 1 | 20 | 18 | Trace | 0 | 15 | 5 | — | 2560 | — | 0 | — | — |
| 55 | | 1 tbsp | 4 | 52 | 10 | Trace | 1 | 1 | Trace | 0 | 1 | Trace | — | 230 | — | 0 | — | — |
| 56 | Powdered, made with whole milk | 1 cup | 75 | 58 | 175 | 3 | 12 | 10 | 1 | Trace | 15 | 62 | Trace | 2330 | 0.02 | 0.08 | 0.1 | Trace |
| 57 | | 1 tbsp | 4 | 58 | 10 | Trace | 1 | 1 | Trace | Trace | 1 | 3 | Trace | 220 | Trace | Trace | Trace | Trace |
| | Milk beverages: | | | | | | | | | | | | | | | | | |
| 58 | Cocoa, homemade | 1 cup | 250 | 79 | 245 | 10 | 12 | 7 | 4 | Trace | 27 | 295 | 1.0 | 400 | 0.10 | 0.45 | 0.5 | 3 |
| 59 | Chocolate-flavored drink made with skim milk and 2% added butterfat | 1 cup | 250 | 83 | 190 | 8 | 6 | 3 | 2 | Trace | 27 | 270 | 0.5 | 210 | 0.10 | 0.40 | 0.3 | 3 |
| | Malted milk: | | | | | | | | | | | | | | | | | |
| 60 | Dry powder, approx. 3 heaping teaspoons per ounce | 1 oz | 28 | 3 | 115 | 4 | 2 | | | | 20 | 82 | 0.6 | 290 | 0.09 | 0.15 | 0.1 | 0 |
| 61 | Beverage | 1 cup | 235 | 78 | 245 | 11 | 10 | | | | 28 | 317 | 0.7 | 590 | 0.14 | 0.49 | 0.2 | 2 |
| | Milk desserts: | | | | | | | | | | | | | | | | | |
| 62 | Custard | 1 cup | 265 | 77 | 305 | 14 | 15 | 7 | 5 | 1 | 29 | 297 | 1.1 | 930 | 0.11 | 0.50 | 0.3 | 1 |
| | Ice cream: | | | | | | | | | | | | | | | | | |
| 63 | Regular (approx. 10% fat) | 1/2 gal | 1,064 | 63 | 2,055 | 48 | 113 | 62 | 37 | 3 | 221 | 1,553 | 0.5 | 4,680 | 0.43 | 2.23 | 1.1 | 11 |
| 64 | | 1 cup | 133 | 63 | 255 | 6 | 14 | 8 | 5 | Trace | 28 | 194 | 0.1 | 590 | 0.05 | 0.28 | 0.1 | 1 |
| 65 | | 3-fl-oz cup | 50 | 63 | 95 | 2 | 5 | 2 | Trace | | 10 | 73 | Trace | 220 | 0.02 | 0.11 | 0.1 | 1 |
| 66 | Rich (approx. 16% fat) | 1/2 gal | 1,188 | 63 | 2,635 | 31 | 191 | 105 | 63 | 6 | 214 | 927 | 0.2 | 7,840 | 0.24 | 1.31 | 1.2 | 2 |
| 67 | | 1 cup | 148 | 63 | 330 | 4 | 24 | 13 | 8 | 1 | 27 | 115 | Trace | 980 | 0.03 | 0.16 | 0.1 | 1 |
| | Ice milk: | | | | | | | | | | | | | | | | | |
| 68 | Hardened | 1/2 gal | 1,048 | 67 | 1,595 | 50 | 53 | 29 | 17 | 2 | 235 | 1,635 | 1.0 | 2,200 | 0.52 | 2.31 | 1.0 | 10 |
| 69 | | 1 cup | 131 | 67 | 200 | 6 | 7 | 4 | 3 | Trace | 29 | 204 | 0.1 | 280 | 0.07 | 0.29 | 0.1 | 1 |
| 70 | Soft-serve | 1 cup | 175 | 67 | 265 | 8 | 9 | 5 | 3 | Trace | 39 | 273 | 0.2 | 370 | 0.09 | 0.39 | 0.2 | 2 |
| | Yoghurt: | | | | | | | | | | | | | | | | | |
| 71 | Made from partially skimmed milk | 1 cup | 245 | 89 | 125 | 8 | 4 | 2 | 1 | Trace | 13 | 294 | 0.1 | 170 | 0.10 | 0.44 | 0.2 | 2 |
| 72 | Made from whole milk | 1 cup | 245 | 88 | 150 | 7 | 8 | 5 | 3 | Trace | 12 | 272 | 0.1 | 340 | 0.07 | 0.39 | 0.2 | 2 |
| | **Eggs** | | | | | | | | | | | | | | | | | |
| | Eggs, large. 24 ounces per dozen: Raw or cooked in shell or with nothing added: | | | | | | | | | | | | | | | | | |
| 73 | Whole, without shell | 1 egg | 50 | 74 | 80 | 6 | 6 | 2 | 3 | Trace | Trace | 27 | 1.1 | 590 | 0.05 | 0.15 | Trace | 0 |
| 74 | White of egg | 1 white | 33 | 88 | 15 | 4 | Trace | | | | Trace | 3 | Trace | 0 | Trace | 0.09 | Trace | 0 |
| 75 | Yolk of egg | 1 yolk | 17 | 51 | 60 | 3 | 5 | 2 | 2 | Trace | Trace | 24 | 0.9 | 580 | 0.04 | 0.07 | Trace | 0 |
| 76 | Scrambled with milk and fat | 1 egg | 64 | 72 | 110 | 7 | 8 | 3 | 3 | Trace | 1 | 51 | 1.1 | 690 | 0.05 | 0.18 | Trace | 0 |
| | **Meat, Poultry, Fish, Shellfish; Related Products** | | | | | | | | | | | | | | | | | |
| 77 | Bacon (20 slices per lb raw), 2 slices broiled or fried crisp | | 15 | 8 | 90 | 5 | 8 | 3 | 4 | 1 | 1 | 2 | 0.5 | 0 | 0.08 | 0.05 | 0.8 | — |
| | Beef,[3] cooked: | | | | | | | | | | | | | | | | | |
| 78 | Cuts braised, simmered, or pot-roasted: Lean and fat | 3 ounces | 85 | 53 | 245 | 23 | 16 | 8 | 7 | Trace | 0 | 10 | 2.9 | 30 | 0.04 | 0.18 | 3.5 | — |

308

| No. | Food, approximate measure | Grams | Water (%) | Food energy (Calories) | Protein (g) | Fat (g) | Saturated (total) (g) | Unsat. Oleic (g) | Unsat. Linoleic (g) | Carbohydrate (g) | Calcium (mg) | Iron (mg) | Vitamin A value (I.U.) | Thiamin (mg) | Riboflavin (mg) | Niacin (mg) | Ascorbic acid (mg) |
|---|---|---|---|---|---|---|---|---|---|---|---|---|---|---|---|---|---|
| 79 | Lean only, 2.5 ounces | 72 | 62 | 140 | 22 | 5 | 2 | 2 | Trace | 0 | 10 | 2.7 | 10 | 0.04 | 0.16 | 3.3 | — |
|  | Hamburger (ground beef), broiled: |  |  |  |  |  |  |  |  |  |  |  |  |  |  |  |  |
| 80 | Lean, 3 ounces | 85 | 60 | 185 | 23 | 10 | 5 | 4 | Trace | 0 | 10 | 3.0 | 20 | 0.08 | 0.20 | 5.1 | — |
| 81 | Regular, 3 ounces | 85 | 54 | 245 | 21 | 17 | 8 | 8 | Trace | 0 | 9 | 2.7 | 30 | 0.07 | 0.18 | 4.6 | — |
|  | Roast, oven-cooked, no liquid added: |  |  |  |  |  |  |  |  |  |  |  |  |  |  |  |  |
|  | Relatively fat, such as rib: |  |  |  |  |  |  |  |  |  |  |  |  |  |  |  |  |
| 82 | Lean and fat, 3 ounces | 85 | 40 | 375 | 17 | 34 | 16 | 15 | 1 | 0 | 8 | 2.2 | 70 | 0.05 | 0.13 | 3.1 | — |
| 83 | Lean only, 1.8 ounces | 51 | 57 | 125 | 14 | 7 | 3 | 3 | Trace | 0 | 6 | 1.8 | 10 | 0.04 | 0.11 | 2.6 | — |
|  | Relatively lean, such as heel of round: |  |  |  |  |  |  |  |  |  |  |  |  |  |  |  |  |
| 84 | Lean and fat, 3 ounces | 85 | 62 | 165 | 25 | 7 | 3 | 3 | Trace | 0 | 11 | 3.2 | 10 | 0.06 | 0.19 | 4.5 | — |
| 85 | Lean only, 2.7 ounces | 78 | 65 | 125 | 24 | 3 | 1 | 1 | Trace | 0 | 10 | 3.0 | Trace | 0.06 | 0.18 | 4.3 | — |
|  | Steak, broiled: |  |  |  |  |  |  |  |  |  |  |  |  |  |  |  |  |
|  | Relatively fat, such as sirloin: |  |  |  |  |  |  |  |  |  |  |  |  |  |  |  |  |
| 86 | Lean and fat, 3 ounces | 85 | 44 | 330 | 20 | 27 | 13 | 12 | 1 | 0 | 9 | 2.5 | 50 | 0.05 | 0.16 | 4.0 | — |
| 87 | Lean only, 2.0 ounces | 56 | 59 | 115 | 18 | 4 | 2 | 2 | Trace | 0 | 7 | 2.2 | 10 | 0.05 | 0.14 | 3.6 | — |
|  | Relatively lean, such as round: |  |  |  |  |  |  |  |  |  |  |  |  |  |  |  |  |
| 88 | Lean and fat, 3 ounces | 85 | 55 | 220 | 24 | 13 | 6 | 6 | Trace | 0 | 10 | 3.0 | 20 | 0.07 | 0.19 | 4.8 | — |
| 89 | Lean only, 2.4 ounces | 68 | 61 | 130 | 21 | 4 | 2 | 2 | Trace | 0 | 9 | 2.5 | 10 | 0.06 | 0.16 | 4.1 | — |
|  | Beef, canned: |  |  |  |  |  |  |  |  |  |  |  |  |  |  |  |  |
| 90 | Corned beef, 3 ounces | 85 | 59 | 185 | 22 | 10 | 5 | 4 | Trace | 0 | 17 | 3.7 | 20 | 0.01 | 0.20 | 2.9 | — |
| 91 | Corned beef hash, 3 ounces | 85 | 67 | 155 | 7 | 10 | 5 | 4 | Trace | 9 | 11 | 1.7 | — | 0.01 | 0.08 | 1.8 | — |
| 92 | Beef, dried or chipped, 2 ounces | 57 | 48 | 115 | 19 | 4 | 2 | 2 | Trace | 0 | 11 | 2.9 | — | 0.04 | 0.18 | 2.2 | — |
| 93 | Beef and vegetable stew, 1 cup | 235 | 82 | 210 | 15 | 10 | 5 | 4 | Trace | 15 | 28 | 2.8 | 2,310 | 0.13 | 0.17 | 4.4 | 15 |
| 94 | Beef potpie, baked, 4 1/4-inch diam., weight before baking about 8 ounces, 1 pie | 227 | 55 | 560 | 23 | 33 | 9 | 20 | 2 | 43 | 32 | 4.1 | 1,860 | 0.25 | 0.27 | 4.5 | 7 |
|  | Chicken, cooked: |  |  |  |  |  |  |  |  |  |  |  |  |  |  |  |  |
| 95 | Flesh only, broiled, 3 ounces | 85 | 71 | 115 | 20 | 3 | 1 | 1 | 1 | 0 | 8 | 1.4 | 80 | 0.05 | 0.16 | 7.4 | — |
|  | Breast, fried, 1/2 breast: |  |  |  |  |  |  |  |  |  |  |  |  |  |  |  |  |
| 96 | With bone, 3.3 ounces | 94 | 58 | 155 | 25 | 5 | 1 | 2 | 1 | 1 | 9 | 1.3 | 70 | 0.04 | 0.17 | 11.2 | — |
| 97 | Flesh and skin only, 2.7 ounces | 76 | 58 | 155 | 25 | 5 | 1 | 2 | 1 | 1 | 9 | 1.3 | 70 | 0.04 | 0.17 | 11.2 | — |
|  | Drumstick, fried: |  |  |  |  |  |  |  |  |  |  |  |  |  |  |  |  |
| 98 | With bone, 2.1 ounces | 59 | 55 | 90 | 12 | 4 | 1 | 2 | 1 | Trace | 6 | 0.9 | 50 | 0.03 | 0.15 | 2.7 | — |
| 99 | Flesh and skin only, 1.3 ounces | 38 | 55 | 90 | 12 | 4 | 1 | 2 | 1 | Trace | 6 | 0.9 | 50 | 0.03 | 0.15 | 2.7 | — |
| 100 | Chicken, canned, boneless, 3 ounces | 85 | 65 | 170 | 18 | 10 | 3 | 4 | 2 | 0 | 18 | 1.3 | 200 | 0.03 | 0.11 | 3.7 | 3 |
| 101 | Chicken potpie, baked 4 1/4-inch diam., weight before baking about 8 ounces, 1 pie | 227 | 57 | 535 | 23 | 31 | 10 | 15 | 3 | 42 | 68 | 3.0 | 3,020 | 0.25 | 0.26 | 4.1 | 5 |
|  | Chili con carne, canned: |  |  |  |  |  |  |  |  |  |  |  |  |  |  |  |  |
| 102 | With beans, 1 cup | 250 | 72 | 335 | 19 | 15 | 7 | 7 | Trace | 30 | 80 | 4.2 | 150 | 0.08 | 0.18 | 3.2 | — |
| 103 | Without beans, 1 cup | 255 | 67 | 510 | 26 | 38 | 18 | 17 | 1 | 15 | 97 | 3.6 | 380 | 0.05 | 0.31 | 5.6 | — |
| 104 | Heart, beef, lean, braised, 3 ounces | 85 | 61 | 160 | 27 | 5 | — | — | — | 1 | 10 | 5.0 | 20 | 0.21 | 1.04 | 6.5 | 1 |
|  | Lamb,[3] cooked: |  |  |  |  |  |  |  |  |  |  |  |  |  |  |  |  |
|  | Chop, thick, with bone, broiled: |  |  |  |  |  |  |  |  |  |  |  |  |  |  |  |  |
| 105 | 1 chop, 4.8 ounces | 137 | 47 | 400 | 25 | 33 | 18 | 12 | 1 | 0 | 10 | 1.5 | — | 0.14 | 0.25 | 5.6 | — |
| 106 | Lean and fat, 4.0 ounces | 112 | 47 | 400 | 25 | 33 | 18 | 12 | 1 | 0 | 10 | 1.5 | — | 0.14 | 0.25 | 5.6 | — |
| 107 | Lean only, 2.6 ounces | 74 | 62 | 140 | 21 | 6 | 3 | 2 | Trace | 0 | 9 | 1.5 | — | 0.11 | 0.20 | 4.5 | — |
|  | Leg, roasted: |  |  |  |  |  |  |  |  |  |  |  |  |  |  |  |  |
| 108 | Lean and fat, 3 ounces | 85 | 54 | 235 | 22 | 16 | 9 | 6 | Trace | 0 | 9 | 1.4 | — | 0.13 | 0.23 | 4.7 | — |
| 109 | Lean only, 2.5 ounces | 71 | 62 | 130 | 20 | 5 | 3 | 2 | Trace | 0 | 9 | 1.4 | — | 0.12 | 0.21 | 4.4 | — |
|  | Shoulder, roasted: |  |  |  |  |  |  |  |  |  |  |  |  |  |  |  |  |
| 110 | Lean and fat, 3 ounces | 85 | 50 | 285 | 18 | 23 | 13 | 8 | 1 | 0 | 9 | 1.0 | — | 0.11 | 0.20 | 4.0 | — |
| 111 | Lean only, 2.3 ounces | 64 | 61 | 130 | 17 | 6 | 3 | 1 | Trace | 0 | 8 | 1.0 | — | 0.10 | 0.18 | 3.7 | — |
| 112 | Liver, beef, fried, 2 ounces | 57 | 57 | 130 | 15 | 6 | — | — | — | 3 | 6 | 5.0 | 30,280 | 0.15 | 2.37 | 9.4 | 15 |

[2] Contributed largely from beta-carotene used for coloring.

[3] Outer layer of fat on the cut was removed to within approximately 1/2-inch of the lean. Deposits of fat within the cut were not removed.

Table A-1. (Cont.)

| | Food, Approximate Measure, and Weight (in grams) | gm | Water per cent | Food Energy calories | Protein gm | Fat gm | Saturated (total) gm | Oleic gm | Linoleic gm | Carbohydrate gm | Calcium mg | Iron mg | Vitamin A Value I.U. | Thiamine mg | Riboflavin mg | Niacin mg | Ascorbic Acid mg |
|---|---|---|---|---|---|---|---|---|---|---|---|---|---|---|---|---|---|
| | | | | | | | **Fatty Acids** | | | | | | | | | | |
| | | | | | | | | Unsaturated | | | | | | | | | |
| 113 | Pork, cured, cooked: Ham, light cure, lean and fat, roasted | 3 ounces | 85 | 54 | 245 | 18 | 19 | 7 | 8 | 2 | 0 | 8 | 2.2 | 0 | 0.40 | 0.16 | 3.1 | — |
| | Luncheon meat: | | | | | | | | | | | | | | | | |
| 114 | Boiled ham, sliced | 2 ounces | 57 | 59 | 135 | 11 | 10 | 4 | 4 | 1 | 0 | 6 | 1.6 | 0 | 0.25 | 0.09 | 1.5 | — |
| 115 | Canned, spiced or unspiced | 2 ounces | 57 | 55 | 165 | 8 | 14 | 5 | 6 | 1 | 1 | 5 | 1.2 | 0 | 0.18 | 0.12 | 1.6 | — |
| 116 | Pork, fresh, cooked: Chop, thick, with bone | 1 chop, 3.5 ounces | 98 | 42 | 260 | 16 | 21 | 8 | 9 | 2 | 0 | 8 | 2.2 | 0 | 0.63 | 0.18 | 3.8 | — |
| 117 | Lean and fat | 2.3 ounces | 66 | 42 | 260 | 16 | 21 | 8 | 9 | 2 | 0 | 8 | 2.2 | 0 | 0.63 | 0.18 | 3.8 | — |
| 118 | Lean only | 1.7 ounces | 48 | 53 | 130 | 15 | 7 | 2 | 3 | 1 | 0 | 7 | 1.9 | 0 | 0.54 | 0.16 | 3.3 | — |
| 119 | Roast, oven-cooked, no liquid added: Lean and fat | 3 ounces | 85 | 46 | 310 | 21 | 24 | 9 | 10 | 2 | 0 | 9 | 2.7 | 0 | 0.78 | 0.22 | 4.7 | — |
| 120 | Lean only | 2.4 ounces | 68 | 55 | 175 | 20 | 10 | 3 | 4 | 1 | 0 | 9 | 2.6 | 0 | 0.73 | 0.21 | 4.4 | — |
| 121 | Cuts, simmered: Lean and fat | 3 ounces | 85 | 46 | 320 | 20 | 26 | 9 | 11 | 2 | 0 | 8 | 2.5 | 0 | 0.46 | 0.21 | 4.1 | — |
| 122 | Lean only | 2.2 ounces | 63 | 60 | 135 | 18 | 6 | 2 | 3 | 1 | 0 | 8 | 2.3 | 0 | 0.42 | 0.19 | 3.7 | — |
| 123 | Sausage: Bologna, slice, 3-in diam. by 1/8 inch | 2 slices | 26 | 56 | 80 | 3 | 7 | — | — | — | Trace | 2 | 0.5 | — | 0.04 | 0.06 | 0.7 | — |
| 124 | Braunschweiger, slice 2-in diam. by 1/4 inch | 2 slices | 20 | 53 | 65 | 3 | 5 | — | — | — | Trace | 2 | 1.2 | 1,310 | 0.03 | 0.29 | 1.6 | — |
| 125 | Deviled ham, canned | 1 tbsp | 13 | 51 | 45 | 2 | 4 | 2 | 2 | Trace | 0 | 1 | 0.3 | — | 0.02 | 0.01 | 0.2 | — |
| 126 | Frankfurter, heated (8 per lb purchased pkg) | 1 frank | 56 | 57 | 170 | 7 | 15 | — | — | — | 1 | 3 | 0.8 | — | 0.08 | 0.11 | 1.4 | — |
| 127 | Pork links, cooked (16 links per lb raw) | 2 links | 26 | 35 | 125 | 5 | 11 | 4 | 5 | 1 | Trace | 2 | 0.6 | 0 | 0.21 | 0.09 | 1.0 | — |
| 128 | Salami, dry type | 1 oz | 28 | 30 | 130 | 7 | 11 | — | — | — | Trace | 4 | 1.0 | — | 0.10 | 0.07 | 1.5 | — |
| 129 | Salami, cooked | 1 oz | 28 | 51 | 90 | 5 | 7 | — | — | — | Trace | 3 | 0.7 | — | 0.07 | 0.07 | 1.2 | — |
| 130 | Vienna, canned (7 sausages per 5-oz can) | 1 sausage | 16 | 63 | 40 | 2 | 3 | — | — | — | Trace | 1 | 0.3 | — | 0.01 | 0.02 | 0.4 | — |
| 131 | Veal, medium fat, cooked, bone removed: Cutlet | 3 oz | 85 | 60 | 185 | 23 | 9 | 5 | 4 | Trace | — | 9 | 2.7 | — | 0.06 | 0.21 | 4.6 | — |
| 132 | Roast | 3 oz | 85 | 55 | 230 | 23 | 14 | 7 | 6 | Trace | 0 | 10 | 2.9 | — | 0.11 | 0.26 | 6.6 | — |
| 133 | Fish and shellfish: Bluefish, baked with table fat | 3 oz | 85 | 68 | 135 | 22 | 4 | — | — | — | 0 | 25 | 0.6 | 40 | 0.09 | 0.08 | 1.6 | — |
| 134 | Clams: Raw, meat only | 3 oz | 85 | 82 | 65 | 11 | 1 | — | — | — | 2 | 59 | 5.2 | 90 | 0.08 | 0.15 | 1.1 | 8 |
| 135 | Canned, solids and liquid | 3 oz | 85 | 86 | 45 | 7 | 1 | — | — | — | 2 | 47 | 3.5 | — | 0.01 | 0.09 | 0.9 | — |
| 136 | Crabmeat, canned | 3 oz | 85 | 77 | 85 | 15 | 2 | — | — | — | 1 | 38 | 0.7 | — | 0.07 | 0.07 | 1.6 | — |
| 137 | Fish sticks, breaded, cooked, frozen; stick 3 3/4 by 1 by 1/2 inch | 10 sticks or 8 oz pkg. | 227 | 66 | 400 | 38 | 20 | 5 | 4 | 10 | 15 | 25 | 0.9 | — | 0.09 | 0.16 | 3.6 | — |
| 138 | Haddock, breaded, fried | 3 oz | 85 | 66 | 140 | 17 | 5 | 1 | 3 | Trace | 5 | 34 | 1.0 | — | 0.03 | 0.06 | 2.7 | 2 |
| 139 | Ocean perch, breaded, fried | 3 oz | 85 | 59 | 195 | 16 | 11 | — | — | — | 6 | 28 | 1.1 | — | 0.08 | 0.09 | 1.5 | — |
| 140 | Oysters, raw, meat only (13–19 med. selects) | 1 cup | 240 | 85 | 160 | 20 | 4 | 1 | — | — | 8 | 226 | 13.2 | 740 | 0.33 | 0.43 | 6.0 | — |

### Mature Dry Beans and Peas, Nuts, Peanuts; Related Products (continued) / Vegetables and Vegetable Products

| No. | Food | Measure | Grams | Water (%) | Food energy (cal) | Protein (g) | Fat (g) | Fatty acids — Saturated (total) (g) | Unsaturated Oleic (g) | Unsaturated Linoleic (g) | Carbohydrate (g) | Calcium (mg) | Iron (mg) | Vitamin A (I.U.) | Thiamin (mg) | Riboflavin (mg) | Niacin (mg) | Ascorbic acid (mg) |
|---|---|---|---|---|---|---|---|---|---|---|---|---|---|---|---|---|---|---|
| 141 | Salmon, pink, canned | 3 oz | 85 | 71 | 120 | 17 | 5 | 1 | 1 | — | 0 | ⁴167 | 0.7 | 60 | 0.03 | 0.16 | 6.8 | — |
| 142 | Sardines, Atlantic, canned in oil, drained solids | 3 oz | 85 | 62 | 175 | 20 | 9 | — | — | — | 0 | 372 | 2.5 | 190 | 0.02 | 0.17 | 4.6 | — |
| 143 | Shad, baked with table fat and bacon | 3 oz | 85 | 64 | 170 | 20 | 10 | — | — | — | 0 | 20 | 0.5 | 20 | 0.11 | 0.22 | 7.3 | — |
| 144 | Shrimp, canned, meat | 3 oz | 85 | 70 | 100 | 21 | 1 | — | — | — | 1 | 98 | 2.6 | 50 | 0.01 | 0.03 | 1.5 | — |
| 145 | Swordfish, broiled with butter or margarine | 3 oz | 85 | 65 | 150 | 24 | 5 | — | — | — | 0 | 23 | 1.1 | 1,750 | 0.03 | 0.04 | 9.3 | — |
| 146 | Tuna, canned in oil, drained solids | 3 oz | 85 | 61 | 170 | 24 | 7 | 2 | 1 | 2 | 0 | 7 | 1.6 | 70 | 0.04 | 0.10 | 10.1 | — |

**Mature Dry Beans and Peas, Nuts, Peanuts; Related Products**

| No. | Food | Measure | Grams | Water (%) | Food energy (cal) | Protein (g) | Fat (g) | Saturated (total) (g) | Oleic (g) | Linoleic (g) | Carbohydrate (g) | Calcium (mg) | Iron (mg) | Vitamin A (I.U.) | Thiamin (mg) | Riboflavin (mg) | Niacin (mg) | Ascorbic acid (mg) |
|---|---|---|---|---|---|---|---|---|---|---|---|---|---|---|---|---|---|---|
| 147 | Almonds, shelled, whole kernels | 1 cup | 142 | 5 | 850 | 26 | 77 | 6 | 52 | 15 | 28 | 332 | 6.7 | 0 | 0.34 | 1.31 | 5.0 | Trace |
| | Beans, dry: Common varieties as Great Northern, navy and others: Cooked, drained: | | | | | | | | | | | | | | | | | |
| 148 | Great Northern | 1 cup | 180 | 69 | 210 | 14 | 1 | — | — | — | 38 | 90 | 4.9 | 0 | 0.25 | 0.13 | 1.3 | 0 |
| 149 | Navy (pea) | 1 cup | 190 | 69 | 225 | 15 | 1 | — | — | — | 40 | 95 | 5.1 | 0 | 0.27 | 0.13 | 1.3 | 0 |
| | Canned, solids and liquid: White with— | | | | | | | | | | | | | | | | | |
| 150 | Frankfurters (sliced) | 1 cup | 255 | 71 | 365 | 19 | 18 | — | — | — | 32 | 94 | 4.8 | 330 | 0.18 | 0.15 | 3.3 | Trace |
| 151 | Pork and tomato sauce | 1 cup | 255 | 71 | 310 | 16 | 7 | — | — | — | 49 | 138 | 4.6 | 330 | 0.20 | 0.08 | 1.5 | 5 |
| 152 | Pork and sweet sauce | 1 cup | 255 | 66 | 385 | 16 | 12 | — | — | — | 54 | 161 | 5.9 | 10 | 0.15 | 0.10 | 1.3 | — |
| 153 | Red kidney | 1 cup | 255 | 76 | 230 | 15 | 1 | — | — | — | 42 | 74 | 4.6 | — | 0.13 | 0.10 | 1.5 | — |
| 154 | Lima, cooked, drained | 1 cup | 190 | 64 | 260 | 16 | 1 | — | — | — | 49 | 55 | 5.9 | — | 0.25 | 0.11 | 1.3 | — |
| 155 | Cashew nuts, roasted | 1 cup | 140 | 5 | 785 | 24 | 64 | 11 | 45 | 4 | 41 | 53 | 5.3 | 140 | 0.60 | 0.35 | 2.5 | — |
| | Coconut, fresh, meat only: | | | | | | | | | | | | | | | | | |
| 156 | Pieces, approx. 2 by 2 by 1/2 inch | 1 piece | 45 | 51 | 155 | 2 | 16 | 14 | 1 | — | 4 | 6 | 0.8 | 0 | 0.02 | 0.01 | 0.2 | 1 |
| 157 | Shredded or grated, firmly packed | 1 cup | 130 | 51 | 450 | 5 | 46 | 39 | 3 | — | 42 | 17 | 2.2 | 0 | 0.07 | 0.03 | 0.7 | 4 |
| 158 | Cowpeas or blackeye peas, dry, cooked | 1 cup | 248 | 80 | 190 | 13 | 1 | — | — | — | 34 | 42 | 3.2 | 20 | 0.41 | 0.11 | 1.1 | Trace |
| 159 | Peanuts, roasted, salted, halves | 1 cup | 144 | 2 | 840 | 37 | 72 | 16 | 31 | 21 | 27 | 107 | 3.0 | — | 0.46 | 0.19 | 24.7 | 0 |
| 160 | Peanut butter | 1 tbsp | 16 | 2 | 95 | 4 | 8 | 2 | 4 | 2 | 3 | 9 | 0.3 | — | 0.02 | 0.02 | 2.4 | 0 |
| 161 | Peas, split, dry, cooked | 1 cup | 250 | 70 | 290 | 20 | 1 | — | — | — | 52 | 28 | 4.2 | 100 | 0.37 | 0.22 | 2.2 | — |
| 162 | Pecans, halves | 1 cup | 108 | 3 | 740 | 10 | 77 | 5 | 48 | 15 | 16 | 79 | 2.6 | 140 | 0.93 | 0.14 | 1.0 | 2 |
| 163 | Walnuts, black or native, chopped | 1 cup | 126 | 3 | 790 | 26 | 75 | 4 | 26 | 36 | 19 | Trace | 7.6 | 380 | 0.28 | 0.14 | 0.9 | — |

**Vegetables and Vegetable Products**

| No. | Food | Measure | Grams | Water (%) | Food energy (cal) | Protein (g) | Fat (g) | Saturated (total) (g) | Oleic (g) | Linoleic (g) | Carbohydrate (g) | Calcium (mg) | Iron (mg) | Vitamin A (I.U.) | Thiamin (mg) | Riboflavin (mg) | Niacin (mg) | Ascorbic acid (mg) |
|---|---|---|---|---|---|---|---|---|---|---|---|---|---|---|---|---|---|---|
| | Asparagus, green: Cooked, drained: | | | | | | | | | | | | | | | | | |
| 164 | Spears, 1/2-in. diam. at base | 4 spears | 60 | 94 | 10 | 1 | Trace | — | — | — | 2 | 13 | 0.4 | 540 | 0.10 | 0.11 | 0.8 | 16 |
| 165 | Pieces, 1 1/2 to 2-in. lengths | 1 cup | 145 | 94 | 30 | 3 | Trace | — | — | — | 5 | 30 | 0.9 | 1,310 | 0.23 | 0.26 | 2.0 | 38 |
| 166 | Canned, solids and liquid | 1 cup | 244 | 94 | 45 | 5 | 1 | — | — | — | 7 | 44 | 4.1 | 1,240 | 0.15 | 0.22 | 2.0 | 37 |

³Outer layer of fat on the cut was removed to within approximately 1/2-inch of the lean. Deposits of fat within the cut were not removed.

⁴If bones are discarded, value will be greatly reduced.

# Table A-1. (Cont.)

| | Food, Approximate Measure, and Weight (in grams) | | gm | Water per cent | Food Energy calories | Pro-tein gm | Fat gm | Fatty Acids Satu-rated (total) gm | Unsaturated Oleic gm | Lin-oleic gm | Carbo-hy-drate gm | Cal-cium mg | Iron mg | Vita-min A Value I.U. | Thia-mine mg | Ribo-flavin mg | Niacin mg | Ascor-bic Acid mg |
|---|---|---|---|---|---|---|---|---|---|---|---|---|---|---|---|---|---|---|
| | Beans: | | | | | | | | | | | | | | | | | |
| 167 | Lima, immature seeds, cooked, drained | 1 cup | 170 | 71 | 190 | 13 | 1 | — | — | — | 34 | 80 | 4.3 | 480 | 0.31 | 0.17 | 2.2 | 29 |
| | Snap: | | | | | | | | | | | | | | | | | |
| | Green: | | | | | | | | | | | | | | | | | |
| 168 | Cooked, drained | 1 cup | 125 | 92 | 30 | 2 | Trace | — | — | — | 7 | 63 | 0.8 | 680 | 0.09 | 0.11 | 0.6 | 15 |
| 169 | Canned, solids and liquid | 1 cup | 239 | 94 | 45 | 2 | Trace | — | — | — | 10 | 81 | 2.9 | 690 | 0.07 | 0.10 | 0.7 | 10 |
| | Yellow or wax: | | | | | | | | | | | | | | | | | |
| 170 | Cooked, drained | 1 cup | 125 | 93 | 30 | 2 | Trace | — | — | — | 6 | 63 | 0.8 | 290 | 0.09 | 0.11 | 0.6 | 16 |
| 171 | Canned, solids and liquid | 1 cup | 239 | 94 | 45 | 2 | 1 | — | — | — | 10 | 81 | 2.9 | 140 | 0.07 | 0.10 | 0.7 | 12 |
| 172 | Sprouted mung beans, cooked, drained | 1 cup | 125 | 91 | 35 | 4 | Trace | — | — | — | 7 | 21 | 1.1 | 30 | 0.11 | 0.13 | 0.9 | 8 |
| | Beets: | | | | | | | | | | | | | | | | | |
| | Cooked, drained, peeled: | | | | | | | | | | | | | | | | | |
| 173 | Whole beets, 2-in. diam. | 2 beets | 100 | 91 | 30 | 1 | Trace | — | — | — | 7 | 14 | 0.5 | 20 | 0.03 | 0.04 | 0.3 | 6 |
| 174 | Diced or sliced | 1 cup | 170 | 91 | 55 | 2 | Trace | — | — | — | 12 | 24 | 0.9 | 30 | 0.05 | 0.07 | 0.5 | 10 |
| 175 | Canned, solids and liquid | 1 cup | 246 | 90 | 85 | 2 | Trace | — | — | — | 19 | 34 | 1.5 | 20 | 0.02 | 0.05 | 0.2 | 7 |
| 176 | Beet greens, leaves and stems, cooked, drained | 1 cup | 145 | 94 | 25 | 3 | Trace | — | — | — | 5 | 144 | 2.8 | 7,400 | 0.10 | 0.22 | 0.4 | 22 |
| | Blackeye peas. See Cowpeas | | | | | | | | | | | | | | | | | |
| | Broccoli, cooked, drained: | | | | | | | | | | | | | | | | | |
| 177 | Whole stalks, medium size | 1 stalk | 180 | 91 | 45 | 6 | 1 | — | — | — | 8 | 158 | 1.4 | 4,500 | 0.16 | 0.36 | 1.4 | 162 |
| 178 | Stalks cut into 1/2-in pieces | 1 cup | 155 | 91 | 40 | 5 | 1 | — | — | — | 7 | 136 | 1.2 | 3,880 | 0.14 | 0.31 | 1.2 | 140 |
| 179 | Chopped, yield from 10-oz frozen pkg | 1 3/8 cups | 250 | 92 | 65 | 7 | 1 | — | — | — | 12 | 135 | 1.8 | 6,500 | 0.15 | 0.30 | 1.3 | 143 |
| 180 | Brussels sprouts, 7–8 sprouts (1 1/4 to 1 1/2 in. diam.) | 1 cup | 155 | 88 | 55 | 7 | 1 | — | — | — | 10 | 50 | 1.7 | 810 | 0.12 | 0.22 | 1.2 | 135 |
| | Cabbage: | | | | | | | | | | | | | | | | | |
| | Common varieties: | | | | | | | | | | | | | | | | | |
| | Raw: | | | | | | | | | | | | | | | | | |
| 181 | Coarsely shredded or sliced | 1 cup | 70 | 92 | 15 | 1 | Trace | — | — | — | 4 | 34 | 0.3 | 90 | 0.04 | 0.04 | 0.2 | 33 |
| 182 | Finely shredded or chopped | 1 cup | 90 | 92 | 20 | 1 | Trace | — | — | — | 5 | 44 | 0.4 | 120 | 0.05 | 0.05 | 0.3 | 42 |
| 183 | Cooked | 1 cup | 145 | 94 | 30 | 2 | Trace | — | — | — | 6 | 64 | 0.4 | 190 | 0.06 | 0.06 | 0.4 | 48 |
| 184 | Red, raw, coarsely shredded | 1 cup | 70 | 90 | 20 | 1 | Trace | — | — | — | 5 | 29 | 0.6 | 30 | 0.06 | 0.04 | 0.3 | 43 |
| 185 | Savoy, raw, coarsely shredded | 1 cup | 70 | 92 | 15 | 2 | Trace | — | — | — | 3 | 47 | 0.6 | 140 | 0.04 | 0.06 | 0.2 | 39 |
| 186 | Cabbage, celery or Chinese raw, cut in 1-in pieces | 1 cup | 75 | 95 | 10 | 1 | Trace | — | — | — | 2 | 32 | 0.5 | 110 | 0.04 | 0.03 | 0.5 | 19 |
| 187 | Cabbage, spoon (or pakchoy), cooked | 1 cup | 170 | 95 | 25 | 2 | Trace | — | — | — | 4 | 252 | 1.0 | 5,270 | 0.07 | 0.14 | 1.2 | 26 |
| | Carrots: | | | | | | | | | | | | | | | | | |
| | Raw: | | | | | | | | | | | | | | | | | |
| 188 | Whole, 5 1/2 by 1 inch, (25 thin strips) | 1 carrot | 50 | 88 | 20 | 1 | Trace | — | — | — | 5 | 18 | 0.4 | 5,500 | 0.03 | 0.03 | 0.3 | 4 |

| No. | Food | Measure | Weight (g) | Water (%) | Food energy (cal) | Protein (g) | Fat (g) | Saturated | Oleic | Linoleic | Carbohydrate (g) | Calcium (mg) | Iron (mg) | Vitamin A (I.U.) | Thiamine (mg) | Riboflavin (mg) | Niacin (mg) | Ascorbic acid (mg) |
|---|---|---|---|---|---|---|---|---|---|---|---|---|---|---|---|---|---|---|
| 189 | Grated | 1 cup | 110 | 88 | 45 | 1 | Trace | — | — | — | 11 | 41 | 0.8 | 12,100 | 0.06 | 0.06 | 0.7 | 9 |
| 190 | Cooked, diced | 1 cup | 145 | 91 | 45 | 1 | Trace | — | — | — | 10 | 48 | 0.9 | 15,220 | 0.08 | 0.07 | 0.7 | 9 |
| 191 | Canned, strained or chopped (baby food) | 1 ounce | 28 | 92 | 10 | Trace | Trace | — | — | — | 2 | 7 | 0.1 | 3,690 | 0.01 | 0.01 | 0.1 | 1 |
| 192 | Cauliflower, cooked, flower-buds | 1 cup | 120 | 93 | 25 | 3 | Trace | — | — | — | 5 | 25 | 0.8 | 70 | 0.11 | 0.10 | 0.7 | 66 |
| 193 | Celery, raw: Stalk, large outer, 8 by about 1 1/2 inches, at root end | 1 stalk | 40 | 94 | 5 | Trace | Trace | — | — | — | 2 | 16 | 0.1 | 100 | 0.01 | 0.01 | 0.1 | 4 |
| 194 | Pieces, diced | 1 cup | 100 | 94 | 15 | 1 | Trace | — | — | — | 4 | 39 | 0.3 | 240 | 0.03 | 0.03 | 0.3 | 9 |
| 195 | Collards, cooked | 1 cup | 190 | 91 | 55 | 5 | 1 | — | — | — | 9 | 289 | 1.1 | 10,260 | 0.27 | 0.37 | 2.4 | 87 |
| 196 | Corn sweet: Cooked, ear 5 by 1 3/4 inches[5] | 1 ear | 140 | 74 | 70 | 3 | 1 | — | — | — | 16 | 2 | 0.5 | [6]310 | 0.09 | 0.08 | 1.0 | 7 |
| 197 | Canned, solids and liquid | 1 cup | 256 | 81 | 170 | 5 | 2 | — | — | — | 40 | 10 | 1.0 | [6]690 | 0.07 | 0.12 | 2.3 | 13 |
| 198 | Cowpeas, cooked immature seeds | 1 cup | 160 | 72 | 175 | 13 | 1 | — | — | — | 29 | 38 | 3.4 | 560 | 0.49 | 0.18 | 2.3 | 28 |
| 199 | Cucumbers, 10-ounce; 7 1/2 by about 2 inches: Raw, pared | 1 cucumber | 207 | 96 | 30 | 1 | Trace | — | — | — | 7 | 35 | 0.6 | Trace | 0.07 | 0.09 | 0.4 | 23 |
| 200 | Raw, pared, center slice 1/8-inch thick | 6 slices | 50 | 96 | 5 | Trace | Trace | — | — | — | 2 | 8 | 0.2 | Trace | 0.02 | 0.02 | 0.1 | 6 |
| 201 | Dandelion greens, cooked | 1 cup | 180 | 90 | 60 | 4 | 1 | — | — | — | 12 | 252 | 3.2 | 21,060 | 0.24 | 0.29 | — | 32 |
| 202 | Endive, curly (including escarole) | 2 ounces | 57 | 93 | 10 | 1 | Trace | — | — | — | 2 | 46 | 1.0 | 1,870 | 0.04 | 0.08 | 0.3 | 6 |
| 203 | Kale, leaves including stems, cooked | 1 cup | 110 | 91 | 30 | 4 | 1 | — | — | — | 4 | 147 | 1.3 | 8,140 | 0.14 | — | — | 68 |
| 204 | Lettuce, raw: Butterhead, as Boston types; head, 4-inch diameter | 1 head | 220 | 95 | 30 | 3 | Trace | — | — | — | 6 | 77 | 4.4 | 2,130 | 0.14 | 0.13 | 0.6 | 18 |
| 205 | Crisphead, as Iceberg; head, 4 3/4 inch diameter | 1 head | 454 | 96 | 60 | 4 | Trace | — | — | — | 13 | 91 | 2.3 | 1,500 | 0.29 | 0.27 | 1.3 | 29 |
| 206 | Looseleaf, or bunching varieties, leaves | 2 large | 50 | 94 | 10 | 1 | Trace | — | — | — | 2 | 34 | 0.7 | 950 | 0.03 | 0.04 | 0.2 | 9 |
| 207 | Mushrooms, canned, solids and liquid | 1 cup | 244 | 93 | 40 | 5 | Trace | — | — | — | 6 | 15 | 1.2 | Trace | 0.04 | 0.60 | 4.8 | 4 |
| 208 | Mustard greens, cooked | 1 cup | 140 | 93 | 35 | 3 | 1 | — | — | — | 6 | 193 | 2.5 | 8,120 | 0.11 | 0.19 | 0.9 | 68 |
| 209 | Okra, cooked, pod 3 by 5/8 inch | 8 pods | 85 | 91 | 25 | 2 | Trace | — | — | — | 5 | 78 | 0.4 | 420 | 0.11 | 0.15 | 0.8 | 17 |
| 210 | Onions: Mature: Raw, onion 2 1/2-inch diameter | 1 onion | 110 | 89 | 40 | 2 | Trace | — | — | — | 10 | 30 | 0.6 | 40 | 0.04 | 0.04 | 0.2 | 11 |
| 211 | Cooked | 1 cup | 210 | 92 | 60 | 3 | Trace | — | — | — | 14 | 50 | 0.8 | 80 | 0.06 | 0.06 | 0.4 | 14 |
| 212 | Young green, small, without tops | 6 onions | 50 | 88 | 20 | 1 | Trace | — | — | — | 5 | 20 | 0.3 | Trace | 0.02 | 0.02 | 0.2 | 12 |
| 213 | Parsley, raw, chopped | 1 tablespoon | 4 | 85 | Trace | Trace | Trace | — | — | — | Trace | 8 | 0.2 | 340 | Trace | 0.01 | Trace | 7 |
| 214 | Parsnips, cooked | 1 cup | 155 | 82 | 100 | 2 | 1 | — | — | — | 23 | 70 | 0.9 | 50 | 0.11 | 0.12 | 0.2 | 16 |
| 215 | Peas, green: Cooked | 1 cup | 160 | 82 | 115 | 9 | 1 | — | — | — | 19 | 37 | 2.9 | 860 | 0.44 | 0.17 | 3.7 | 33 |
| 216 | Canned, solids and liquid | 1 cup | 249 | 83 | 165 | 9 | 1 | — | — | — | 31 | 50 | 4.2 | 1,120 | 0.23 | 0.13 | 2.2 | 22 |
| 217 | Canned, strained (baby food) | 1 ounce | 28 | 86 | 15 | 1 | Trace | — | — | — | 3 | 3 | 0.4 | 140 | 0.02 | 0.02 | 0.4 | 3 |

[5] Measure and weight apply to entire vegetable or fruit including parts not usually eaten.

[6] Based on yellow varieties; white varieties contain only a trace of cryptoxanthin and carotenes, the pigments in corn that have biologic activity.

**Table A-1. (Cont.)**

| | Food, Approximate Measure, and Weight (in grams) | | Water per cent | Food Energy calories | Pro-tein gm | Fat gm | Fatty Acids | | | Carbo-hy-drate gm | Cal-cium mg | Iron mg | Vita-min A Value I.U. | Thia-mine mg | Ribo-flavin mg | Niacin mg | Ascor-bic Acid mg |
| | | | | | | | Satu-rated (total) gm | Unsaturated Oleic gm | Lin-oleic gm | | | | | | | | |
|---|---|---|---|---|---|---|---|---|---|---|---|---|---|---|---|---|---|
| | | gm | | | | | | | | | | | | | | | |
| 218 | Peppers, hot, red, without seeds, dried (ground chili powder, added seasonings) | 1 tablespoon | 15 | 8 | 50 | 2 | 2 | — | — | — | 8 | 40 | 2.3 | 9,750 | 0.03 | 0.17 | 1.3 | 2 |
| | Peppers, sweet: | | | | | | | | | | | | | | | | | |
| | Raw, about 5 per pound: | | | | | | | | | | | | | | | | | |
| 219 | Green pod without stem and seeds | 1 pod | 74 | 93 | 15 | 1 | Trace | — | — | — | 4 | 7 | 0.5 | 310 | 0.06 | 0.06 | 0.4 | 94 |
| 220 | Cooked, boiled, drained | 1 pod | 73 | 95 | 15 | 1 | Trace | — | — | — | 3 | 7 | 0.4 | 310 | 0.05 | 0.05 | 0.4 | 70 |
| | Potatoes, medium (about 3 per pound raw): | | | | | | | | | | | | | | | | | |
| 221 | Baked, peeled after baking | 1 potato | 99 | 75 | 90 | 3 | Trace | — | — | — | 21 | 9 | 0.7 | Trace | 0.10 | 0.04 | 1.7 | 20 |
| | Boiled: | | | | | | | | | | | | | | | | | |
| 222 | Peeled after boiling | 1 potato | 136 | 80 | 105 | 3 | Trace | — | — | — | 23 | 10 | 0.8 | Trace | 0.13 | 0.05 | 2.0 | 22 |
| 223 | Peeled before boiling | 1 potato | 122 | 83 | 80 | 2 | Trace | — | — | — | 18 | 7 | 0.6 | Trace | 0.11 | 0.04 | 1.4 | 20 |
| | French-fried, piece 2 by 1/2 by 1/2 inch: | | | | | | | | | | | | | | | | | |
| 224 | Cooked in deep fat | 10 pieces | 57 | 45 | 155 | 2 | 7 | 2 | 2 | 4 | 20 | 9 | 0.7 | Trace | 0.07 | 0.04 | 1.8 | 12 |
| 225 | Frozen, heated | 10 pieces | 57 | 53 | 125 | 2 | 5 | 1 | 1 | 2 | 19 | 5 | 1.0 | Trace | 0.08 | 0.01 | 1.5 | 12 |
| | Mashed: | | | | | | | | | | | | | | | | | |
| 226 | Milk added | 1 cup | 195 | 83 | 125 | 4 | 1 | — | — | — | 25 | 47 | 0.8 | 50 | 0.16 | 0.10 | 2.0 | 19 |
| 227 | Milk and butter added | 1 cup | 195 | 80 | 185 | 4 | 8 | 4 | 3 | Trace | 24 | 47 | 0.8 | 330 | 0.16 | 0.10 | 1.9 | 18 |
| 228 | Potato chips, medium, 2-inch diameter | 10 chips | 20 | 2 | 115 | 1 | 8 | 2 | 2 | 4 | 10 | 8 | 0.4 | Trace | 0.04 | 0.01 | 1.0 | 3 |
| 229 | Pumpkin, canned | 1 cup | 228 | 90 | 75 | 2 | 1 | — | — | — | 18 | 57 | 0.9 | 14,590 | 0.07 | 0.12 | 1.3 | 12 |
| 230 | Radishes, raw, small, without tops | 4 radishes | 40 | 94 | 5 | Trace | Trace | — | — | — | 1 | 12 | 0.4 | Trace | 0.01 | 0.01 | 0.1 | 10 |
| 231 | Sauerkraut, canned, solids and liquid | 1 cup | 235 | 93 | 45 | 2 | Trace | — | — | — | 9 | 85 | 1.2 | 120 | 0.07 | 0.09 | 0.4 | 33 |
| | Spinach: | | | | | | | | | | | | | | | | | |
| 232 | Cooked | 1 cup | 180 | 92 | 40 | 5 | 1 | — | — | — | 6 | 167 | 4.0 | 14,580 | 0.13 | 0.25 | 1.0 | 50 |
| 233 | Canned, drained solids | 1 cup | 180 | 91 | 45 | 5 | 1 | — | — | — | 6 | 212 | 4.7 | 14,400 | 0.03 | 0.21 | 0.6 | 24 |
| | Squash: | | | | | | | | | | | | | | | | | |
| | Cooked: | | | | | | | | | | | | | | | | | |
| 234 | Summer, diced | 1 cup | 210 | 96 | 30 | 2 | Trace | — | — | — | 7 | 52 | 0.8 | 820 | 0.10 | 0.16 | 1.6 | 21 |
| 235 | Winter, baked, mashed | 1 cup | 205 | 81 | 130 | 4 | 1 | — | — | — | 32 | 57 | 1.6 | 8,610 | 0.10 | 0.27 | 1.4 | 27 |
| | Sweetpotatoes: | | | | | | | | | | | | | | | | | |
| | Cooked, medium, 5 by 2 inches, weight raw about 6 ounces: | | | | | | | | | | | | | | | | | |
| 236 | Baked, peeled after baking | 1 sweet-potato | 110 | 64 | 155 | 2 | 1 | — | — | — | 36 | 44 | 1.0 | 8,910 | 0.10 | 0.07 | 0.7 | 24 |
| 237 | Boiled, peeled after boiling | 1 sweet-potato | 147 | 71 | 170 | 2 | 1 | — | — | — | 39 | 47 | 1.0 | 11,610 | 0.13 | 0.09 | 0.9 | 25 |
| 238 | Candied, 3 1/2 by 2 1/4 inches | 1 sweet-potato | 175 | 60 | 295 | 2 | 6 | 2 | 3 | 1 | 60 | 65 | 1.6 | 11,030 | 0.10 | 0.08 | 0.8 | 17 |
| 239 | Canned, vacuum or solid pack | 1 cup | 218 | 72 | 235 | 4 | Trace | — | — | — | 54 | 54 | 1.7 | 17,000 | 0.10 | 0.10 | 1.4 | 30 |
| | Tomatoes: | | | | | | | | | | | | | | | | | |
| 240 | Raw, approx. 3-in diam. 2 1/8 in high; wt. 7 oz | 1 tomato | 200 | 94 | 40 | 2 | Trace | — | — | — | 9 | 24 | 0.9 | 1,640 | 0.11 | 0.07 | 1.3 | 42 |
| 241 | Canned, solids and liquid | 1 cup | 241 | 94 | 50 | 2 | 1 | — | — | — | 10 | 14 | 1.2 | 2,170 | 0.12 | 0.07 | 1.7 | 41 |

## Fruits and Fruit Products

| No. | Food | Measure | Grams | Water (%) | Food energy (Cal) | Protein (g) | Fat (g) | Saturated (g) | Oleic (g) | Linoleic (g) | Carbohydrate (g) | Calcium (mg) | Iron (mg) | Vitamin A (I.U.) | Thiamin (mg) | Riboflavin (mg) | Niacin (mg) | Ascorbic acid (mg) |
|---|---|---|---|---|---|---|---|---|---|---|---|---|---|---|---|---|---|---|
| | Tomato catsup: | | | | | | | | | | | | | | | | | |
| 242 | Cup | 1 cup | 273 | 69 | 290 | 6 | 1 | — | — | — | 69 | 60 | 2.2 | 3,820 | 0.25 | 0.19 | 4.4 | 41 |
| 243 | Tablespoon | 1 tbsp. | 15 | 69 | 15 | Trace | Trace | — | — | — | 4 | 3 | 0.1 | 210 | 0.01 | 0.01 | 0.2 | 2 |
| | Tomato juice, canned: | | | | | | | | | | | | | | | | | |
| 244 | Cup | 1 cup | 243 | 94 | 45 | 2 | Trace | — | — | — | 10 | 17 | 2.2 | 1,940 | 0.12 | 0.07 | 1.9 | 39 |
| 245 | Glass (6 fl oz) | 1 glass | 182 | 94 | 35 | 2 | Trace | — | — | — | 8 | 13 | 1.6 | 1,460 | 0.09 | 0.05 | 1.5 | 29 |
| 246 | Turnips, cooked, diced | 1 cup | 155 | 94 | 35 | 1 | Trace | — | — | — | 8 | 54 | 0.6 | Trace | 0.06 | 0.08 | 0.5 | 34 |
| 247 | Turnips greens, cooked | 1 cup | 145 | 94 | 30 | 3 | Trace | — | — | — | 5 | 252 | 1.5 | 8,270 | 0.15 | 0.33 | 0.7 | 68 |
| **Fruits and Fruit Products** | | | | | | | | | | | | | | | | | | |
| 248 | Apples, raw (about 3 per lb)5 | 1 apple | 150 | 85 | 70 | Trace | Trace | — | — | — | 18 | 8 | 0.4 | 50 | 0.04 | 0.02 | 0.1 | 3 |
| 249 | Apple juice, bottled or canned | 1 cup | 248 | 88 | 120 | Trace | Trace | — | — | — | 30 | 15 | 1.5 | — | 0.02 | 0.05 | 0.2 | 2 |
| | Applesauce, canned: | | | | | | | | | | | | | | | | | |
| 250 | Sweetened | 1 cup | 255 | 76 | 230 | 1 | Trace | — | — | — | 61 | 10 | 1.3 | 100 | 0.05 | 0.03 | 0.1 | 83 |
| 251 | Unsweetened or artificially sweetened | 1 cup | 244 | 88 | 100 | 1 | Trace | — | — | — | 26 | 10 | 1.2 | 100 | 0.05 | 0.02 | 0.1 | 82 |
| | Apricots: | | | | | | | | | | | | | | | | | |
| 252 | Raw (about 12 per lb)5 | 3 apricots | 114 | 85 | 55 | 1 | Trace | — | — | — | 14 | 18 | 0.5 | 2,890 | 0.03 | 0.04 | 0.7 | 10 |
| 253 | Canned in heavy syrup | 1 cup | 259 | 77 | 220 | 2 | Trace | — | — | — | 57 | 28 | 0.8 | 4,510 | 0.05 | 0.06 | 0.9 | 10 |
| 254 | Dried, uncooked (40 halves per cup) | 1 cup | 150 | 25 | 390 | 8 | 1 | — | — | — | 100 | 100 | 8.2 | 16,350 | 0.02 | 0.23 | 4.9 | 19 |
| 255 | Cooked, unsweetened, fruit and liquid | 1 cup | 285 | 76 | 240 | 5 | Trace | — | — | — | 62 | 63 | 5.1 | 8,550 | 0.01 | 0.13 | 2.8 | 8 |
| 256 | Apricot nectar, canned | 1 cup | 251 | 85 | 140 | 1 | Trace | — | — | — | 37 | 23 | 0.5 | 2,380 | 0.03 | 0.03 | 0.5 | 88 |
| 257 | Avocados, whole fruit, raw:5 California (mid- and late-winter; diam. 3 1/8 in) | 1 avocado | 284 | 74 | 370 | 5 | 37 | 5 | 17 | 7 | 13 | 22 | 1.3 | 630 | 0.24 | 0.43 | 3.5 | 30 |
| 258 | Florida (late summer, fall; diam. 3 5/8 in) | 1 avocado | 454 | 78 | 390 | 4 | 33 | 4 | 15 | 7 | 27 | 30 | 1.8 | 880 | 0.33 | 0.61 | 4.9 | 43 |
| 259 | Bananas, raw, medium size5 | 1 banana | 175 | 76 | 100 | 1 | Trace | — | — | — | 26 | 10 | 0.8 | 230 | 0.06 | 0.07 | 0.8 | 12 |
| 260 | Banana flakes | 1 cup | 100 | 3 | 340 | 4 | 1 | — | — | — | 89 | 32 | 2.8 | 760 | 0.18 | 0.24 | 2.8 | 7 |
| 261 | Blackberries, raw | 1 cup | 144 | 84 | 85 | 2 | 1 | — | — | — | 19 | 46 | 1.3 | 290 | 0.05 | 0.06 | 0.5 | 30 |
| 262 | Blueberries, raw | 1 cup | 140 | 83 | 85 | 1 | 1 | — | — | — | 21 | 21 | 1.4 | 140 | 0.04 | 0.08 | 0.6 | 20 |
| 263 | Cantaloups, raw; medium; 5-inch diameter about 1 2/3 pounds5 | 1/2 melon | 385 | 91 | 60 | 1 | Trace | — | — | — | 14 | 27 | 0.8 | 96,540 | 0.08 | 0.06 | 1.2 | 63 |
| 264 | Cherries, canned, red, sour, pitted, water pack | 1 cup | 244 | 88 | 105 | 2 | Trace | — | — | — | 26 | 37 | 0.7 | 1,660 | 0.07 | 0.05 | 0.5 | 12 |
| 265 | Cranberry juice cocktail, canned | 1 cup | 250 | 83 | 165 | Trace | Trace | — | — | — | 42 | 13 | 0.8 | Trace | 0.03 | 0.03 | 0.1 | 1040 |
| 266 | Cranberry sauce, sweetened, canned, strained | 1 cup | 277 | 62 | 405 | Trace | 1 | — | — | — | 104 | 17 | 0.6 | 60 | 0.03 | 0.03 | 0.1 | 6 |
| 267 | Dates, pitted, cut | 1 cup | 178 | 22 | 490 | 4 | 1 | — | — | — | 130 | 105 | 5.3 | 90 | 0.16 | 0.17 | 3.9 | 0 |
| 268 | Figs, dried, large, 2 by 1 in | 1 fig | 21 | 23 | 60 | 1 | Trace | — | — | — | 15 | 26 | 0.6 | 20 | 0.02 | 0.02 | 0.1 | 0 |
| 269 | Fruit cocktail, canned, in heavy syrup | 1 cup | 256 | 80 | 195 | 1 | Trace | — | — | — | 50 | 23 | 1.0 | 360 | 0.05 | 0.03 | 1.3 | 5 |
| | Grapefruit: | | | | | | | | | | | | | | | | | |
| 270 | Raw, medium, 3 3/4-in diam.5 White | 1/2 grapefruit | 241 | 88 | 45 | 1 | Trace | — | — | — | 12 | 19 | 0.5 | 10 | 0.05 | 0.02 | 0.2 | 44 |
| 271 | Pink or red | 1/2 grapefruit | 241 | 89 | 50 | 1 | Trace | — | — | — | 13 | 20 | 0.5 | 540 | 0.05 | 0.02 | 0.2 | 44 |
| 272 | Canned, syrup pack | 1 cup | 254 | 81 | 180 | 2 | Trace | — | — | — | 45 | 33 | 0.8 | 30 | 0.08 | 0.05 | 0.5 | 76 |

5 Measure and weight apply to entire vegetable or fruit including parts not usually eaten.
7 Year-round average. Samples marketed from November through May, average 20 milligrams per 200-gram tomato; from June through October, around 52 milligrams.
8 This is the amount from the fruit. Additional ascorbic acid may be added by the manufacturer. Refer to the label for this information.
9 Value for varieties with orange-colored flesh; value for varieties with green flesh would be about 540 I.U.
10 Value listed is based on products with label stating 30 mg per 6-fl-oz serving.

# Table A-1. (Cont.)

| | Food, Approximate Measure, and Weight (in grams) | | gm | Water per cent | Food Energy calories | Protein gm | Fat gm | Fatty Acids Saturated (total) gm | Unsaturated Oleic gm | Linoleic gm | Carbohydrate gm | Calcium mg | Iron mg | Vitamin A Value I.U. | Thiamine mg | Riboflavin mg | Niacin mg | Ascorbic Acid mg |
|---|---|---|---|---|---|---|---|---|---|---|---|---|---|---|---|---|---|---|
| 273 | Grapefruit juice: Fresh | 1 cup | 246 | 90 | 95 | 1 | Trace | — | — | — | 23 | 22 | 0.5 | (11) | 0.09 | 0.04 | 0.4 | 92 |
| 274 | Canned, white: Unsweetened | 1 cup | 247 | 89 | 100 | 1 | Trace | — | — | — | 24 | 20 | 1.0 | 20 | 0.07 | 0.04 | 0.4 | 84 |
| 275 | Sweetened | 1 cup | 250 | 86 | 130 | 1 | Trace | — | — | — | 32 | 20 | 1.0 | 20 | 0.07 | 0.04 | 0.4 | 78 |
| 276 | Frozen, concentrate, unsweetened: Undiluted, can, 6 fluid ounces | 1 can | 207 | 62 | 300 | 4 | 1 | — | — | — | 72 | 70 | 0.8 | 60 | 0.29 | 0.12 | 1.4 | 286 |
| 277 | Diluted with 3 parts water, by volume | 1 cup | 247 | 89 | 100 | 1 | Trace | — | — | — | 24 | 25 | 0.2 | 20 | 0.10 | 0.04 | 0.5 | 96 |
| 278 | Dehydrated crystals | 4 oz | 113 | 1 | 410 | 6 | 1 | — | — | — | 102 | 100 | 1.2 | 80 | 0.40 | 0.20 | 2.0 | 396 |
| 279 | Prepared with water (1 pound yields about 1 gallon) | 1 cup | 247 | 90 | 100 | 1 | Trace | — | — | — | 24 | 22 | 0.2 | 20 | 0.10 | 0.05 | 0.5 | 91 |
| | Grapes, raw:[5] | | | | | | | | | | | | | | | | | |
| 280 | American type (slip skin) | 1 cup | 153 | 82 | 65 | 1 | 1 | — | — | — | 15 | 15 | 0.4 | 100 | 0.05 | 0.03 | 0.2 | 3 |
| 281 | European type (adherent skin) | 1 cup | 160 | 81 | 95 | 1 | Trace | — | — | — | 25 | 17 | 0.6 | 140 | 0.07 | 0.04 | 0.4 | 6 |
| | Grapejuice: | | | | | | | | | | | | | | | | | |
| 282 | Canned or bottled | 1 cup | 253 | 83 | 165 | 1 | Trace | — | — | — | 42 | 28 | 0.8 | — | 0.10 | 0.05 | 0.5 | Trace |
| 283 | Frozen concentrate, sweetened: Undiluted, can, 6 fluid ounces | 1 can | 216 | 53 | 395 | 1 | Trace | — | — | — | 100 | 22 | 0.9 | 40 | 0.13 | 0.22 | 1.5 | (12) |
| 284 | Diluted with 3 parts water, by volume | 1 cup | 250 | 86 | 135 | 1 | Trace | — | — | — | 33 | 8 | 0.3 | 10 | 0.05 | 0.08 | 0.5 | (12) |
| 285 | Grapejuice drink, canned | 1 cup | 250 | 86 | 135 | Trace | Trace | — | — | — | 35 | 8 | 0.3 | — | 0.03 | 0.03 | 0.3 | (12) |
| 286 | Lemons, raw, 2 1/8-in diam., size 165.[5] Used for juice | 1 lemon | 110 | 90 | 20 | 1 | Trace | — | — | — | 6 | 19 | 0.4 | 10 | 0.03 | 0.01 | 0.1 | 39 |
| 287 | Lemon juice, raw | 1 cup | 244 | 91 | 60 | 1 | Trace | — | — | — | 20 | 17 | 0.5 | 50 | 0.07 | 0.02 | 0.2 | 112 |
| | Lemonade concentrate: | | | | | | | | | | | | | | | | | |
| 288 | Frozen, 6 fl oz per can | 1 can | 219 | 48 | 430 | Trace | Trace | — | — | — | 112 | 9 | 0.4 | 40 | 0.04 | 0.07 | 0.7 | 66 |
| 289 | Diluted with 4 1/3 parts water, by volume | 1 cup | 248 | 88 | 110 | Trace | Trace | — | — | — | 28 | 2 | Trace | Trace | Trace | 0.02 | 0.2 | 17 |
| | Lime juice: | | | | | | | | | | | | | | | | | |
| 290 | Fresh | 1 cup | 246 | 90 | 65 | 1 | Trace | — | — | — | 22 | 22 | 0.5 | 20 | 0.05 | 0.02 | 0.2 | 79 |
| 291 | Canned, unsweetened | 1 cup | 246 | 90 | 65 | 1 | Trace | — | — | — | 22 | 22 | 0.5 | 20 | 0.05 | 0.02 | 0.2 | 52 |
| 292 | Limeade concentrate, frozen: Undiluted, can, 6 fluid ounces | 1 can | 218 | 50 | 410 | Trace | Trace | — | — | — | 108 | 11 | 0.2 | Trace | 0.02 | 0.02 | 0.2 | 26 |
| 293 | Diluted with 4 1/3 parts water, by volume | 1 cup | 247 | 90 | 100 | Trace | Trace | — | — | — | 27 | 2 | Trace | Trace | Trace | Trace | Trace | 5 |
| 294 | Oranges, raw, 2 5/8-in diam., all commercial varieties[5] | 1 orange | 180 | 86 | 65 | 1 | Trace | — | — | — | 16 | 54 | 0.5 | 260 | 0.13 | 0.05 | 0.5 | 66 |
| 295 | Orange juice, fresh, all varieties | 1 cup | 248 | 88 | 110 | 2 | 1 | — | — | — | 26 | 27 | 0.5 | 500 | 0.22 | 0.07 | 1.0 | 124 |
| 296 | Canned, unsweetened | 1 cup | 249 | 87 | 120 | 2 | Trace | — | — | — | 28 | 25 | 1.0 | 500 | 0.17 | 0.05 | 0.7 | 100 |
| 297 | Frozen concentrate: Undiluted, can, 6 fluid ounces | 1 can | 213 | 55 | 360 | 5 | Trace | — | — | — | 87 | 75 | 0.9 | 1,620 | 0.68 | 0.11 | 2.8 | 360 |

| No. | Food, approximate measure | Measure | Grams | Water (%) | Food energy (cal.) | Protein (g) | Fat (g) | Saturated | Oleic | Linoleic | Carbohydrate (g) | Calcium (mg) | Iron (mg) | Vitamin A (I.U.) | Thiamin (mg) | Riboflavin (mg) | Niacin (mg) | Ascorbic acid (mg) |
|---|---|---|---|---|---|---|---|---|---|---|---|---|---|---|---|---|---|---|
| 298 | Diluted with 3 parts water, by volume | 1 cup | 249 | 87 | 120 | 2 | Trace | — | — | — | 29 | 25 | 0.2 | 550 | 0.22 | 0.02 | 1.0 | 120 |
| 299 | Dehydrated crystals | 4 oz | 113 | 1 | 430 | 6 | 2 | — | — | — | 100 | 95 | 1.9 | 1,900 | 0.76 | 0.24 | 3.3 | 408 |
| 300 | Prepared with water (1 pound yields about 1 gallon) | 1 cup | 248 | 88 | 115 | 2 | 1 | — | — | — | 27 | 25 | 0.5 | 500 | 0.20 | 0.07 | 1.0 | 109 |
| 301 | Orange-apricot juice drink | 1 cup | 249 | 87 | 125 | 1 | Trace | — | — | — | 32 | 12 | 0.2 | 1,440 | 0.05 | 0.02 | 0.5 | [10]40 |
| | Orange and grapefruit juice: Frozen concentrate: | | | | | | | | | | | | | | | | | |
| 302 | Undiluted, can, 6 fluid ounces | 1 can | 210 | 59 | 330 | 4 | 1 | — | — | — | 78 | 61 | 0.8 | 800 | 0.48 | 0.06 | 2.3 | 302 |
| 303 | Diluted with 3 parts water, by volume | 1 cup | 248 | 88 | 110 | 1 | Trace | — | — | — | 26 | 20 | 0.2 | 270 | 0.16 | 0.02 | 0.8 | 102 |
| 304 | Papayas, raw, 1/2-inch cubes | 1 cup | 182 | 89 | 70 | 1 | Trace | — | — | — | 18 | 36 | 0.5 | 3,190 | 0.07 | 0.08 | 0.5 | 102 |
| | Peaches: Raw: | | | | | | | | | | | | | | | | | |
| 305 | Whole, medium, 2-inch diameter, about 4 per pound[5] | 1 peach | 114 | 89 | 35 | 1 | Trace | — | — | — | 10 | 9 | 0.5 | [13]1,320 | 0.02 | 0.05 | 1.0 | 7 |
| 306 | Sliced | 1 cup | 168 | 89 | 65 | 1 | Trace | — | — | — | 16 | 15 | 0.8 | [13]2,230 | 0.03 | 0.08 | 1.6 | 12 |
| | Canned, yellow-fleshed, solids and liquid: Syrup pack, heavy: | | | | | | | | | | | | | | | | | |
| 307 | Halves or slices | 1 cup | 257 | 79 | 200 | 1 | Trace | — | — | — | 52 | 10 | 0.8 | 1,100 | 0.02 | 0.06 | 1.4 | 7 |
| 308 | Water pack | 1 cup | 245 | 91 | 75 | 1 | Trace | — | — | — | 20 | 10 | 0.7 | 1,100 | 0.02 | 0.06 | 1.4 | 7 |
| 309 | Dried, uncooked | 1 cup | 160 | 25 | 420 | 5 | 1 | — | — | — | 109 | 77 | 9.6 | 6,240 | 0.02 | 0.31 | 8.5 | 28 |
| 310 | Cooked, unsweetened, 10–12 halves and juice | 1 cup | 270 | 77 | 220 | 3 | 1 | — | — | — | 58 | 41 | 5.1 | 3,290 | 0.01 | 0.15 | 4.2 | 6 |
| | Frozen: | | | | | | | | | | | | | | | | | |
| 311 | Carton, 12 ounces, not thawed | 1 carton | 340 | 76 | 300 | 1 | Trace | — | — | — | 77 | 14 | 1.7 | 2,210 | 0.03 | 0.14 | 2.4 | [14]135 |
| | Pears: | | | | | | | | | | | | | | | | | |
| 312 | Raw, 3 by 2 1/2-inch diameter[5] | 1 pear | 182 | 83 | 100 | 1 | 1 | — | — | — | 25 | 13 | 0.5 | 30 | 0.04 | 0.07 | 0.2 | 7 |
| | Canned, solids, and liquid: Syrup pack, heavy: | | | | | | | | | | | | | | | | | |
| 313 | Halves or slices | 1 cup | 255 | 80 | 195 | 1 | 1 | — | — | — | 50 | 13 | 0.5 | Trace | 0.03 | 0.05 | 0.3 | 4 |
| | Pineapple: | | | | | | | | | | | | | | | | | |
| 314 | Raw, diced | 1 cup | 140 | 85 | 75 | 1 | Trace | — | — | — | 19 | 24 | 0.7 | 100 | 0.12 | 0.04 | 0.3 | 24 |
| | Canned, heavy syrup pack, solids and liquids: | | | | | | | | | | | | | | | | | |
| 315 | Crushed | 1 cup | 260 | 80 | 195 | 1 | Trace | — | — | — | 50 | 29 | 0.8 | 120 | 0.20 | 0.06 | 0.5 | 17 |
| 316 | Sliced, slices and juice | 2 small or 1 large | 122 | 80 | 90 | Trace | Trace | — | — | — | 24 | 13 | 0.4 | 50 | 0.09 | 0.03 | 0.2 | 8 |
| 317 | Pineapple juice, canned | 1 cup | 249 | 86 | 135 | 1 | Trace | — | — | — | 34 | 37 | 0.7 | 120 | 0.12 | 0.04 | 0.5 | [8]22 |
| | Plums, all except prunes: | | | | | | | | | | | | | | | | | |
| 318 | Raw, 2-inch diameter, about 2 ounces[5] | 1 plum | 60 | 87 | 25 | Trace | Trace | — | — | — | 7 | 7 | 0.3 | 140 | 0.02 | 0.02 | 0.3 | 3 |
| | Canned, syrup pack (Italian prunes): | | | | | | | | | | | | | | | | | |
| 319 | Plums (with pits) and juice[5] | 1 cup | 256 | 77 | 205 | 1 | Trace | — | — | — | 53 | 22 | 2.2 | 2,970 | 0.05 | 0.05 | 0.9 | 4 |

[5] Measure and weight may apply to entire vegetable or fruit including parts not usually eaten.
[8] This is the amount from the fruit. Additional ascorbic acid may be added by the manufacturer. Refer to the label for this information.
[10] Value listed is based on product with label stating 30 milligrams per 6-fl-oz serving.
[11] For white-fleshed varieties value is about 20 I.U. per cup; for red-fleshed varieties, 1,080 I.U. per cup.
[12] Present only if added by the manufacturer. Refer to the label for this information.
[13] Based on yellow-fleshed varieties; for white-fleshed varieties value is about 50 I.U. per 114-gm peach and 80 I.U. per cup of sliced peaches.
[14] This value includes ascorbic acid added by manufacturer.

**Table A–1. (Cont.)**

| # | Food, Approximate Measure, and Weight (in grams) | Weight gm | Water per cent | Food Energy calories | Protein gm | Fat gm | Satu-rated (total) gm | Oleic gm | Lin-oleic gm | Carbo-hy-drate gm | Cal-cium mg | Iron mg | Vita-min A Value I.U. | Thia-mine mg | Ribo-flavin mg | Niacin mg | Ascor-bic Acid mg |
|---|---|---|---|---|---|---|---|---|---|---|---|---|---|---|---|---|---|
| | Prunes, dried, "softenized," medium: | | | | | | | | | | | | | | | | |
| 320 | Uncooked[5] 4 prunes | 32 | 28 | 70 | 1 | Trace | — | — | — | 18 | 14 | 1.1 | 440 | 0.02 | 0.04 | 0.4 | 1 |
| 321 | Cooked, unsweetened, 17–18 1 cup prunes and 1/3 cup liquid[5] | 270 | 66 | 295 | 2 | 1 | — | — | — | 78 | 60 | 4.5 | 1,860 | 0.08 | 0.18 | 1.7 | 2 |
| 322 | Prune juice, canned or bottled 1 cup | 256 | 80 | 200 | 1 | Trace | — | — | — | 49 | 36 | 10.5 | — | 0.03 | 0.03 | 1.0 | 85 |
| | Raisins, seedless: | | | | | | | | | | | | | | | | |
| 323 | Packaged, 1/2 oz or 1 1/2 1 pkg tbsp per pkg. | 14 | 18 | 40 | Trace | Trace | — | — | — | 11 | 9 | 0.5 | Trace | 0.02 | 0.01 | 0.1 | Trace |
| 324 | Cup, pressed down 1 cup | 165 | 18 | 480 | 4 | Trace | — | — | — | 128 | 102 | 5.8 | 30 | 0.18 | 0.13 | 0.8 | 2 |
| | Raspberries, red: | | | | | | | | | | | | | | | | |
| 325 | Raw 1 cup | 123 | 84 | 70 | 1 | 1 | — | — | — | 17 | 27 | 1.1 | 160 | 0.04 | 0.11 | 1.1 | 31 |
| 326 | Frozen, 10-ounce carton, 1 carton not thawed | 284 | 74 | 275 | 2 | 1 | — | — | — | 70 | 37 | 1.7 | 200 | 0.06 | 0.17 | 1.7 | 59 |
| 327 | Rhubarb, cooked, sugar added 1 cup | 272 | 63 | 385 | 1 | Trace | — | — | — | 98 | 212 | 1.6 | 220 | 0.06 | 0.15 | 0.7 | 17 |
| | Strawberries: | | | | | | | | | | | | | | | | |
| 328 | Raw, capped 1 cup | 149 | 90 | 55 | 1 | 1 | — | — | — | 13 | 31 | 1.5 | 90 | 0.04 | 0.10 | 1.0 | 88 |
| 329 | Frozen, 10-ounce carton, 1 carton not thawed | 284 | 71 | 310 | 1 | 1 | — | — | — | 79 | 40 | 2.0 | 90 | 0.06 | 0.17 | 1.5 | 150 |
| 330 | Tangerines, raw, medium, 1 tangerine 2 3/8-in diam., size 176[5] | 116 | 87 | 40 | 1 | Trace | — | — | — | 10 | 34 | 0.3 | 360 | 0.05 | 0.02 | 0.1 | 27 |
| 331 | Tangerine juice, canned, 1 cup sweetened | 249 | 87 | 125 | 1 | 1 | — | — | — | 30 | 45 | 0.5 | 1,050 | 0.15 | 0.05 | 0.2 | 55 |
| 332 | Watermelon, raw, wedge, 1 wedge 4 by 8 inches (1/16 of 10 by 16-inch melon, about 2 pounds with rind)[5] | 925 | 93 | 115 | 2 | 1 | — | — | — | 27 | 30 | 2.1 | 2,510 | 0.13 | 0.13 | 0.7 | 30 |
| | **Grain Products** | | | | | | | | | | | | | | | | |
| | Bagel, 3-in diam.: | | | | | | | | | | | | | | | | |
| 333 | Egg 1 bagel | 55 | 32 | 165 | 6 | 2 | — | — | — | 28 | 9 | 1.2 | 30 | 0.14 | 0.10 | 1.2 | 0 |
| 334 | Water 1 bagel | 55 | 29 | 165 | 6 | 2 | — | — | — | 30 | 8 | 1.2 | 0 | 0.15 | 0.11 | 1.4 | 0 |
| 335 | Barley, pearled, light, 1 cup uncooked | 200 | 11 | 700 | 16 | 2 | Trace | 1 | 1 | 158 | 32 | 4.0 | 0 | 0.24 | 0.10 | 6.2 | 0 |
| 336 | Biscuits, baking powder from 1 biscuit home recipe with enriched flour, 2-in diam. | 28 | 27 | 105 | 2 | 5 | 1 | 2 | 1 | 13 | 34 | 0.4 | Trace | 0.06 | 0.06 | 0.1 | Trace |
| 337 | Biscuits, baking powder from 1 biscuit mix, 2-in diam. | 28 | 28 | 90 | 2 | 3 | 1 | 1 | 1 | 15 | 19 | 0.6 | Trace | 0.08 | 0.07 | 0.6 | Trace |
| 338 | Bran flakes (40% bran), 1 cup added thiamine and iron | 35 | 3 | 105 | 4 | 1 | — | — | — | 28 | 25 | 1.2 | 0 | 0.14 | 0.06 | 2.2 | 0 |
| 339 | Bran flakes with raisins, 1 cup added thiamine and iron | 50 | 7 | 145 | 4 | 1 | — | — | — | 40 | 28 | 1.4 | Trace | 0.16 | 0.07 | 2.7 | 0 |
| 340 | Boston brown bread, slice 1 slice 3 by 3/4 in | 48 | 45 | 100 | 3 | 1 | — | — | — | 22 | 43 | 0.9 | 0 | 0.05 | 0.03 | 0.6 | 0 |
| | Breads: Cracked-wheat bread: | | | | | | | | | | | | | | | | |
| 341 | Loaf, 1 lb 1 loaf | 454 | 35 | 1,190 | 40 | 10 | 2 | 5 | 2 | 236 | 399 | 5.0 | Trace | 0.53 | 0.41 | 5.9 | Trace |
| 342 | Slice, 18 slices per loaf 1 slice | 25 | 35 | 65 | 2 | 1 | — | — | — | 13 | 22 | 0.3 | Trace | 0.03 | 0.02 | 0.3 | Trace |

| No. | Food | Measure | Weight (g) | Water (%) | Food energy (cal.) | Protein (g) | Fat (g) | Saturated (g) | Oleic (g) | Linoleic (g) | Carbohydrate (g) | Calcium (mg) | Iron (mg) | Vitamin A (IU) | Thiamine (mg) | Riboflavin (mg) | Niacin (mg) | Ascorbic acid (mg) |
|---|---|---|---|---|---|---|---|---|---|---|---|---|---|---|---|---|---|---|
| | **French or Vienna bread:** | | | | | | | | | | | | | | | | | |
| 343 | Enriched, 1-lb loaf | 1 loaf | 454 | 31 | 1,315 | 41 | 14 | 3 | 8 | 2 | 251 | 195 | 10.0 | Trace | 1.27 | 1.00 | 11.3 | Trace |
| 344 | Unenriched, 1-lb loaf | 1 loaf | 454 | 31 | 1,315 | 41 | 14 | 3 | 8 | 2 | 251 | 195 | 3.2 | Trace | 0.36 | 0.36 | 3.6 | Trace |
| | **Italian bread:** | | | | | | | | | | | | | | | | | |
| 345 | Enriched, 1-lb loaf | 1 loaf | 454 | 32 | 1,250 | 41 | 4 | Trace | 1 | 2 | 256 | 77 | 10.0 | 0 | 1.32 | 0.91 | 11.8 | 0 |
| 346 | Unenriched, 1-lb loaf | 1 loaf | 454 | 32 | 1,250 | 41 | 4 | Trace | 1 | 2 | 256 | 77 | 3.2 | 0 | 0.41 | 0.27 | 3.6 | 0 |
| | **Raisin bread:** | | | | | | | | | | | | | | | | | |
| 347 | Loaf, 1 lb | 1 loaf | 454 | 35 | 1,190 | 30 | 13 | 3 | 8 | 2 | 243 | 322 | 5.9 | Trace | 0.23 | 0.41 | 3.2 | Trace |
| 348 | Slice, 18 slices per loaf | 1 slice | 25 | 35 | 65 | 2 | 1 | — | — | — | 13 | 18 | 0.3 | Trace | 0.01 | 0.02 | 0.2 | Trace |
| | **Rye bread:** | | | | | | | | | | | | | | | | | |
| | American, light (1/3 rye, 2/3 wheat): | | | | | | | | | | | | | | | | | |
| 349 | Loaf, 1 lb | 1 loaf | 454 | 36 | 1,100 | 41 | 5 | — | — | — | 236 | 340 | 7.3 | 0 | 0.82 | 0.32 | 6.4 | 0 |
| 350 | Slice, 18 slices per loaf | 1 slice | 25 | 36 | 60 | 2 | Trace | — | — | — | 13 | 19 | 0.4 | 0 | 0.05 | 0.02 | 0.4 | 0 |
| 351 | Pumpernickel, loaf, 1 lb | 1 loaf | 454 | 34 | 1,115 | 41 | 5 | — | — | — | 241 | 381 | 10.9 | 0 | 1.04 | 0.64 | 5.4 | 0 |
| | **White bread, enriched:**[15] | | | | | | | | | | | | | | | | | |
| | Soft-crumb type: | | | | | | | | | | | | | | | | | |
| 352 | Loaf, 1 lb | 1 loaf | 454 | 36 | 1,225 | 39 | 15 | 3 | 8 | 2 | 229 | 381 | 11.3 | Trace | 1.13 | 0.95 | 10.9 | Trace |
| 353 | Slice, 18 slices per loaf | 1 slice | 25 | 36 | 70 | 2 | 1 | — | — | — | 13 | 21 | 0.6 | Trace | 0.06 | 0.05 | 0.6 | Trace |
| 354 | Slice, toasted | 1 slice | 22 | 25 | 70 | 2 | 1 | — | — | — | 13 | 21 | 0.6 | Trace | 0.06 | 0.05 | 0.6 | Trace |
| 355 | Slice, 22 slices per loaf | 1 slice | 20 | 36 | 55 | 2 | 1 | — | — | — | 10 | 17 | 0.5 | Trace | 0.05 | 0.04 | 0.5 | Trace |
| 356 | Slice, toasted | 1 slice | 17 | 25 | 55 | 2 | 1 | — | — | — | 10 | 17 | 0.5 | Trace | 0.05 | 0.04 | 0.5 | Trace |
| 357 | Loaf, 1 1/2 lb | 1 loaf | 680 | 36 | 1,835 | 59 | 22 | 5 | 12 | 3 | 343 | 571 | 17.0 | Trace | 1.70 | 1.43 | 16.3 | Trace |
| 358 | Slice, 24 slices per loaf | 1 slice | 28 | 36 | 75 | 2 | 1 | — | — | — | 14 | 24 | 0.7 | Trace | 0.07 | 0.06 | 0.7 | Trace |
| 359 | Slice, toasted | 1 slice | 24 | 25 | 75 | 2 | 1 | — | — | — | 14 | 24 | 0.7 | Trace | 0.07 | 0.06 | 0.7 | Trace |
| 360 | Slice, 28 slices per loaf | 1 slice | 24 | 36 | 65 | 2 | 1 | — | — | — | 12 | 20 | 0.6 | Trace | 0.06 | 0.05 | 0.6 | Trace |
| 361 | Slice, toasted | 1 slice | 21 | 25 | 65 | 2 | 1 | — | — | — | 12 | 20 | 0.6 | Trace | 0.06 | 0.05 | 0.6 | Trace |
| | Firm-crumb type: | | | | | | | | | | | | | | | | | |
| 362 | Loaf, 1 lb | 1 loaf | 454 | 35 | 1,245 | 41 | 17 | 4 | 10 | 2 | 228 | 435 | 11.3 | Trace | 1.22 | 0.91 | 10.9 | Trace |
| 363 | Slice, 20 slices per loaf | 1 slice | 23 | 35 | 65 | 2 | 1 | — | — | — | 12 | 22 | 0.6 | Trace | 0.06 | 0.05 | 0.6 | Trace |
| 364 | Slice, toasted | 1 slice | 20 | 24 | 65 | 2 | 1 | — | — | — | 12 | 22 | 0.6 | Trace | 0.06 | 0.05 | 0.6 | Trace |
| 365 | Loaf, 2 lb | 1 loaf | 907 | 35 | 2,495 | 82 | 34 | 8 | 20 | 4 | 455 | 871 | 22.7 | Trace | 2.45 | 1.81 | 21.8 | Trace |
| 366 | Slice, 34 slices per loaf | 1 slice | 27 | 35 | 75 | 2 | 1 | — | — | — | 14 | 26 | 0.7 | Trace | 0.07 | 0.05 | 0.6 | Trace |
| 367 | Slice, toasted | 1 slice | 23 | 25 | 75 | 2 | 1 | — | — | — | 14 | 26 | 0.7 | Trace | 0.07 | 0.05 | 0.6 | Trace |
| | **Whole-wheat bread, soft-crumb type:** | | | | | | | | | | | | | | | | | |
| 368 | Loaf, 1 lb | 1 loaf | 454 | 36 | 1,095 | 41 | 12 | 2 | 6 | 2 | 224 | 381 | 13.6 | Trace | 1.36 | 0.45 | 12.7 | Trace |
| 369 | Slice, 16 slices per loaf | 1 slice | 28 | 36 | 65 | 3 | 1 | — | — | — | 14 | 24 | 0.8 | Trace | 0.09 | 0.03 | 0.8 | Trace |
| 370 | Slice, toasted | 1 slice | 24 | 24 | 65 | 3 | 1 | — | — | — | 14 | 24 | 0.8 | Trace | 0.09 | 0.03 | 0.8 | Trace |
| | **Whole-wheat bread, firm-crumb type:** | | | | | | | | | | | | | | | | | |
| 371 | Loaf, 1 lb | 1 loaf | 454 | 36 | 1,100 | 48 | 14 | 3 | 6 | 3 | 216 | 449 | 13.6 | Trace | 1.18 | 0.54 | 12.7 | Trace |
| 372 | Slice, 18 slices per loaf | 1 slice | 25 | 36 | 60 | 3 | 1 | — | — | — | 12 | 25 | 0.8 | Trace | 0.06 | 0.03 | 0.7 | Trace |
| 373 | Slice, toasted | 1 slice | 21 | 24 | 60 | 3 | 1 | — | — | — | 12 | 25 | 0.8 | Trace | 0.06 | 0.03 | 0.7 | Trace |
| 374 | Breadcrumbs, dry, grated | 1 cup | 100 | 6 | 390 | 13 | 5 | 1 | 2 | 1 | 73 | 122 | 3.6 | Trace | 0.22 | 0.30 | 3.5 | Trace |
| 375 | Buckwheat flour, light, sifted | 1 cup | 98 | 12 | 340 | 6 | 1 | — | — | — | 78 | 11 | 1.0 | 0 | 0.08 | 0.04 | 0.4 | 0 |
| 376 | Bulgur, canned, seasoned | 1 cup | 135 | 56 | 245 | 8 | 4 | — | — | — | 44 | 27 | 1.9 | 0 | 0.08 | 0.05 | 4.1 | 0 |
| | **Cakes made from cake mixes:** | | | | | | | | | | | | | | | | | |
| | Angel food: | | | | | | | | | | | | | | | | | |
| 377 | Whole cake | 1 cake | 635 | 34 | 1,645 | 36 | 1 | — | — | — | 377 | 603 | 1.9 | 0 | 0.03 | 0.70 | 0.6 | 0 |
| 378 | Piece, 1/12 of 10-in diam. cake | 1 piece | 53 | 34 | 135 | 3 | Trace | — | — | — | 32 | 50 | 0.2 | 0 | Trace | 0.06 | 0.1 | 0 |

[5] Measure and weight apply to entire vegetable or fruit including parts not usually eaten.

[8] This is the amount from the fruit. Additionhl ascorbic acid may be added by the manufacturer. Refer to the label for this information.

[15] Values for iron, thiamine, riboflavin, and niacin per pound of unenriched white bread would be as follows:

| | Iron | Thiamine | Riboflavin | Niacin |
|---|---|---|---|---|
| | mg | mg | mg | mg |
| Soft crumb | 3.2 | .31 | .39 | 5.0 |
| Firm crumb | 3.2 | .32 | .59 | 4.1 |

# Table A–1. (Cont.)

| Food, Approximate Measure, and Weight (in grams) | | gm | Water per cent | Food Energy calories | Protein gm | Fat gm | Fatty Acids | | | Carbo-hy-drate gm | Cal-cium mg | Iron mg | Vita-min A Value I.U. | Thia-mine mg | Ribo-flavin mg | Niacin mg | Ascor-bic Acid mg |
|---|---|---|---|---|---|---|---|---|---|---|---|---|---|---|---|---|---|
| | | | | | | | Satu-rated (total) gm | Unsaturated | | | | | | | | | |
| | | | | | | | | Oleic gm | Lin-oleic gm | | | | | | | | |
| | Cakes made from cake mixes (cont.) | | | | | | | | | | | | | | | | |
| | Cupcakes, small, 2 1/2 in diam.: | | | | | | | | | | | | | | | | |
| 379 | Without icing | 1 cupcake | 25 | 26 | 90 | 1 | 3 | 1 | 1 | 1 | 14 | 40 | 0.1 | 40 | 0.01 | 0.03 | 0.1 | Trace |
| 380 | With chocolate icing | 1 cupcake | 36 | 22 | 130 | 2 | 5 | 2 | 2 | 1 | 21 | 47 | 0.3 | 60 | 0.01 | 0.04 | 0.1 | Trace |
| | Devil's food, 2-layer, with chocolate icing: | | | | | | | | | | | | | | | | |
| 381 | Whole cake | 1 cake | 1,107 | 24 | 3,755 | 49 | 136 | 54 | 58 | 16 | 645 | 653 | 8.9 | 1,660 | 0.33 | 0.89 | 3.3 | 1 |
| 382 | Piece, 1/16 of 9-in diam. cake | 1 piece | 69 | 24 | 235 | 3 | 9 | 3 | 4 | 1 | 40 | 41 | 0.6 | 100 | 0.02 | 0.06 | 0.2 | Trace |
| 383 | Cupcake, small, 2 1/2-in diam | 1 cupcake | 35 | 24 | 120 | 2 | 4 | 1 | 2 | Trace | 20 | 21 | 0.3 | 50 | 0.01 | 0.03 | 0.1 | Trace |
| | Gingerbread: | | | | | | | | | | | | | | | | |
| 384 | Whole cake | 1 cake | 570 | 37 | 1,575 | 18 | 39 | 10 | 19 | 9 | 291 | 513 | 9.1 | Trace | 0.17 | 0.51 | 4.6 | 2 |
| 385 | Piece, 1/9 of 8-in square cake | 1 piece | 63 | 37 | 175 | 2 | 4 | 1 | 2 | 1 | 32 | 57 | 1.0 | Trace | 0.02 | 0.06 | 0.5 | Trace |
| | White, 2-layer, with chocolate icing: | | | | | | | | | | | | | | | | |
| 386 | Whole cake | 1 cake | 1,140 | 21 | 4,000 | 45 | 122 | 45 | 54 | 17 | 716 | 1,129 | 5.7 | 680 | 0.23 | 0.91 | 2.3 | 2 |
| 387 | Piece, 1/16 of 9-in diam. cake | 1 piece | 71 | 21 | 250 | 3 | 8 | 3 | 3 | 1 | 45 | 70 | 0.4 | 40 | 0.01 | 0.06 | 0.1 | Trace |
| | Cakes made from home recipes:[16] | | | | | | | | | | | | | | | | |
| 388 | Boston cream pie; piece 1/12 of 8-in diam. | 1 piece | 69 | 35 | 210 | 4 | 6 | 2 | 3 | 1 | 34 | 46 | 0.3 | 140 | 0.02 | 0.08 | 0.1 | Trace |
| | Fruitcake, dark, made with enriched flour: | | | | | | | | | | | | | | | | |
| 389 | Loaf, 1 lb | 1 loaf | 454 | 18 | 1,720 | 22 | 69 | 15 | 37 | 13 | 271 | 327 | 11.8 | 540 | 0.59 | 0.64 | 3.6 | 2 |
| 390 | Slice, 1/30 of 8-in loaf | 1 slice | 15 | 18 | 55 | 1 | 2 | Trace | 1 | Trace | 9 | 11 | 0.4 | 20 | 0.02 | 0.02 | 0.1 | Trace |
| | Plain sheet cake: | | | | | | | | | | | | | | | | |
| | Without icing: | | | | | | | | | | | | | | | | |
| 391 | Whole cake | 1 cake | 777 | 25 | 2,830 | 35 | 108 | 30 | 52 | 21 | 434 | 497 | 3.1 | 1,320 | 0.16 | 0.70 | 1.6 | 2 |
| 392 | Piece, 1/9 of 9-in square cake | 1 piece | 86 | 25 | 315 | 4 | 12 | 3 | 6 | 2 | 48 | 55 | 0.3 | 150 | 0.02 | 0.08 | 0.2 | Trace |
| 393 | With boiled white icing, piece, 1/9 of 9-in square cake | 1 piece | 114 | 23 | 400 | 4 | 12 | 3 | 6 | 2 | 71 | 56 | 0.3 | 150 | 0.02 | 0.08 | 0.2 | Trace |
| | Pound: | | | | | | | | | | | | | | | | |
| 394 | Loaf, 8 1/2 by 3 1/2 by 3 in | 1 loaf | 514 | 17 | 2,430 | 29 | 152 | 34 | 68 | 17 | 242 | 108 | 4.1 | 1,440 | 0.15 | 0.46 | 1.0 | 0 |
| 395 | Slice, 1/2-in thick | 1 slice | 30 | 17 | 140 | 2 | 9 | 2 | 4 | 1 | 14 | 6 | 0.2 | 80 | 0.01 | 0.03 | 0.1 | 0 |
| | Sponge: | | | | | | | | | | | | | | | | |
| 396 | Whole cake | 1 cake | 790 | 32 | 2,345 | 60 | 45 | 14 | 20 | 4 | 427 | 237 | 9.5 | 3,560 | 0.40 | 1.11 | 1.6 | Trace |
| 397 | Piece, 1/12 of 10-in diam. cake | 1 piece | 66 | 32 | 195 | 5 | 4 | 1 | 2 | Trace | 36 | 20 | 0.8 | 300 | 0.03 | 0.09 | 0.1 | Trace |
| | Yellow, 2 layer, without icing: | | | | | | | | | | | | | | | | |
| 398 | Whole cake | 1 cake | 870 | 24 | 3,160 | 39 | 111 | 31 | 53 | 22 | 506 | 618 | 3.5 | 1,310 | 0.17 | 0.70 | 1.7 | 2 |
| 399 | Piece, 1/16 of 9-in diam. cake | 1 piece | 54 | 24 | 200 | 2 | 7 | 2 | 3 | 1 | 32 | 39 | 0.2 | 80 | 0.01 | 0.04 | 0.1 | Trace |
| | Yellow, 2-layer, with chocolate icing: | | | | | | | | | | | | | | | | |
| 400 | Whole cake | 1 cake | 1,203 | 21 | 4,390 | 51 | 156 | 55 | 69 | 23 | 727 | 818 | 7.2 | 1,920 | 0.24 | 0.96 | 2.4 | 2 |
| 401 | Piece, 1/16 of 9-in diam. cake | 1 piece | 75 | 21 | 275 | 3 | 10 | 3 | 4 | 1 | 45 | 51 | 0.5 | 120 | 0.02 | 0.06 | 0.2 | Trace |
| | Cake icings. See Sugars, Sweets | | | | | | | | | | | | | | | | |

| No. | Food | Measure | Grams | Water (%) | Food energy (cal) | Protein (g) | Fat (g) | Saturated (g) | Oleic (g) | Linoleic (g) | Carbohydrate (g) | Calcium (mg) | Iron (mg) | Vitamin A (IU) | Thiamine (mg) | Riboflavin (mg) | Niacin (mg) | Ascorbic acid (mg) |
|---|---|---|---|---|---|---|---|---|---|---|---|---|---|---|---|---|---|---|
| | **Cookies:** | | | | | | | | | | | | | | | | | |
| 402 | Brownies with nuts: Made from home recipe with enriched flour | 1 brownie | 20 | 10 | 95 | 1 | 6 | 1 | 3 | 1 | 10 | 8 | 0.4 | 40 | 0.04 | 0.02 | 0.1 | Trace |
| 403 | Made from mix | 1 brownie | 20 | 11 | 85 | 1 | 4 | 1 | 2 | 1 | 13 | 9 | 0.4 | 20 | 0.03 | 0.02 | 0.1 | Trace |
| 404 | Chocolate chip: Made from home recipe with enriched flour | 1 cookie | 10 | 3 | 50 | 1 | 3 | 1 | 1 | 1 | 6 | 4 | 0.2 | 10 | 0.01 | 0.01 | 0.1 | Trace |
| 405 | Commercial | 1 cookie | 10 | 3 | 50 | 1 | 2 | Trace | 1 | 1 | 7 | 4 | 0.2 | 10 | Trace | Trace | Trace | Trace |
| 406 | Fig bars, commercial | 1 cookie | 14 | 14 | 50 | 1 | 1 | — | 1 | Trace | 11 | 11 | 0.2 | 20 | Trace | 0.01 | 0.1 | Trace |
| 407 | Sandwich, chocolate or vanilla, commercial | 1 cookie | 10 | 2 | 50 | 1 | 2 | Trace | 1 | 1 | 7 | 2 | 0.1 | 0 | Trace | Trace | 0.1 | 0 |
| 408 | Corn flakes, added nutrients: Plain | 1 cup | 25 | 4 | 100 | 2 | Trace | — | — | — | 21 | 4 | 0.4 | 0 | 0.11 | 0.02 | 0.5 | 0 |
| 409 | Sugar-covered | 1 cup | 40 | 2 | 155 | 2 | Trace | — | — | — | 36 | 5 | 0.4 | 0 | 0.16 | 0.02 | 0.8 | 0 |
| | Corn (hominy) grits, degermed, cooked: | | | | | | | | | | | | | | | | | |
| 410 | Enriched | 1 cup | 245 | 87 | 125 | 3 | Trace | — | — | — | 27 | 2 | 0.7 | [17]150 | 0.10 | 0.07 | 1.0 | 0 |
| 411 | Unenriched | 1 cup | 245 | 87 | 125 | 3 | Trace | — | — | — | 27 | 2 | 0.2 | [17]150 | 0.05 | 0.02 | 0.5 | 0 |
| | Cornmeal: | | | | | | | | | | | | | | | | | |
| 412 | Whole-ground, unbolted, dry | 1 cup | 122 | 12 | 435 | 11 | 5 | 1 | 2 | 2 | 90 | 24 | 2.9 | [17]620 | 0.46 | 0.13 | 2.4 | 0 |
| 413 | Bolted (nearly whole-grain) dry | 1 cup | 122 | 12 | 440 | 11 | 4 | Trace | 1 | 2 | 91 | 21 | 2.2 | [17]590 | 0.37 | 0.10 | 2.3 | 0 |
| | Degermed, enriched: | | | | | | | | | | | | | | | | | |
| 414 | Dry form | 1 cup | 138 | 12 | 500 | 11 | 2 | — | — | — | 108 | 8 | 4.0 | [17]610 | 0.61 | 0.36 | 4.8 | 0 |
| 415 | Cooked | 1 cup | 240 | 88 | 120 | 3 | 1 | — | — | — | 26 | 2 | 1.0 | [17]140 | 0.14 | 0.10 | 1.2 | 0 |
| | Degermed, unenriched: | | | | | | | | | | | | | | | | | |
| 416 | Dry form | 1 cup | 138 | 12 | 500 | 11 | 2 | — | — | — | 108 | 8 | 1.5 | [17]610 | 0.19 | 0.07 | 1.4 | 0 |
| 417 | Cooked | 1 cup | 240 | 88 | 120 | 3 | 1 | — | — | — | 26 | 2 | 0.5 | [17]140 | 0.05 | 0.02 | 0.2 | 0 |
| 418 | Corn muffins, made with enriched degermed cornmeal and enriched flour; muffin 2 3/8-in diam. | 1 muffin | 40 | 33 | 125 | 3 | 4 | 2 | 1 | 2 | 19 | 42 | 0.7 | [17]120 | 0.08 | 0.09 | 0.6 | Trace |
| 419 | Corn muffins, made with mix, egg, and milk; muffin 2 3/8-in diam. | 1 muffin | 40 | 30 | 130 | 3 | 4 | 1 | 2 | 1 | 20 | 96 | 0.6 | 100 | 0.07 | 0.08 | 0.6 | Trace |
| 420 | Corn, puffed, presweetened, added nutrients | 1 cup | 30 | 2 | 115 | 1 | Trace | — | — | — | 27 | 3 | 0.5 | 0 | 0.13 | 0.05 | 0.6 | 0 |
| 421 | Corn, shredded, added nutrients | 1 cup | 25 | 3 | 100 | 2 | Trace | — | — | — | 22 | 1 | 0.6 | 0 | 0.11 | 0.05 | 0.5 | 0 |
| | Crackers: | | | | | | | | | | | | | | | | | |
| 422 | Graham, 2 1/2-in square | 4 crackers | 28 | 6 | 110 | 2 | 3 | — | — | — | 21 | 11 | 0.4 | 0 | 0.01 | 0.06 | 0.4 | 0 |
| 423 | Saltines | 4 crackers | 11 | 4 | 50 | 1 | 1 | — | — | — | 8 | 2 | 0.1 | 0 | Trace | Trace | 0.1 | 0 |
| | Danish pastry, plain (without fruit or nuts): | | | | | | | | | | | | | | | | | |
| 424 | Packaged ring, 12 ounces | 1 ring | 340 | 22 | 1,435 | 25 | 80 | 24 | 37 | 15 | 155 | 170 | 3.1 | 1,050 | 0.24 | 0.51 | 2.7 | Trace |
| 425 | Round piece, approx. 4 1/4-in diam. by 1 in | 1 pastry | 65 | 22 | 275 | 5 | 15 | 5 | 7 | 3 | 30 | 33 | 0.6 | 200 | 0.05 | 0.10 | 0.5 | Trace |
| | Doughnuts, cake type | | | | | | | | | | | | | | | | | |
| 426 | Ounce | 1 oz | 28 | 22 | 120 | 2 | 7 | 2 | 3 | 1 | 13 | 14 | 0.3 | 90 | 0.02 | 0.04 | 0.2 | Trace |
| 427 | | 1 doughnut | 32 | 24 | 125 | 1 | 6 | 1 | 1 | Trace | 16 | 13 | [18]0.4 | 30 | [18]0.05 | [18]0.05 | [18]0.4 | Trace |
| 428 | Farina, quick-cooking, enriched, cooked | 1 cup | 245 | 89 | 105 | 3 | Trace | — | — | — | 22 | 147 | [19]0.7 | 0 | [19]0.12 | [19]0.07 | [19]1.0 | 0 |

[16] Unenriched cake flour used unless otherwise specified.

[17] This value is based on product made from yellow varieties of corn; white varieties contain only a trace.

[18] Based on product made with enriched flour. With unenriched flour, approximate values per doughnut are: iron, 0.2 mg; thiamine, 0.01 mg; riboflavin, 0.03 mg; niacin, 0.2 mg.

[19] Iron, thiamine, riboflavin, and niacin are based on the minimum levels of enrichment specified in standards of identity promulgated under the Federal Food, Drug, and Cosmetic Act.

**Table A-1. (Cont.)**

| | Food, Approximate Measure, and Weight (in grams) | | Water per cent | Food Energy calories | Pro-tein gm | Fat gm | Satu-rated (total) gm | Oleic gm | Lin-oleic gm | Carbo-hy-drate gm | Cal-cium mg | Iron mg | Vita-min A Value I.U. | Thia-mine mg | Ribo-flavin mg | Niacin mg | Ascor-bic Acid mg |
|---|---|---|---|---|---|---|---|---|---|---|---|---|---|---|---|---|---|
| | | gm | | | | | | | | | | | | | | | |
| | Macaroni; cooked: | | | | | | | | | | | | | | | | |
| | Enriched: | | | | | | | | | | | | | | | | |
| 429 | Cooked, firm stage (undergoes additional cooking in a food mixture) | 1 cup / 130 | 64 | 190 | 6 | 1 | — | — | — | 39 | 14 | 191.4 | 0 | 190.23 | 190.14 | 191.8 | 0 |
| 430 | Cooked until tender | 1 cup / 140 | 72 | 155 | 5 | 1 | — | — | — | 32 | 8 | 191.3 | 0 | 190.20 | 190.11 | 191.5 | 0 |
| | Unenriched: | | | | | | | | | | | | | | | | |
| 431 | Cooked, firm stage (undergoes additional cooking in a food mixture) | 1 cup / 130 | 64 | 190 | 6 | 1 | — | — | — | 39 | 14 | 0.7 | 0 | 0.03 | 0.03 | 0.5 | 0 |
| 432 | Cooked until tender | 1 cup / 140 | 72 | 155 | 5 | 1 | — | — | — | 32 | 11 | 0.6 | 0 | 0.01 | 0.01 | 0.4 | 0 |
| 433 | Macaroni (enriched) and cheese, baked | 1 cup / 200 | 58 | 430 | 17 | 22 | 10 | 9 | 2 | 40 | 362 | 1.8 | 860 | 0.20 | 0.40 | 1.8 | Trace |
| 434 | Canned | 1 cup / 240 | 80 | 230 | 9 | 10 | 4 | 3 | 1 | 26 | 199 | 1.0 | 260 | 0.12 | 0.24 | 1.0 | Trace |
| 435 | Muffins, with enriched white flour; muffin, 3-inch diam. | 1 muffin / 40 | 38 | 120 | 3 | 4 | 1 | 2 | 1 | 17 | 42 | 0.6 | 40 | 0.07 | 0.09 | 0.6 | Trace |
| | Noodles (egg noodles), cooked: | | | | | | | | | | | | | | | | |
| 436 | Enriched | 1 cup / 160 | 70 | 200 | 7 | 2 | 1 | 1 | Trace | 37 | 16 | 191.4 | 110 | 190.22 | 190.13 | 191.9 | 0 |
| 437 | Unenriched | 1 cup / 160 | 70 | 200 | 7 | 2 | 1 | 1 | Trace | 37 | 16 | 1.0 | 110 | 0.05 | 0.03 | 0.6 | 0 |
| 438 | Oats (with or without corn) puffed, added nutrients | 1 cup / 25 | 3 | 100 | 3 | 1 | — | — | — | 19 | 44 | 1.2 | 0 | 0.24 | 0.04 | 0.5 | 0 |
| 439 | Oatmeal or rolled oats, cooked | 1 cup / 240 | 87 | 130 | 5 | 2 | — | — | 1 | 23 | 22 | 1.4 | 0 | 0.19 | 0.05 | 0.2 | 0 |
| | Pancakes, 4-inch diam.: | | | | | | | | | | | | | | | | |
| 440 | Wheat, enriched flour (home recipe) | 1 cake / 27 | 50 | 60 | 2 | 2 | Trace | 1 | Trace | 9 | 27 | 0.4 | 30 | 0.05 | 0.06 | 0.4 | Trace |
| 441 | Buckwheat (made from mix with egg and milk) | 1 cake / 27 | 58 | 55 | 2 | 2 | 1 | 1 | Trace | 6 | 59 | 0.4 | 60 | 0.03 | 0.04 | 0.2 | Trace |
| 442 | Plain or buttermilk (made from mix with egg and milk) | 1 cake / 27 | 51 | 60 | 2 | 2 | 1 | 1 | Trace | 9 | 58 | 0.3 | 70 | 0.04 | 0.06 | 0.2 | Trace |
| | Pie (piecrust made with unenriched flour): Sector, 4-in, 1/7 of 9-in-diam. pie: | | | | | | | | | | | | | | | | |
| 443 | Apple (2-crust) | 1 sector / 135 | 48 | 350 | 3 | 15 | 4 | 7 | 3 | 51 | 11 | 0.4 | 40 | 0.03 | 0.03 | 0.5 | 1 |
| 444 | Butterscotch (1-crust) | 1 sector / 130 | 45 | 350 | 6 | 14 | 5 | 6 | 3 | 50 | 98 | 1.2 | 340 | 0.04 | 0.13 | 0.3 | Trace |
| 445 | Cherry (2-crust) | 1 sector / 135 | 47 | 350 | 4 | 15 | 4 | 7 | 3 | 52 | 19 | 0.4 | 590 | 0.03 | 0.03 | 0.7 | Trace |
| 446 | Custard (1-crust) | 1 sector / 130 | 58 | 285 | 8 | 14 | 5 | 7 | 2 | 30 | 125 | 0.8 | 300 | 0.07 | 0.21 | 0.4 | 0 |
| 447 | Lemon meringue (1-crust) | 1 sector / 120 | 47 | 305 | 4 | 12 | 4 | 6 | 2 | 45 | 17 | 0.6 | 200 | 0.04 | 0.10 | 0.2 | 4 |
| 448 | Mince (2-crust) | 1 sector / 135 | 43 | 365 | 3 | 16 | 4 | 8 | 3 | 56 | 38 | 1.4 | Trace | 0.09 | 0.05 | 0.5 | 1 |
| 449 | Pecan (1-crust) | 1 sector / 118 | 20 | 490 | 6 | 27 | 4 | 16 | 5 | 60 | 55 | 3.3 | 190 | 0.19 | 0.08 | 0.4 | Trace |
| 450 | Pineapple chiffon (1-crust) | 1 sector / 93 | 41 | 265 | 6 | 11 | 3 | 5 | 2 | 36 | 22 | 0.8 | 320 | 0.04 | 0.08 | 0.4 | 1 |
| 451 | Pumpkin (1-crust) | 1 sector / 130 | 59 | 275 | 5 | 15 | 5 | 6 | 2 | 32 | 66 | 0.7 | 3,210 | 0.04 | 0.13 | 0.7 | Trace |
| | Piecrust, baked shell for pie made with: | | | | | | | | | | | | | | | | |
| 452 | Enriched flour | 1 shell / 180 | 15 | 900 | 11 | 60 | 16 | 28 | 12 | 79 | 25 | 3.1 | 0 | 0.36 | 0.25 | 3.2 | 0 |
| 453 | Unenriched flour | 1 shell / 180 | 15 | 900 | 11 | 60 | 16 | 28 | 12 | 79 | 25 | 0.9 | 0 | 0.05 | 0.05 | 0.9 | 0 |

| No. | Food (measure) | | | | | | | | | | | | | | | | |
|---|---|---|---|---|---|---|---|---|---|---|---|---|---|---|---|---|---|
| 454 | Piecrust mix including stick form: Package, 10 oz, for double crust (1 pkg.) | 284 | 9 | 1,480 | 20 | 93 | 23 | 46 | 21 | 141 | 131 | 1.4 | 0 | 0.11 | 0.11 | 2.0 | 0 |
| 455 | Pizza (cheese) 5 1/2-in sector; 1/8 of 14-in diam. pie (1 sector) | 75 | 45 | 185 | 7 | 6 | 2 | 3 | Trace | 27 | 107 | 0.7 | 290 | 0.04 | 0.12 | 0.7 | 4 |
| | Popcorn, popped: | | | | | | | | | | | | | | | | |
| 456 | Plain, large kernel (1 cup) | 6 | 4 | 25 | 1 | Trace | — | Trace | — | 5 | 1 | 0.2 | — | — | 0.01 | 0.1 | 0 |
| 457 | With oil and salt (1 cup) | 9 | 3 | 40 | 1 | 2 | — | — | — | 5 | 1 | 0.2 | — | — | 0.01 | 0.2 | 0 |
| 458 | Sugar coated (1 cup) | 35 | 4 | 135 | 2 | 1 | — | — | — | 30 | 2 | 0.5 | — | 0.02 | 0.02 | 0.4 | 0 |
| | Pretzels: | | | | | | | | | | | | | | | | |
| 459 | Dutch, twisted (1 pretzel) | 16 | 5 | 60 | 2 | 1 | — | — | — | 12 | 4 | 0.2 | 0 | Trace | Trace | 0.1 | 0 |
| 460 | Thin, twisted (1 pretzel) | 6 | 5 | 25 | 1 | Trace | — | — | — | 5 | 1 | 0.1 | 0 | Trace | Trace | Trace | 0 |
| 461 | Sticks, small 2 1/4 inches (10 sticks) | 3 | 5 | 10 | Trace | Trace | — | — | — | 2 | 1 | Trace | 0 | Trace | Trace | Trace | 0 |
| 462 | Sticks, regular, 3 1/8 inches (5 sticks) | 3 | 5 | 10 | Trace | Trace | — | — | — | 2 | 1 | Trace | 0 | Trace | Trace | Trace | 0 |
| | Rice, white: Enriched: | | | | | | | | | | | | | | | | |
| 463 | Raw (1 cup) | 185 | 12 | 670 | 12 | 1 | — | — | — | 149 | 44 | 5.4[20] | 0 | 0.81[20] | 0.06[20] | 6.5[20] | 0 |
| 464 | Cooked (1 cup) | 205 | 73 | 225 | 4 | Trace | — | — | — | 50 | 21 | 1.8[20] | 0 | 0.23[20] | 0.02[20] | 2.1[20] | 0 |
| 465 | Instant, ready to serve (1 cup) | 165 | 73 | 180 | 4 | Trace | — | — | — | 40 | 5 | 1.3[20] | 0 | 0.21[20] | [20]— | 1.7[20] | 0 |
| 466 | Unenriched, cooked (1 cup) | 205 | 73 | 225 | 4 | Trace | — | — | — | 50 | 21 | 0.4 | 0 | 0.04 | [20]— | 0.8 | 0 |
| 467 | Parboiled, cooked (1 cup) | 175 | 73 | 185 | 4 | Trace | — | — | — | 41 | 33 | 1.4[20] | 0 | 0.19[20] | 0.02 | 2.1[20] | 0 |
| 468 | Rice, puffed, added nutrients (1 cup) | 15 | 4 | 60 | 1 | Trace | — | — | — | 13 | 3 | 0.3 | 0 | 0.07 | 0.01 | 0.7 | 0 |
| | Rolls, enriched: Cloverleaf or pan: | | | | | | | | | | | | | | | | |
| 469 | Home recipe (1 roll) | 35 | 26 | 120 | 3 | 3 | 1 | 1 | Trace | 20 | 16 | 0.7 | 30 | 0.09 | 0.09 | 0.8 | Trace |
| 470 | Commercial (1 roll) | 28 | 31 | 85 | 2 | 2 | Trace | 1 | Trace | 15 | 21 | 0.5 | Trace | 0.08 | 0.05 | 0.6 | Trace |
| 471 | Frankfurter or hamburger (1 roll) | 40 | 31 | 120 | 3 | 2 | 1 | 1 | Trace | 21 | 30 | 0.8 | Trace | 0.11 | 0.07 | 0.9 | Trace |
| 472 | Hard, round or rectangular (1 roll) | 50 | 25 | 155 | 5 | 2 | 1 | 1 | Trace | 30 | 24 | 1.2 | Trace | 0.13 | 0.12 | 1.4 | Trace |
| 473 | Rye wafers, whole-grain, 1 7/8 by 3 1/2 inches (2 wafers) | 13 | 6 | 45 | 2 | Trace | — | 1 | — | 10 | 7 | 0.5 | 0 | 0.04 | 0.03 | 0.2 | 0 |
| 474 | Spaghetti, cooked, tender stage, enriched (1 cup) | 140 | 72 | 155 | 5 | 1 | — | — | — | 32 | 11 | 1.3[19] | 0 | 0.20[19] | 0.11[19] | 1.5[19] | 0 |
| | Spaghetti with meat balls, and tomato sauce: | | | | | | | | | | | | | | | | |
| 475 | Home recipe (1 cup) | 248 | 70 | 330 | 19 | 12 | 4 | 6 | 1 | 39 | 124 | 3.7 | 1,590 | 0.25 | 0.30 | 4.0 | 22 |
| 476 | Canned (1 cup) | 250 | 78 | 260 | 12 | 10 | 2 | 3 | 4 | 28 | 53 | 3.3 | 1,000 | 0.15 | 0.18 | 2.3 | 5 |
| | Spaghetti in tomato sauce with cheese: | | | | | | | | | | | | | | | | |
| 477 | Home recipe (1 cup) | 250 | 77 | 260 | 9 | 9 | 2 | 5 | 1 | 37 | 80 | 2.3 | 1,080 | 0.25 | 0.18 | 2.3 | 13 |
| 478 | Canned (1 cup) | 250 | 80 | 190 | 6 | 2 | 1 | 1 | 1 | 38 | 40 | 2.8 | 930 | 0.35 | 0.28 | 4.5 | 10 |
| 479 | Waffles, with enriched flour, 7-in diam. (1 waffle) | 75 | 41 | 210 | 7 | 7 | 2 | 4 | 1 | 28 | 85 | 1.3 | 250 | 0.13 | 0.19 | 1.0 | Trace |
| 480 | Waffles, made from mix, enriched, egg and milk added, 7-in diam. (1 waffle) | 75 | 42 | 205 | 7 | 8 | 3 | 3 | 1 | 27 | 179 | 1.0 | 170 | 0.11 | 0.17 | 0.7 | Trace |
| 481 | Wheat, puffed, added nutrients (1 cup) | 15 | 3 | 55 | 2 | Trace | — | — | — | 12 | 4 | 0.6 | 0 | 0.08 | 0.03 | 1.2 | 0 |
| 482 | Wheat, shredded, plain (1 biscuit) | 25 | 7 | 90 | 2 | 1 | — | — | — | 20 | 11 | 0.9 | 0 | 0.06 | 0.03 | 1.1 | 0 |
| 483 | Wheat flakes, added nutrients (1 cup) | 30 | 4 | 105 | 3 | Trace | — | — | — | 24 | 12 | 1.3 | 0 | 0.19 | 0.04 | 1.5 | 0 |
| | Wheat flours: | | | | | | | | | | | | | | | | |
| 484 | Whole wheat, from hard wheats, stirred (1 cup) | 120 | 12 | 400 | 16 | 2 | Trace | 1 | 1 | 85 | 49 | 4.0 | 0 | 0.66 | 0.14 | 5.2 | 0 |

[19]Iron, thiamine, riboflavin, and niacin are based on the minimum levels of enrichment specified in standards of identity promulgated under the Federal Food, Drug, and Cosmetic Act.

[20]Iron, thiamine, and niacin are based on the minimum levels of enrichment specified in standards of identity promulgated under the Federal Food, Drug, and Cosmetic Act. Riboflavin is based on unenriched rice. When the minimum level of enrichment specified in the standards of identity becomes effective the value will be 0.12 mg per cup of parboiled rice and of white rice.

Table A–1. (Cont.)

| | Food, Approximate Measure, and Weight (in grams) | | Water per cent | Food Energy calories | Pro-tein gm | Fat gm | Fatty Acids Satu-rated (total) gm | Unsaturated Oleic gm | Lin-oleic gm | Carbo-hy-drate gm | Cal-cium mg | Iron mg | Vita-min A Value I.U. | Thia-mine mg | Ribo-flavin mg | Niacin mg | Ascor-bic Acid mg |
|---|---|---|---|---|---|---|---|---|---|---|---|---|---|---|---|---|---|
| | | gm | | | | | | | | | | | | | | | |
| | **Wheat flours (cont.)** | | | | | | | | | | | | | | | | |
| | All-purpose or family flour, enriched: | | | | | | | | | | | | | | | | |
| 485 | Sifted 1 cup | 115 | 12 | 420 | 12 | 1 | — | — | — | 88 | 18 | 193.3 | 0 | 190.51 | 190.30 | 194.0 | 0 |
| 486 | Unsifted 1 cup | 125 | 12 | 455 | 13 | 1 | — | — | — | 95 | 20 | 193.6 | 0 | 190.55 | 190.33 | 194.4 | 0 |
| 487 | Self-rising, enriched 1 cup | 125 | 12 | 440 | 12 | 1 | — | — | — | 93 | 331 | 193.6 | 0 | 190.55 | 190.33 | 194.4 | 0 |
| 488 | Cake or pastry flour, sifted 1 cup | 96 | 12 | 350 | 7 | 1 | — | — | — | 76 | 16 | 0.5 | 0 | 0.03 | 0.03 | 0.7 | 0 |
| | **Fats, Oils** | | | | | | | | | | | | | | | | |
| | Butter: | | | | | | | | | | | | | | | | |
| | Regular, 4 sticks per pound: | | | | | | | | | | | | | | | | |
| 489 | Stick 1/2 cup | 113 | 16 | 810 | 1 | 92 | 51 | 30 | 3 | Trace | 23 | 0 | 213,750 | — | — | — | 0 |
| 490 | Tablespoon (approx. 1/8 stick) 1 tbsp. | 14 | 16 | 100 | Trace | 12 | 6 | 4 | Trace | 1 | 3 | 0 | 21470 | — | — | — | 0 |
| 491 | Pat (1-in sq. 1/3-in high; 90 per lb) 1 pat | 5 | 16 | 35 | Trace | 4 | 2 | 1 | Trace | Trace | 1 | 0 | 21170 | — | — | — | 0 |
| | Whipped, 6 sticks or 2, 8-oz containers per pound: | | | | | | | | | | | | | | | | |
| 492 | Stick 1/2 cup | 76 | 16 | 540 | 1 | 61 | 34 | 20 | 2 | Trace | 15 | 0 | 212,500 | — | — | — | 0 |
| 493 | Tablespoon (approx. 1/8 stick) 1 tbsp. | 9 | 16 | 65 | Trace | 8 | 4 | 3 | Trace | Trace | 2 | 0 | 21310 | — | — | — | 0 |
| 494 | Pat (1 1/4-in sq 1/3-in high; 120 per lb) 1 pat | 4 | 16 | 25 | Trace | 3 | 2 | 1 | Trace | Trace | 1 | 0 | 21130 | — | — | — | 0 |
| | Fats, cooking: | | | | | | | | | | | | | | | | |
| 495 | Lard 1 cup | 205 | 0 | 1,850 | 0 | 205 | 78 | 94 | 20 | 0 | 0 | 0 | 0 | 0 | 0 | 0 | 0 |
| 496 | 1 tbsp. | 13 | 0 | 115 | 0 | 13 | 5 | 6 | 1 | 0 | 0 | 0 | 0 | 0 | 0 | 0 | 0 |
| 497 | Vegetable fats 1 cup | 200 | 0 | 1,770 | 0 | 200 | 50 | 100 | 44 | 0 | 0 | 0 | — | 0 | 0 | 0 | 0 |
| 498 | 1 tbsp | 13 | 0 | 110 | 0 | 13 | 3 | 6 | 3 | 0 | 0 | 0 | — | 0 | 0 | 0 | 0 |
| | Margarine: | | | | | | | | | | | | | | | | |
| | Regular, 4 sticks per pound: | | | | | | | | | | | | | | | | |
| 499 | Stick 1/2 cup | 113 | 16 | 815 | 1 | 92 | 17 | 46 | 25 | 1 | 23 | 0 | 223,750 | — | — | — | 0 |
| 500 | Tablespoon (approx. 1/8 stick) 1 tbsp | 14 | 16 | 100 | Trace | 12 | 2 | 6 | 3 | Trace | 3 | 0 | 22470 | — | — | — | 0 |
| 501 | Pat (1-in sq 1/3-in high; 90 per lb) 1 pat | 5 | 16 | 35 | Trace | 4 | 1 | 2 | 1 | Trace | 1 | 0 | 22170 | — | — | — | 0 |
| | Whipped, 6 sticks per pound: | | | | | | | | | | | | | | | | |
| 502 | Stick 1/2 cup | 76 | 16 | 545 | 1 | 61 | 11 | 31 | 17 | Trace | 15 | 0 | 222,500 | — | — | — | 0 |
| | Soft, 2 8-oz tubs per pound: | | | | | | | | | | | | | | | | |
| 503 | Tub 1 tub | 227 | 16 | 1,635 | 1 | 184 | 34 | 68 | 68 | 1 | 45 | 0 | 227,500 | — | — | — | 0 |
| 504 | 1 tbsp | 14 | 16 | 100 | Trace | 11 | 2 | 4 | 4 | Trace | 3 | 0 | 22470 | — | — | — | 0 |
| | Oils, salad or cooking: | | | | | | | | | | | | | | | | |
| 505 | Corn 1 cup | 220 | 0 | 1,945 | 0 | 220 | 22 | 62 | 117 | 0 | 0 | 0 | — | — | — | — | 0 |
| 506 | 1 tbsp | 14 | 0 | 125 | 0 | 14 | 2 | 4 | 7 | 0 | 0 | 0 | — | — | — | — | 0 |
| 507 | Cottonseed 1 cup | 220 | 0 | 1,945 | 0 | 220 | 55 | 46 | 110 | 0 | 0 | 0 | — | — | — | — | 0 |
| 508 | 1 tbsp | 14 | 0 | 125 | 0 | 14 | 4 | 3 | 7 | 0 | 0 | 0 | — | — | — | — | 0 |
| 509 | Olive 1 cup | 220 | 0 | 1,945 | 0 | 220 | 24 | 167 | 15 | 0 | 0 | 0 | — | — | — | — | 0 |
| 510 | 1 tbsp | 14 | 0 | 125 | 0 | 14 | 2 | 11 | 1 | 0 | 0 | 0 | — | — | — | — | 0 |
| 511 | Peanut 1 cup | 220 | 0 | 1,945 | 0 | 220 | 40 | 103 | 64 | 0 | 0 | 0 | — | — | — | — | 0 |
| 512 | 1 tbsp | 14 | 0 | 125 | 0 | 14 | 3 | 7 | 4 | 0 | 0 | 0 | — | — | — | — | 0 |

| No. | Food | Measure | Weight (g) | Water (%) | Food energy (cal) | Protein (g) | Fat (g) | Saturated (g) | Oleic (g) | Linoleic (g) | Carbohydrate (g) | Calcium (mg) | Iron (mg) | Vitamin A (I.U.) | Thiamin (mg) | Riboflavin (mg) | Niacin (mg) | Ascorbic acid (mg) |
|---|---|---|---|---|---|---|---|---|---|---|---|---|---|---|---|---|---|---|
| 513 | Safflower | 1 cup | 220 | 0 | 1,945 | 0 | 220 | 18 | 37 | 165 | 0 | 0 | 0 | — | 0 | 0 | 0 | 0 |
| 514 | Soybean | 1 tbsp | 14 | 0 | 125 | 0 | 14 | 1 | 2 | 10 | 0 | 0 | 0 | — | 0 | 0 | 0 | 0 |
| 515 | | 1 cup | 220 | 0 | 1,945 | 0 | 220 | 33 | 44 | 114 | 0 | 0 | 0 | — | 0 | 0 | 0 | 0 |
| 516 | | 1 tbsp | 14 | 0 | 125 | 0 | 14 | 2 | 3 | 7 | 0 | 0 | 0 | — | 0 | 0 | 0 | 0 |
| | **Salad dressing:** | | | | | | | | | | | | | | | | | |
| 517 | Blue cheese | 1 tbsp | 15 | 32 | 75 | 1 | 8 | 2 | 2 | 4 | 1 | 12 | Trace | 30 | Trace | 0.02 | Trace | Trace |
| | Commercial, mayonnaise type: | | | | | | | | | | | | | | | | | |
| 518 | Regular | 1 tbsp | 15 | 41 | 65 | Trace | 6 | 1 | 1 | 3 | 2 | 2 | Trace | 30 | Trace | Trace | Trace | Trace |
| 519 | Special dietary, low calorie | 1 tbsp | 16 | 81 | 20 | Trace | 2 | Trace | Trace | 1 | 1 | 3 | Trace | 40 | Trace | Trace | Trace | Trace |
| | French: | | | | | | | | | | | | | | | | | |
| 520 | Regular | 1 tbsp | 16 | 39 | 65 | Trace | 6 | 1 | 1 | 3 | 3 | 2 | 0.1 | — | — | — | — | Trace |
| 521 | Special dietary, low fat with artificial sweeteners | 1 tbsp | 15 | 95 | Trace | Trace | Trace | — | — | Trace | Trace | 2 | 0.1 | — | — | — | — | Trace |
| 522 | Home cooked, boiled | 1 tbsp | 16 | 68 | 25 | 1 | 2 | 1 | 1 | Trace | 2 | 14 | 0.1 | 80 | 0.01 | 0.03 | Trace | Trace |
| 523 | Mayonnaise | 1 tbsp | 14 | 15 | 100 | Trace | 11 | 2 | 2 | 6 | Trace | 3 | 0.1 | 40 | Trace | 0.01 | Trace | Trace |
| 524 | Thousand island | 1 tbsp | 16 | 32 | 80 | Trace | 8 | 2 | 2 | 4 | 3 | 2 | 0.1 | 50 | Trace | Trace | Trace | Trace |
| | **Sugars, Sweets** | | | | | | | | | | | | | | | | | |
| | Cake icings: | | | | | | | | | | | | | | | | | |
| 525 | Chocolate made with milk and table fat | 1 cup | 275 | 14 | 1,035 | 9 | 38 | 21 | 14 | 1 | 185 | 165 | 3.3 | 580 | 0.06 | 0.28 | 0.6 | 1 |
| 526 | Coconut (with boiled icing) | 1 cup | 166 | 15 | 605 | 3 | 13 | 11 | 1 | Trace | 124 | 10 | 0.8 | 0 | 0.02 | 0.07 | 0.3 | 0 |
| 527 | Creamy fudge from mix with water only | 1 cup | 245 | 15 | 830 | 7 | 16 | 5 | 8 | 3 | 183 | 96 | 2.7 | Trace | 0.05 | 0.20 | 0.7 | Trace |
| 528 | White, boiled | 1 cup | 94 | 18 | 300 | 0 | 0 | — | — | — | 76 | 2 | Trace | 0 | Trace | 0.03 | Trace | 0 |
| | Candy: | | | | | | | | | | | | | | | | | |
| 529 | Carmels, plain or chocolate | 1 oz | 28 | 8 | 115 | 1 | 3 | 2 | 1 | Trace | 22 | 42 | 0.4 | Trace | 0.01 | 0.05 | 0.1 | Trace |
| 530 | Chocolate, milk, plain | 1 oz | 28 | 1 | 145 | 2 | 9 | 5 | 3 | Trace | 16 | 65 | 0.3 | 80 | 0.02 | 0.10 | 0.1 | Trace |
| 531 | Chocolate-coated peanuts | 1 oz | 28 | 1 | 160 | 5 | 12 | 3 | 6 | 2 | 11 | 33 | 0.4 | Trace | 0.10 | 0.05 | 2.1 | Trace |
| 532 | Fondant; mints, uncoated; candy corn | 1 oz | 28 | 8 | 105 | Trace | 1 | — | — | — | 25 | 4 | 0.3 | 0 | Trace | Trace | Trace | 0 |
| 533 | Fudge, plain | 1 oz | 28 | 8 | 115 | 1 | 4 | 2 | 1 | Trace | 21 | 22 | 0.3 | Trace | 0.01 | 0.03 | 0.1 | Trace |
| 534 | Gum drops | 1 oz | 28 | 12 | 100 | Trace | Trace | — | — | — | 25 | 2 | 0.1 | 0 | 0 | Trace | Trace | 0 |
| 535 | Hard | 1 oz | 28 | 1 | 110 | 0 | Trace | — | — | — | 28 | 6 | 0.5 | 0 | 0 | 0 | 0 | 0 |
| 536 | Marshmallows | 1 oz | 28 | 17 | 90 | 1 | Trace | — | — | — | 23 | 5 | 0.5 | 0 | 0 | Trace | Trace | 0 |
| | Chocolate-flavored syrup or topping: | | | | | | | | | | | | | | | | | |
| 537 | Thin type | 1 fl oz | 38 | 32 | 90 | 1 | 1 | Trace | Trace | Trace | 24 | 6 | 0.6 | Trace | 0.01 | 0.03 | 0.2 | 0 |
| 538 | Fudge type | 1 fl oz | 38 | 25 | 125 | 2 | 5 | 3 | 2 | Trace | 20 | 48 | 0.5 | 60 | 0.02 | 0.08 | 0.2 | Trace |
| 539 | Chocolate-flavored beverage powder (approx. 4 heaping teaspoons per oz): With nonfat dry milk | 1 oz | 28 | 2 | 100 | 5 | 1 | Trace | Trace | Trace | 20 | 167 | 0.5 | 10 | 0.04 | 0.21 | 0.2 | 1 |
| 540 | Without nonfat dry milk | 1 oz | 28 | 1 | 100 | 1 | 0 | Trace | Trace | Trace | 25 | 9 | 0.6 | 0 | 0.01 | 0.03 | 0.1 | 0 |
| 541 | Honey, strained or extracted | 1 tbsp | 21 | 17 | 65 | Trace | 0 | — | — | — | 17 | 1 | 0.1 | Trace | Trace | 0.01 | 0.1 | Trace |
| 542 | Jams and preserves | 1 tbsp | 20 | 29 | 55 | Trace | Trace | — | — | — | 14 | 4 | 0.2 | Trace | Trace | 0.01 | Trace | Trace |
| 543 | Jellies | 1 tbsp | 18 | 29 | 50 | Trace | Trace | — | — | — | 13 | 4 | 0.3 | Trace | Trace | 0.01 | Trace | 1 |
| | Molasses, cane: | | | | | | | | | | | | | | | | | |
| 544 | Light (first extraction) | 1 tbsp | 20 | 24 | 50 | — | — | — | — | — | 13 | 33 | 0.9 | — | 0.01 | 0.01 | Trace | — |
| 545 | Blackstrap (third extraction) | 1 tbsp | 20 | 24 | 45 | — | — | — | — | — | 11 | 137 | 3.2 | — | 0.02 | 0.04 | 0.4 | — |
| | Syrups: | | | | | | | | | | | | | | | | | |
| 546 | Sorghum | 1 tbsp | 21 | 23 | 55 | — | — | — | — | — | 14 | 35 | 2.6 | — | — | 0.02 | Trace | — |

[19] Iron, thiamine, riboflavin, and niacin are based on the minimum levels of enrichment specified in standards of identity promulgated under the Federal Food, Drug, and Cosmetic Act.

[21] Year-round average.

[22] Based on the average vitamin A content of fortified margarine. Federal specifications for fortified margarine require a minimum of 15,000 I.U. of vitamin A per pound.

# Table A-1. (Cont.)

| | Food, Approximate Measure, and Weight (in grams) | | gm | Water per cent | Food Energy calories | Protein gm | Fat gm | Fatty Acids | | | Carbohydrate gm | Calcium mg | Iron mg | Vitamin A Value I.U. | Thiamine mg | Riboflavin mg | Niacin mg | Ascorbic Acid mg |
|---|---|---|---|---|---|---|---|---|---|---|---|---|---|---|---|---|---|---|
| | | | | | | | | Saturated (total) gm | Unsaturated Oleic gm | Linoleic gm | | | | | | | | |
| | Syrups (cont.) | | | | | | | | | | | | | | | | | |
| 547 | Table blends, chiefly corn, light and dark | 1 tbsp | 21 | 24 | 60 | 0 | 0 | — | — | — | 15 | 9 | 0.8 | 0 | 0 | 0 | 0 | 0 |
| | Sugars: | | | | | | | | | | | | | | | | | |
| 548 | Brown, firm packed | 1 cup | 220 | 2 | 820 | 0 | 0 | — | — | — | 212 | 187 | 7.5 | 0 | 0.02 | 0.07 | 0.4 | 0 |
| | White: | | | | | | | | | | | | | | | | | |
| 549 | Granulated | 1 cup | 200 | Trace | 770 | 0 | 0 | — | — | — | 199 | 0 | 0.2 | 0 | 0 | 0 | 0 | 0 |
| 550 | | 1 tbsp | 11 | Trace | 40 | 0 | 0 | — | — | — | 11 | 0 | Trace | 0 | 0 | 0 | 0 | 0 |
| 551 | Powdered, stirred before measuring | 1 cup | 120 | Trace | 460 | 0 | 0 | — | — | — | 119 | 0 | 0.1 | 0 | 0 | 0 | 0 | 0 |
| | **Miscellaneous Items** | | | | | | | | | | | | | | | | | |
| 552 | Barbecue sauce | 1 cup | 250 | 81 | 230 | 4 | 17 | 2 | 5 | 9 | 20 | 53 | 2.0 | 900 | 0.03 | 0.03 | 0.8 | 13 |
| | Beverages, alcoholic: | | | | | | | | | | | | | | | | | |
| 553 | Beer | 12 fl oz | 360 | 92 | 150 | 1 | 0 | — | — | — | 14 | 18 | Trace | — | 0.01 | 0.11 | 2.2 | — |
| | Gin, rum, vodka, whiskey: | | | | | | | | | | | | | | | | | |
| 554 | 80 proof | 1 1/2 fl oz jigger | 42 | 67 | 100 | — | — | — | — | — | Trace | — | — | — | — | — | — | — |
| 555 | 86 proof | 1 1/2 fl oz jigger | 42 | 64 | 105 | — | — | — | — | — | Trace | — | — | — | — | — | — | — |
| 556 | 90 proof | 1 1/2 fl oz jigger | 42 | 62 | 110 | — | — | — | — | — | Trace | — | — | — | — | — | — | — |
| 557 | 94 proof | 1 1/2 fl oz jigger | 42 | 60 | 115 | — | — | — | — | — | Trace | — | — | — | — | — | — | — |
| 558 | 100 proof | 1 1/2 fl oz jigger | 42 | 58 | 125 | — | — | — | — | — | Trace | — | — | — | — | — | — | — |
| | Wines: | | | | | | | | | | | | | | | | | |
| 559 | Dessert | 3 1/2 fl oz glass | 103 | 77 | 140 | Trace | 0 | — | — | — | 8 | 8 | — | — | 0.01 | 0.02 | 0.2 | — |
| 560 | Table | 3 1/2 fl oz glass | 102 | 86 | 85 | Trace | 0 | — | — | — | 4 | 9 | 0.4 | — | Trace | 0.01 | 0.1 | — |
| | Beverages, carbonated, sweetened, nonalcoholic: | | | | | | | | | | | | | | | | | |
| 561 | Carbonated water | 12 fl oz | 366 | 92 | 115 | 0 | 0 | — | — | — | 29 | — | — | — | — | — | — | — |
| 562 | Cola type | 12 fl oz | 369 | 90 | 145 | 0 | 0 | — | — | — | 37 | — | — | 0 | 0 | 0 | 0 | 0 |
| 563 | Fruit-flavored sodas and Tom Collins mixes | 12 fl oz | 372 | 88 | 170 | 0 | 0 | — | — | — | 45 | — | — | 0 | 0 | 0 | 0 | 0 |
| 564 | Ginger ale | 12 fl oz | 366 | 92 | 115 | 0 | 0 | — | — | — | 29 | — | — | 0 | 0 | 0 | 0 | 0 |
| 565 | Root beer | 12 fl oz | 370 | 90 | 150 | 0 | 0 | — | — | — | 39 | — | — | 0 | 0 | 0 | 0 | 0 |
| 566 | Bouillon cubes, approx. 1/2 in | 1 cube | 4 | 4 | 5 | 1 | Trace | — | — | — | Trace | — | — | — | — | — | — | — |
| | Chocolate: | | | | | | | | | | | | | | | | | |
| 567 | Bitter or baking | 1 oz | 28 | 2 | 145 | 3 | 15 | 8 | 6 | Trace | 8 | 22 | 1.9 | 20 | 0.01 | 0.07 | 0.4 | 0 |
| 568 | Semisweet, small pieces | 1 cup | 170 | 1 | 860 | 7 | 61 | 34 | 22 | 1 | 97 | 51 | 4.4 | 30 | 0.02 | 0.14 | 0.9 | 0 |
| | Gelatin: | | | | | | | | | | | | | | | | | |
| 569 | Plain, dry powder in envelope | 1 envelope | 7 | 13 | 25 | 6 | Trace | — | — | — | 0 | — | — | — | — | — | — | — |
| 570 | Dessert powder, 3-oz package | 1 pkg | 85 | 2 | 315 | 8 | 0 | — | — | — | 75 | — | — | — | — | — | — | — |
| 571 | Gelatin dessert, prepared with water | 1 cup | 240 | 84 | 140 | 4 | 0 | — | — | — | 34 | — | — | — | — | — | — | — |

| No. | Food, approximate measure | Measure | Grams | Water (%) | Food energy (cal.) | Protein (g) | Fat (g) | Saturated (g) | Oleic (g) | Linoleic (g) | Carbohydrate (g) | Calcium (mg) | Iron (mg) | Vitamin A (IU) | Thiamin (mg) | Riboflavin (mg) | Niacin (mg) | Ascorbic acid (mg) |
|---|---|---|---|---|---|---|---|---|---|---|---|---|---|---|---|---|---|---|
| | Olives, pickled: | | | | | | | | | | | | | | | | | |
| 572 | Green | 4 medium or 3 extra large or 2 giant | 16 | 78 | 15 | Trace | 2 | Trace | 2 | Trace | Trace | 8 | 0.2 | 40 | — | — | — | — |
| 573 | Ripe: Mission | 3 small or 2 large | 10 | 73 | 15 | Trace | 2 | Trace | 2 | Trace | Trace | 9 | 0.1 | 10 | — | Trace | — | — |
| | Pickles, cucumber: | | | | | | | | | | | | | | | | | |
| 574 | Dill, medium, whole, 3 3/4 in long, 1 1/4 in diam. | 1 pickle | 65 | 93 | 10 | 1 | Trace | — | — | — | 1 | 17 | 0.7 | 70 | Trace | 0.01 | Trace | 4 |
| 575 | Fresh, sliced, 1 1/2 in diam, 1/4 in thick | 2 slices | 15 | 79 | 10 | Trace | Trace | — | — | — | Trace | 5 | 0.3 | 20 | Trace | Trace | Trace | 1 |
| 576 | Sweet, gherkin, small, whole, approx. 2 1/2 in long, 3/4 in diam. | 1 pickle | 15 | 61 | 20 | Trace | Trace | — | — | — | 5 | 2 | 0.2 | 10 | Trace | Trace | Trace | 1 |
| 577 | Relish, finely chopped, sweet | 1 tbsp | 15 | 63 | 20 | Trace | Trace | — | — | — | 5 | 3 | 0.1 | — | — | — | — | — |
| | Popcorn. See Grain Products | | | | | | | | | | | | | | | | | |
| 578 | Popsicle, 3-fl oz size | 1 popsicle | 95 | 80 | 70 | 0 | 0 | 0 | 0 | 0 | 18 | 0 | Trace | 0 | 0 | 0 | 0 | 0 |
| | Pudding, home recipe with starch base: | | | | | | | | | | | | | | | | | |
| 579 | Chocolate | 1 cup | 260 | 66 | 385 | 8 | 12 | 7 | 4 | Trace | 67 | 250 | 1.3 | 390 | 0.05 | 0.36 | 0.3 | 1 |
| 580 | Vanilla (blanc mange) | 1 cup | 255 | 76 | 285 | 9 | 10 | 5 | 3 | Trace | 41 | 298 | Trace | 410 | 0.08 | 0.41 | 0.3 | 2 |
| 581 | Pudding mix, dry form, 4-oz package | 1 pkg | 113 | 2 | 410 | 3 | 2 | 1 | 1 | Trace | 103 | 23 | 1.8 | Trace | 0.02 | 0.08 | 0.5 | 0 |
| 582 | Sherbet | 1 cup | 193 | 67 | 260 | 2 | 2 | — | — | — | 59 | 31 | Trace | 120 | 0.02 | 0.06 | Trace | 4 |
| | Soups: | | | | | | | | | | | | | | | | | |
| | Canned, condensed, ready-to-serve: | | | | | | | | | | | | | | | | | |
| | Prepared with an equal volume of milk: | | | | | | | | | | | | | | | | | |
| 583 | Cream of chicken | 1 cup | 245 | 85 | 180 | 7 | 10 | 3 | 3 | 3 | 15 | 172 | 0.5 | 610 | 0.05 | 0.27 | 0.7 | 2 |
| 584 | Cream of mushroom | 1 cup | 245 | 83 | 215 | 7 | 14 | 4 | 4 | 5 | 16 | 191 | 0.5 | 250 | 0.05 | 0.34 | 0.7 | 1 |
| 585 | Tomato | 1 cup | 250 | 84 | 175 | 7 | 7 | 3 | 2 | 1 | 23 | 168 | 0.8 | 1,200 | 0.10 | 0.25 | 1.3 | 15 |
| | Prepared with an equal volume of water: | | | | | | | | | | | | | | | | | |
| 586 | Bean with pork | 1 cup | 250 | 84 | 170 | 8 | 6 | 1 | 2 | 2 | 22 | 63 | 2.3 | 650 | 0.13 | 0.08 | 1.0 | 3 |
| 587 | Beef broth, bouillon consommé | 1 cup | 240 | 96 | 30 | 5 | 0 | — | — | — | 3 | Trace | 0.5 | Trace | Trace | 0.02 | 1.2 | — |
| 588 | Beef noodle | 1 cup | 240 | 93 | 70 | 4 | 3 | 1 | 1 | 1 | 7 | 7 | 1.0 | 50 | 0.05 | 0.07 | 1.0 | Trace |
| 589 | Clam chowder, Manhattan type (with tomatoes, without milk) | 1 cup | 245 | 92 | 80 | 2 | 3 | — | — | — | 12 | 34 | 1.0 | 880 | 0.02 | 0.02 | 1.0 | — |
| 590 | Cream of chicken | 1 cup | 240 | 92 | 95 | 3 | 6 | 2 | 2 | 3 | 8 | 24 | 0.5 | 410 | 0.02 | 0.05 | 0.5 | Trace |
| 591 | Cream of mushroom | 1 cup | 240 | 90 | 135 | 2 | 10 | 3 | 3 | 5 | 10 | 41 | 0.5 | 70 | 0.02 | 0.12 | 0.7 | Trace |
| 592 | Minestrone | 1 cup | 245 | 90 | 105 | 5 | 3 | — | — | — | 14 | 37 | 1.0 | 2,350 | 0.07 | 0.05 | 1.0 | — |
| 593 | Split pea | 1 cup | 245 | 85 | 145 | 9 | 3 | 1 | 2 | Trace | 21 | 29 | 1.5 | 440 | 0.25 | 0.15 | 1.5 | 1 |
| 594 | Tomato | 1 cup | 245 | 90 | 90 | 2 | 2 | Trace | 1 | 1 | 16 | 15 | 0.7 | 1,000 | 0.05 | 0.05 | 1.2 | 12 |
| 595 | Vegetable beef | 1 cup | 245 | 92 | 80 | 5 | 2 | — | — | — | 10 | 12 | 0.7 | 2,700 | 0.05 | 0.05 | 1.0 | — |
| 596 | Vegetarian | 1 cup | 245 | 92 | 80 | 2 | 2 | — | — | — | 13 | 20 | 1.0 | 2,940 | 0.05 | 0.05 | 1.0 | — |
| | Dehydrated, dry form: | | | | | | | | | | | | | | | | | |
| 597 | Chicken noodle (2-oz package) | 1 pkg | 57 | 6 | 220 | 8 | 6 | 2 | 3 | 3 | 33 | 34 | 1.4 | 190 | 0.30 | 0.15 | 2.4 | 3 |
| 598 | Onion mix (1 1/2-oz package) | 1 pkg | 43 | 3 | 150 | 6 | 5 | 1 | 2 | 5 | 23 | 42 | 0.6 | 30 | 0.05 | 0.03 | 0.3 | 6 |
| 599 | Tomato vegetable with noodles (2 1/2-oz pkg) | 1 pkg | 71 | 4 | 245 | 6 | 6 | 2 | 3 | Trace | 45 | 33 | 1.4 | 1,700 | 0.21 | 0.13 | 1.8 | 18 |
| | Frozen, condensed: | | | | | | | | | | | | | | | | | |
| | Clam chowder, New England type (with milk, without tomatoes): | | | | | | | | | | | | | | | | | |
| 600 | Prepared with equal volume of milk | 1 cup | 245 | 83 | 210 | 9 | 12 | — | — | — | 16 | 240 | 1.0 | 250 | 0.07 | 0.29 | 0.5 | Trace |

**Table A–1. (Cont.)**

| Food, Approximate Measure, and Weight (in grams) | | gm | Water per cent | Food Energy calories | Protein gm | Fat gm | Saturated (total) gm | Oleic gm | Linoleic gm | Carbohydrate gm | Calcium mg | Iron mg | Vitamin A Value I.U. | Thiamine mg | Riboflavin mg | Niacin mg | Ascorbic Acid mg |
|---|---|---|---|---|---|---|---|---|---|---|---|---|---|---|---|---|---|
| | | | | | | | | Unsaturated | Fatty Acids | | | | | | | | |
| **Soups, frozen (cont.)** | | | | | | | | | | | | | | | | | |
| 601 | Clam chowder, New England type Prepared with equal volume of water | 1 cup | 240 | 89 | 130 | 4 | 8 | — | — | — | 11 | 91 | 1.0 | 50 | 0.05 | 0.10 | 0.5 | — |
| 602 | Cream of potato: Prepared with equal volume of milk | 1 cup | 245 | 83 | 185 | 8 | 10 | 5 | 3 | Trace | 18 | 208 | 1.0 | 590 | 0.10 | 0.27 | 0.5 | Trace |
| 603 | Prepared with equal volume of water | 1 cup | 240 | 90 | 105 | 3 | 5 | 3 | 2 | Trace | 12 | 58 | 1.0 | 410 | 0.05 | 0.05 | 0.5 | — |
| 604 | Cream of shrimp: Prepared with equal volume of milk | 1 cup | 245 | 82 | 245 | 9 | 16 | — | — | — | 15 | 189 | 0.5 | 290 | 0.07 | 0.27 | 0.5 | Trace |
| 605 | Prepared with equal volume of water | 1 cup | 240 | 88 | 160 | 5 | 12 | — | — | — | 8 | 38 | 0.5 | 120 | 0.05 | 0.05 | 0.5 | — |
| 606 | Oyster stew: Prepared with equal volume of milk | 1 cup | 240 | 83 | 200 | 10 | 12 | — | — | — | 14 | 305 | 1.4 | 410 | 0.12 | 0.41 | 0.5 | Trace |
| 607 | Prepared with equal volume of water | 1 cup | 240 | 90 | 120 | 6 | 8 | — | — | — | 8 | 158 | 1.4 | 240 | 0.07 | 0.19 | 0.5 | — |
| 608 | Tapioca, dry, quick cooking | 1 cup | 152 | 13 | 535 | 1 | Trace | — | — | — | 131 | 15 | 0.6 | 0 | 0 | 0 | 0 | 0 |
| | **Tapioca desserts:** | | | | | | | | | | | | | | | | | |
| 609 | Apple | 1 cup | 250 | 70 | 295 | 1 | Trace | — | — | — | 74 | 8 | 0.5 | 30 | Trace | Trace | Trace | Trace |
| 610 | Cream pudding | 1 cup | 165 | 72 | 220 | 8 | 8 | 4 | 3 | Trace | 28 | 173 | 0.7 | 480 | 0.07 | 0.30 | 0.2 | 2 |
| 611 | Tartar sauce | 1 tbsp | 14 | 34 | 75 | Trace | 8 | 1 | 1 | 4 | 1 | 3 | 0.1 | 30 | Trace | Trace | Trace | Trace |
| 612 | Vinegar | 1 tbsp | 15 | 94 | Trace | Trace | 0 | — | — | — | 1 | 1 | 0.1 | — | — | — | — | — |
| 613 | White sauce, medium | 1 cup | 250 | 73 | 405 | 10 | 31 | 10 | 10 | 1 | 22 | 288 | 0.5 | 1,150 | 0.10 | 0.43 | 0.5 | 2 |
| | **Yeast:** | | | | | | | | | | | | | | | | | |
| 614 | Bakers', dry, active | 1 pkg | 7 | 5 | 20 | 3 | Trace | — | — | — | 3 | 3 | 1.1 | Trace | 0.16 | 0.38 | 2.6 | Trace |
| 615 | Brewers', dry | 1 tbsp | 8 | 5 | 25 | 3 | Trace | — | — | — | 3 | 17 | 1.4 | Trace | 1.25 | 0.34 | 3.0 | Trace |
| | Yogurt. See Milk, Cheese, Cream, Imitation Cream | | | | | | | | | | | | | | | | | |

Foods are divided into six groups, according to their composition.

| Food Exchange | Measure | Weight (gm) | Carbo-hydrate (gm) | Protein (gm) | Fat (gm) | Calories |
|---|---|---|---|---|---|---|
| | | Quantity for One Exchange | | | | |
| Milk | 8 oz | 240 | 12 | 8 | 10 | 170 |
| Vegetables—A | As desired | — | — | — | — | — |
| Vegetables—B | ½ cup | 100 | 7 | 2 | — | 36 |
| Fruit | Varies | — | 10 | — | — | 40 |
| Bread | Varies | — | 15 | 2 | — | 68 |
| Meat | 1 oz | 30 | — | 7 | 5 | 73 |
| Fat | 1 teaspoon | 5 | — | — | 5 | 45 |

* Caso, E. K.: "Calculation of Diabetic Diets," *J. Amer. Diet. Assoc.*, **26**:575, 1950.

## LIST 1—MILK EXCHANGES

PER EXCHANGE: CARBOHYDRATE, 12 GM; PROTEIN, 8 GM; FAT 10 GM.

| | Measure |
|---|---|
| Milk, whole (plain or homogenized) | 1 cup (8 ounces) |
| Milk, skim, liquid * | 1 cup |
| Milk, evaporated | ½ cup |
| Milk, powdered whole | 3–5 tablespoons † |
| Milk, nonfat dry * | 3–5 tablespoons † |
| Buttermilk (from whole milk) | 1 cup |
| Buttermilk (from skim milk) * | 1 cup |

* Because these forms of milk contain no fat, two fat exchanges may be added to the diet when they are used; or one exchange of these forms of milk may be calculated as carbohydrate, 12; protein, 8; and fat, 0.

† The amount of milk powder to use depends upon the brand used; read package direction for the equivalent for 1 cup liquid milk.

## LIST 2—VEGETABLE EXCHANGES

GROUP A VEGETABLES—NEGLIGIBLE CARBOHYDRATE, PROTEIN, AND FAT IF 1 CUP (200 GM) OR LESS IS USED. COUNT EACH ADDITIONAL CUP AS ONE EXCHANGE OF GROUP B VEGETABLE.

Asparagus
Beans, string, young
Broccoli * †
Brussels sprouts †
Cabbage †
Cauliflower †
Celery
Chicory * †
Cucumbers
Escarole * †

Eggplant
Greens *
  beet greens
  chard, Swiss
  collard †
  dandelion
  kale †
  mustard †
  spinach †
  turnip greens †

Lettuce
Mushrooms
Okra
Pepper * †
Radish
Sauerkraut
Squash, summer
Tomatoes * †
Watercress *

GROUP B VEGETABLES—PER EXCHANGE: CARBOHYDRATE, 7 GM; PROTEIN, 2 GM; FAT, NEGLIGIBLE. ONE EXCHANGE = ½ CUP = 100 GM.

| | | |
|---|---|---|
| Beets | Peas, green | Squash, winter * |
| Carrots * | Pumpkin * | Turnip |
| Onion | Rutabaga | |

 * These vegetables have high vitamin A value. At least one serving should be included in the diet each day.

 † These vegetables are good sources of ascorbic acid.

## LIST 3—FRUIT EXCHANGES

PER EXCHANGE: CARBOHYDRATE, 10 GM; PROTEIN, AND FAT, NEGLIGIBLE. FRUITS MAY BE USED FRESH, COOKED, CANNED, OR FROZEN, UNSWEETENED.

| | *Measure* |
|---|---|
| Apple | 1 small, 2-in. diameter |
| Applesauce | ½ cup |
| Apricots, dried * | 4 halves |
| Apricots, fresh * | 2 medium |
| Banana | ½ small |
| Blackberries | 1 cup |
| Blueberries | ⅔ cup |
| Cantaloupe †* | ¼, 6-in. diameter |
| Cherries | 10 large |
| Dates | 2 |
| Figs, dried | 1 small |
| Figs, fresh | 2 large |
| Grapefruit † | ½ small |
| Grapefruit juice † | ½ cup |
| Grape juice | ¼ cup |
| Grapes | 12 |
| Honeydew melon † | ⅛, 7-in. diameter |
| Mango | ½ small |
| Nectarines | 1 medium |
| Orange †* | 1 small |
| Orange juice †* | ½ cup |
| Papaya * | ⅓ medium |
| Peach * (yellow) | 1 medium |
| Pear | 1 small |
| Pineapple | ½ cup cubed |
| Pineapple juice | ⅓ cup |
| Plums * | 2 medium |
| Prunes, dried * | 2 medium |
| Raisins | 2 tablespoons |
| Raspberries | 1 cup |
| Strawberries † | 1 cup |
| Tangerine * | 1 large |
| Watermelon | 1 cup diced |

 * These fruits are good sources of vitamin A.

 † These fruits are rich sources of ascorbic acid. Include at least one exchange daily.

PER EXCHANGE: CARBOHYDRATE, 15 GM; PROTEIN, 2 GM; FAT, NEGLIGIBLE.

|  | *Measure* |
|---|---|
| Bread | 1 slice |
| biscuit, roll (2-in. diameter) | 1 |
| muffin | 1 medium |
| cornbread | 1½-inch cube |
| Cereal, cooked | ½ cup |
| Cereal, dry | ¾ cup |
| Crackers, graham | 2 |
| oyster | 20 (½ cup) |
| saltines (2-in. square) | 5 |
| soda (2½-in square) | 3 |
| round, thin (1½-in. diameter) | 6–8 |
| Flour | 2½ tablespoons |
| Grits | ½ cup cooked |
| Ice cream, vanilla (omit two fat exchanges) | ⅛ quart |
| Macaroni | ½ cup cooked |
| Matzoth | ½ (6½-in. square) |
| Noodles | ½ cup cooked |
| Rice | ½ cup cooked |
| Spaghetti | ½ cup cooked |
| Sponge cake, no icing | 1½-inch cube |
| Vegetables |  |
| beans, baked; no pork | ¼ cup |
| beans, and peas, dried (includes kidney, Lima, navy beans, black-eyed, split, and cowpeas, etc.) | ½ cup cooked |
| beans, Lima, fresh | ½ cup |
| corn, popped | 1 cup |
| corn, fresh | ⅓ cup or ½ small ear |
| parsnips | ⅔ cup |
| potatoes, white | 1 small (2-in. diameter) |
| potatoes, white, mashed | ½ cup |
| potatoes, sweet or yam | ¼ cup |

## List 5—Meat Exchanges

PER EXCHANGE: CABOHYDRATE, NEGLIGIBLE; PROTEIN, 7 GM; FAT, 5 GM.
MEASURES AND WEIGHTS ARE FOR COOKED MEAT.

|  | *Measure* |
|---|---|
| Meat, fish, and poultry (medium fat) (beef, lamb, pork, veal, liver, chicken, turkey, etc.) | 1 oz |
| cold cuts (bologna, liver sausage, luncheon loaf, boiled ham, salami, etc.) | 1 slice, ⅛-in. thick |
| frankfurt | 1 |

| | |
|---|---|
| cod, haddock, halibut, herring, etc. | 1 oz |
| crab, lobster, salmon, tuna | ¼ cup |
| clams, oysters, shrimp | 5 small |
| sardines | 3 medium |
| Cheese, Cheddar | 1 oz |
| cottage | ¼ cup |
| Egg | 1 |
| Peanut butter * | 2 tablespoons |

* Limit to one exchange daily, or adjust for carbohydrate. Deduct 5 gm carbohydrate for each additional exchange.

## List 6—Fat Exchanges

Per Exchange: fat, 5 gm; protein and carbohydrate, negligible.

| | Measure |
|---|---|
| Butter or margarine | 1 teaspoon |
| Bacon, crisp | 1 slice |
| Cream, light, 20 per cent | 2 tablespoons |
| Cream, heavy, 35–40 per cent | 1 tablespoon |
| Cream cheese | 1 tablespoon |
| French dressing | 1 tablespoon |
| Mayonnaise | 1 teaspoon |
| Nuts | 6 small |
| Oil or cooking fat | 1 teaspoon |
| Olives | 5 small |
| Avocado | ⅛, 4-in. diameter |

## Foods Allowed As Desired

Protein, Fat, and Carbohydrate Negligible.

| | | |
|---|---|---|
| Coffee | Gelatin, unsweetened | Vinegar |
| Tea | Rennet tablets | Cranberries, unsweetened |
| Clear broth | Saccharin | Lemon |
| Bouillon | Spices | Mustard, dry |
| (fat-free) | | Pickle, dill, unsweetened |
| Herbs | | Rhubarb, unsweetened |

TABLE A-3 SUGGESTED WEIGHTS FOR HEIGHTS FOR MEN AND WOMEN *

| Height (without shoes) | | Weight (without clothing) | | | | | |
| cm | in. | Low | | Median | | High | |
| | | kg | lb | kg | lb | kg | lb |
|---|---|---|---|---|---|---|---|
| | | | Men | | | | |
| 160 | 63 | 54 | 118 | 59 | 129 | 64 | 141 |
| 163 | 64 | 55 | 122 | 60 | 133 | 66 | 145 |
| 165 | 65 | 57 | 126 | 62 | 137 | 68 | 149 |
| 167 | 66 | 59 | 130 | 65 | 142 | 70 | 155 |
| 170 | 67 | 61 | 134 | 67 | 147 | 73 | 161 |
| 173 | 68 | 63 | 139 | 69 | 151 | 75 | 166 |
| 175 | 69 | 65 | 143 | 70 | 155 | 77 | 170 |
| 178 | 70 | 67 | 147 | 72 | 159 | 80 | 174 |
| 180 | 71 | 68 | 150 | 74 | 163 | 81 | 178 |
| 183 | 72 | 70 | 154 | 76 | 167 | 83 | 183 |
| 185 | 73 | 72 | 158 | 77 | 171 | 85 | 188 |
| 188 | 74 | 74 | 162 | 80 | 175 | 87 | 192 |
| 191 | 75 | 75 | 165 | 81 | 178 | 89 | 195 |
| | | | Women | | | | |
| 152 | 60 | 45 | 100 | 50 | 109 | 54 | 118 |
| 155 | 61 | 47 | 104 | 51 | 112 | 55 | 121 |
| 157 | 62 | 49 | 107 | 52 | 115 | 57 | 125 |
| 160 | 63 | 50 | 110 | 54 | 118 | 58 | 128 |
| 163 | 64 | 51 | 113 | 55 | 122 | 60 | 132 |
| 165 | 65 | 53 | 116 | 57 | 125 | 61 | 135 |
| 167 | 66 | 55 | 120 | 59 | 129 | 63 | 139 |
| 170 | 67 | 56 | 123 | 60 | 132 | 65 | 142 |
| 173 | 68 | 57 | 126 | 62 | 136 | 66 | 146 |
| 175 | 69 | 59 | 130 | 64 | 140 | 69 | 151 |
| 178 | 70 | 60 | 133 | 65 | 144 | 71 | 156 |
| 180 | 71 | 62 | 137 | 67 | 148 | 73 | 161 |
| 183 | 72 | 64 | 141 | 69 | 152 | 75 | 166 |

* Data for heights in inches and weights in pounds taken from: Hathaway, M. L., and Foard, E. D.; *Heights and Weights of Adults in the United States*. Home Economics Research Report No. 10, U.S. Department of Agriculture, Washington, D.C., Table 80, p. 111.
Conversions to centimeters and kilograms were rounded off to the nearest whole number.

## TABLE A-4 Recommended Daily Nutrient Intakes—Canada, Revised 1974
### (Committee for Revision of the Canadian Dietary Standard, Bureau of Nutritional Sciences, Health and Welfare, Ottawa, Canada)

| Age (years) | Sex | Weight (kg) | Height (cm) | Energy[a] (kcal) | Protein (gm) | Thiamin (mg) | Niacin[e] (mg) | Riboflavin (mg) | Vitamin B$_6$[f] (mg) | Folate[g] (mcg) | Vitamin B$_{12}$ (mcg) | Ascorbic Acid (mg) |
|---|---|---|---|---|---|---|---|---|---|---|---|---|
| | | | | | | | | Water-Soluble Vitamins | | | | |
| 0– 6 mos. | both | 6 | | kg × 117 | kg × 2.2 (2.0)[d] | 0.3 | 5 | 0.4 | 0.3 | 40 | 0.3 | 20[h] |
| 1–11 mos. | both | 9 | | kg × 108 | kg × 1.4 | 0.5 | 6 | 0.6 | 0.4 | 60 | 0.3 | 20 |
| 1– 3 | both | 13 | 90 | 1400 | 22 | 0.7 | 9 | 0.8 | 0.8 | 100 | 0.9 | 20 |
| 4– 6 | both | 19 | 110 | 1800 | 27 | 0.9 | 12 | 1.1 | 1.3 | 100 | 1.5 | 30 |
| 7– 9 | M | 27 | 129 | 2200 | 33 | 1.1 | 14 | 1.3 | 1.6 | 100 | 1.5 | 30 |
| | F | 27 | 128 | 2000 | 33 | 1.0 | 13 | 1.2 | 1.4 | 100 | 1.5 | 30 |
| 10–12 | M | 36 | 144 | 2500 | 41 | 1.2 | 17 | 1.5 | 1.8 | 100 | 3.0 | 30 |
| | F | 38 | 145 | 2300 | 40 | 1.1 | 15 | 1.4 | 1.5 | 100 | 3.0 | 30 |
| 13–15 | M | 51 | 162 | 2800 | 52 | 1.4 | 19 | 1.7 | 2.0 | 200 | 3.0 | 30 |
| | F | 49 | 159 | 2200 | 43 | 1.1 | 15 | 1.4 | 1.5 | 200 | 3.0 | 30 |
| 16–18 | M | 64 | 172 | 3200 | 54 | 1.6 | 21 | 2.0 | 2.0 | 200 | 3.0 | 30 |
| | F | 54 | 161 | 2100 | 43 | 1.1 | 14 | 1.3 | 1.5 | 200 | 3.0 | 30 |
| 19–35 | M | 70 | 176 | 3000 | 56 | 1.5 | 20 | 1.8 | 2.0 | 200 | 3.0 | 30 |
| | F | 56 | 161 | 2100 | 41 | 1.1 | 14 | 1.3 | 1.5 | 200 | 3.0 | 30 |
| 36–50 | M | 70 | 176 | 2700 | 56 | 1.4 | 18 | 1.7 | 2.0 | 200 | 3.0 | 30 |
| | F | 56 | 161 | 1900 | 41 | 1.0 | 13 | 1.2 | 1.5 | 200 | 3.0 | 30 |
| 51+ | M | 70 | 176 | 2300[b] | 56 | 1.4 | 18 | 1.7 | 2.0 | 200 | 3.0 | 30 |
| | F | 56 | 161 | 1800[b] | 41 | 1.0 | 13 | 1.2 | 1.5 | 200 | 3.0 | 30 |
| Pregnant | | | | +300[c] | +20 | +0.2 | +2 | +0.3 | +0.5 | +50 | +1.0 | +20 |
| Lactating | | | | +500 | +24 | +0.4 | +7 | +0.6 | +0.6 | +50 | +0.5 | +30 |

[a] Recommendations assume characteristic activity pattern for each age group.

[b] Recommended energy allowance for age 66+ years reduced to 2000 for men and 1500 for women.

[c] Increased energy allowance recommended during second and third trimesters. An increase of 100 kcal per day is recommended during the first trimester.

[d] Recommended protein allowance of 2.2 gm per kg body weight for infants age 0–2 mos., and 2.0 gm per kg body weight for those age 3–5 mos. Protein recommendation for infants, 0–11 mos., assumes consumption of breast milk or protein of equivalent quality.

[e] Approximately 1 mg of niacin is derived from each 60 mg of dietary tryptophan.

[f] Recommendations are based on the estimated average daily protein intake of Canadians.

[g] Recommendations given in terms of free folate.

[h] Considerably higher levels may be prudent for infants during the first week of life to guard against neonatal tyrosinemia.

| Age (years) | Fat-Soluble Vitamins | | | Minerals | | | | | |
|---|---|---|---|---|---|---|---|---|---|
| | Vitamin A (mcg RE)[l] | Vitamin D (mcg cholecalciferol)[j] | Vitamin E (mg α-tocopherol) | Calcium (mg) | Phosphorus (mg) | Magnesium (mg) | Iodine (mcg) | Iron (mg) | Zinc (mg) |
| 0– 6 mos. | 400 | 10 | 3 | 500[l] | 250[l] | 50[l] | 35[l] | 7[l] | 4[l] |
| 7–11 mos. | 400 | 10 | 3 | 500 | 400 | 50 | 50 | 7 | 5 |
| 1– 3 | 400 | 10 | 4 | 500 | 500 | 75 | 70 | 8 | 5 |
| 4– 6 | 500 | 5 | 5 | 500 | 500 | 100 | 90 | 9 | 6 |
| 7– 9 M | 700 | 2.5[k] | 6 | 700 | 700 | 150 | 110 | 10 | 7 |
| 7– 9 F | 700 | 2.5[k] | 6 | 700 | 700 | 150 | 100 | 10 | 7 |
| 10–12 M | 800 | 2.5[k] | 7 | 900 | 900 | 175 | 130 | 11 | 8 |
| 10–12 F | 800 | 2.5[k] | 7 | 1000 | 1000 | 200 | 120 | 11 | 9 |
| 13–15 M | 1000 | 2.5[k] | 9 | 1200 | 1200 | 250 | 140 | 13 | 10 |
| 13–15 F | 800 | 2.6[k] | 7 | 800 | 800 | 250 | 110 | 14 | 10 |
| 16–18 M | 1000 | 2.5[k] | 10 | 1000 | 1000 | 300 | 160 | 14 | 12 |
| 16–18 F | 800 | 2.5[k] | 6 | 700 | 700 | 250 | 110 | 14 | 11 |
| 19–35 M | 1000 | 2.5[k] | 9 | 800 | 800 | 300 | 150 | 10 | 10 |
| 19–35 F | 800 | 2.5[k] | 6 | 700 | 700 | 250 | 110 | 14 | 9 |
| 36–50 M | 1000 | 2.5[k] | 8 | 800 | 800 | 300 | 140 | 10 | 10 |
| 36–50 F | 800 | 2.5[k] | 6 | 700 | 700 | 250 | 100 | 14 | 9 |
| +51 M | 1000 | 2.5[k] | 8 | 800 | 800 | 300 | 140 | 10 | 10 |
| 51 + F | 800 | 2.5[k] | 6 | 700 | 700 | 250 | 100 | 9 | 9 |
| Pregnant | +100 | +2.5[k] | +1 | +500 | +500 | +25 | +15 | +1 [m] | +3 |
| Lactating | +400 | +2.5[k] | +2 | +500 | +500 | +75 | +25 | +1 [m] | +7 |

[l] One mcg retinol equivalent (1 mcg RE) corresponds to a biological activity in humans equal to 1 mcg retinol (3.33 IU) and 6 mcg β-carotene (10 IU).

[j] One mcg cholecalciferol is equivalent to 40 IU vitamin D activity.

[k] Most older children and adults receive enough vitamin D from irradiation but 2.5 mcg daily is recommended. This recommended allowance increases to 5.0 mcg daily for pregnant and lactating women and for those who are confined indoors or otherwise deprived of sunlight for extended periods.

[l] The intake of breast-fed infants may be less than the recommendation but is considered to be adequate.

[m] A recommended total intake of 15 mg daily during pregnancy and lactation assumes the presence of adequate stores of iron. If stores are suspected of being inadequate, additional iron as a supplement is recommended.

TABLE A–5    APPROXIMATE CONVERSIONS TO AND FROM METRIC MEASURES

| If Measure Is in | Multiply by | To Find |
|---|---|---|
| *Length* | | |
| inches | 2.5 | centimeters |
| feet | 30 | centimeters |
| centimeters | 0.4 | inches |
| meters | 3.3 | feet |
| *Weight* | | |
| ounces | 28 | grams |
| pounds | 0.45 | kilograms |
| grams | 0.035 | ounces |
| kilograms | 2.2 | pounds |
| *Volume* | | |
| teaspoons | 5 | milliliters |
| tablespoons | 15 | milliliters |
| fluid ounces | 30 | milliliters |
| cups | 0.24 | liters |
| pints | 0.47 | liters |
| quarts | 0.95 | liters |
| milliliters | 0.03 | fluid ounces |
| liters | 2.1 | pints |
| liters | 1.06 | quarts |
| *Temperature* | | |
| Fahrenheit | subtract 32; then multiply by 5/9 | Celsius |
| Celsius | 9/5; then add 32 | Fahrenheit |

# Appendix B

# B-1 A LIST OF REFERENCE MATERIALS

**BOOKS**

Anderson, L., et al.: Nutrition in Nursing. Philadelphia: J. B. Lippincott Company, 1972.

Howe, P. S.: Basic Nutrition in Health and Disease. Philadelphia: W. B. Saunders Company, 1971.

Krause, M. V., and Hunscher, M. A.: Food, Nutrition and Diet Therapy, 5th ed. Philadelphia: W. B. Saunders Company, 1972.

Leverton, R. M.: Food Becomes You, 3rd ed. Ames: Iowa State University Press, 1965.

Lowenberg, M., et al.: Food and Man. New York: John Wiley & Sons, Inc., 1968.

Martin, E. A.: Nutrition in Action, 3rd ed. New York: Holt, Rinehart and Winston, Inc., 1971.

Mason, M. A.: Basic Medical-Surgical Nursing, 3rd ed. New York: Macmillan Publishing Co., Inc., 1974.

Robinson, C. H.: Normal and Therapeutic Nutrition, 14th ed. New York: Macmillan Publishing Co., Inc., 1972.

Shackelton, A. D.: Practical Nurse Nutrition Education, 3rd ed. Philadelphia: W. B. Saunders Company, 1972.

Stare, F. J., and McWilliams, M.: Living Nutrition. New York: John Wiley & Sons, Inc., 1973.

U.S. Department of Agriculture: Food for Us All: Yearbook of Agriculture. Washington, D.C.: Government Printing Office, 1969.

Williams, S. R.: Nutrition and Diet Therapy, 2nd ed. St. Louis: The C. V. Mosby Company, 1973.

## JOURNALS

*American Journal of Nursing*
*American Journal of Public Health*
*Hospitals*
*Journal of the American Dietetic Association*
*Journal of the American Medical Association*
*Journal of Nutrition Education*
*Modern Medicine*
*Nursing Care*
*Nursing Clinics of North America*
*Nursing Outlook*
*Nursing Times*
*Nutrition Today*
*Today's Health*

## SOURCES OF NUTRITION EDUCATION MATERIALS

In your own state or city:

Cooperative Extension Services, state university or regional office

Division of Nutrition, Department of Health, state or regional office

American Dental Association. 222 East Superior Street, Chicago, Ill. 60611.

American Diabetes Association. 18 East 48th Street, New York, N.Y. 10017.

American Dietetic Association. 430 North Michigan Avenue, Chicago, Ill. 60611.

American Heart Association. 44 East 23rd Street, New York, N.Y. 10010.

American Home Economics Association. 1600 Twentieth Street, N.W., Washington, D.C. 20009.

American Institute of Baking. Consumer Service Department, 400 East Ontario Street, Chicago, Ill. 60611.

American Public Health Association. 1790 Broadway, New York, N.Y. 10019.

American School Food Service Association. P.O. Box 10095, Denver, Colo. 80210.

The Borden Company. 350 Madison Avenue, New York, N.Y. 10017.

The Campbell Soup Company, Home Economics Department. 385 Memorial Avenue, Camden, N.J. 08101.

Cereal Institute, Inc., Educational Director. 135 South LaSalle Street, Chicago. Ill. 60603.

Chicago Dietetic Supply House, Inc. 405 E. Shawnut Ave., P.O. Box 529, La Grange, Ill. 60525.

Children's Bureau. Department of Health, Education, and Welfare. Washington, D.C. 20201.

Council on Foods and Nutrition. American Medical Association. 535 North Dearborn Street, Chicago, Ill. 60610.

Doyle Pharmaceutical Company, Minneapolis, Minn. 55416.

Evaporated Milk Association. 228 N. LaSalle Street, Chicago, Ill. 60601.

Food and Drug Administration. Department of Health, Education, and Welfare. Washington, D.C. 20204.

Food and Nutrition Board, National Research Council. 2101 Constitution Avenue, Washington, D.C. 20037.

General Foods Corporation. 250 North Street, White Plains, N.Y. 10602.

General Mills, Inc., Public Relations Department. 9200 Wayzata Boulevard, Minneapolis, Minn. 55440.

Gerber Products. Department of Nutrition. Fremont, Mich. 49412.

John Hancock Life Insurance Company. 200 Berkeley Street, Boston, Mass. 02117.

Kellogg Company, Department of Home Economics Services. 215 Porter Street, Battle Creek, Mich. 49016.

Maternal and Child Health Services, Department of Health, Education, and Welfare. Rockville, Md. 20852.

Mead Johnson & Company. Evansville, Ind. 47721.

Metropolitan Life Insurance Company, Health Education Director. One Madison Avenue, New York, N.Y. 10010.

National Dairy Council. 111 North Canal Street, Chicago, Ill. 60606 (or check with your local dairy council).

National Live Stock and Meat Board, Home Economics Department. 36 S. Wabash Avenue, Chicago, Ill. 60603.

The Nutrition Foundation, Inc. 99 Park Avenue, New York, N.Y. 10016.

Poultry and Egg National Board. 250 W. 57th Street, New York, N. Y. 10019.

Ross Laboratories. 625 Cleveland Avenue, Columbus, Ohio 43216.

School Lunch Branch, Agricultural Marketing Service. U.S. Department of Agriculture, Washington, D.C. 20250.

Sunkist Growers. Box 2706, Terminal Annex, Los Angeles, Calif. 90005.

U.S. Department of Agriculture, Office of Communication. Washington, D.C. 20250.

Wheat Flour Institute. 14 E. Jackson Boulevard, Chicago, Ill. 60604.

# B-2 A LIST OF AUDIOVISUAL MATERIALS

Films, filmstrips, or slides enrich the teaching of nutrition. They are useful for an overview of the subject, for review, or for illustrating a point. As the course plan is set up the instructor should include several films, filmstrips, or slide presentations.

A representative list of audiovisual materials follows together with suggested correlations with chapters of the text. The content is described when the title does not indicate the scope of the topics covered. Many filmstrips and slide sets are so inexpensive that even the school with a very limited budget can make gradual additions to its collection. Approximate prices have been listed for many of these. Most movies are available for free loan or on a rental basis. The instructor should consult local groups for availability of films, filmstrips, and slides that are available on a loan basis: the audiovisual department of local or state divisions of public education, departments of health; Dairy Council; district heart association; Modern Talking Picture Service, Associated Film Services, and other film services. Films should be ordered at least a month in advance of the expected showing.

FILMS (16 mm, color, sound, unless otherwise noted)

*Chapter
Correlation*

1. "Food, the Color of Life" (1965)                                                    1
   Content: life continues through self replacing cycle of
   which food is a part; motivational film toward better
   diet

Chapter
Correlation

22½ minutes, National Dairy Council: free loan, Association-Sterling Films, 866 Third Avenue, New York, N.Y. 10022

2. "Food for a Modern World"  1, 2, 17
   Content: development of U.S. food technology for past 50 years; compares our ability to produce food with other parts of world
   22 minutes, California Dairy Council; rental from Perennial Education, Inc., 1825 Willow Road, Northfield, Ill. 60693

3. "Hungry Angels" (1961)  2, 5
   Content: nutritional problems related to poverty, ignorance; case studies shown; need for low-cost proteins
   20 minutes, rental: Association Films, Inc., 347 Madison Ave., New York, N.Y. 10017

4. "Prescription: Food" (1973)  2, 14
   Content: problem of malnutrition in low-income area; home visits by nurse practitioners; classes for pregnant mothers; supervised play and meals
   26 minutes, free loan: Director of Public Health Services, Ross Laboratories, Columbus, Ohio 43216

5. "Food for Life" (1969)  2, 14
   Content: food selections by four teen-agers; two Americans choose poor diet even with abundant food supply; South American lacks variety; Asian lacks quantity, variety
   22 minutes, California Dairy Council; rental from Perennial Education, Inc. (# 2 above) *

6. "Nutrition Quackery" (1973)  2, 17
   Content: food faddist giving TV lecture; film gives answer by showing scenes in food production; explains food safety, regulation
   20 minutes, free loan: AIMS Instructional Media Services, Inc., P.O. Box 1010, Hollywood, Calif. 90028

7. "The Human Body: Digestive System"  3
   Content: animation, x-rays, live action scenes; digestion of complex substances to simple; role and relationship of digestive organs
   13½ minutes, produced by Coronet Films: free loan, preview prints, J.P. Lilley and Son, Inc., Box 3035, 2009 N. Third St., Harrisburg, Pa. 17105

8. "How a Hamburger Turns Into You"  3, 5
   Content: 12-year-old learns how protein is digested and resynthesized in cells according to DNA direction

* Numbers in parentheses indicate where the full address is given.

20 minutes, California Dairy Council: rental from Perennial Education, Inc. (# 2)

9. "The Big Dinner Table"          4
Content: nutrition for people all over the world comes from four food groups; family mealtime in 35 world locations
11 minutes, California Dairy Council: rental from Perennial Education, Inc. (# 2)

10. "Food, Energy and You" (1972)    8
Content: animated scenes showing process by which plants store energy; ATP-ADP system as control of energy in body
21 minutes, California Dairy Council: rental from Perennial Education, Inc. (# 2)

11. "Calcium and Phosphorus Metabolism" (1964)  9, 23
Content: sources calcium and phosphorus; regulation of absorption, blood levels, excretion; diagnosis and treatment of metabolic disorders
Part 1, 24 min; part 2, 23 minutes, black and white: loan, National Medical Audiovisual Center, Station "K," Atlanta, Ga. 30324

12. "Vitamins and Some Deficiency Diseases" (1955 revised)  11, 12
Content: laboratory scenes show deficiency in animals; clinical deficiency such as cheilosis, rickets, pellagra, scurvy, vitamin K
35 minutes, free loan: Lederle Laboratories, Division of American Cyanamid Co., Pearl River, N.Y. 10965

13. "Vitamins from Food"  11, 12
Content: Dr. Lind cures scurvy; Dr. Eijkman cures beriberi; vitamins as coenzymes in animated scenes
21 minutes, California Dairy Council: rental from Perennial Education, Inc. (# 2)

14. "The Rights of Age"  13
Content: story of elderly widow, cut off from society, living alone, meager diet; film brings out various protective services
28 minutes: rental from International Film Bureau, Inc., 332 South Michigan Ave., Chicago, Ill. 60604

15. "Eating for Two" (1968)  13
Content: public health nurse helping young black mother learn nutritional needs; meal patterns for family, meal planning, economic shopping; food patterns typical of southeastern United States
22 minutes: check local source for loan; purchase, Bureau of Audio Visual Instruction, 1327 University Ave., Box 2093, Madison, Wis. 53701

Chapter<br>Correlation

16. "What You Eat, You Are" (1970)     13, 15, 16, 17
    Content: situations in black families; planning, purchasing, preparing, serving food; protection against parasites
    15 minutes, free loan: Audio Visual Aids, University of South Carolina, College of General Studies, Carolina Coliseum, Columbia, S.C. 29208

17. "Jenny Is a Good Thing" (1969)     14
    Content: Head Start Centers; linking nutrition practices to play, learning, social experiences, language, development of self-concept
    18 minutes, free loan: Modern Talking Picture Service, Inc., 2323 New Hyde Park Road, New Hyde Park, N.Y. 11140

18. "Looking at Children"     14
    Content: teachers and school nurses alerted to physical health problems of children; discusses anemia, obesity, malnutrition
    24 minutes, free loan: Health and Welfare Division, Metropolitan Life Insurance Company, One Madison Avenue, New York, N.Y. 10010

19. "Nutrition: To Baby with Love" (1973)     14
    Content: young parents with babies from different ethnic backgrounds; which foods, how much, when
    10 minutes, Gerber Products Company: free loan, West Glen Films, 565 Fifth Ave., New York, N.Y. 10017

20. "Food or Famine"     16, 17
    Content: methods of using fertilizers, controlling pests, raising better cattle; Europe, S.E. Asia, India, South America
    28 minutes, free loan: Shell Film Library, 450 N. Meridian St., Indianapolis, Ind. 46204

21. "The Health Fraud Racket" (1967)     16, 17
    Content: traps of the quack; economic waste, risk to health of worthless products
    28 minutes, Food and Drug Administration: free loan, National Medical Audiovisual Center (# 11)

22. "More than Food" (1965)     18
    Content: filmed in nursing home; shows role of all personnel in meeting nutritional, physical, psychological needs
    23 minutes, check local source for loan: purchase, Colorado State Department of Public Health, Denver, Colo. 80203

23. "Feeding the Patient" (1959)     18
    Content: appetite, digestion, feeding ambulatory and

recumbent patients; physical, psychological preparation for meals

15 minutes, black and white: rental, American Hospital Association, 840 N. Lake Shore Drive, Chicago, Ill. 60611

24. "The Missing Millions" (1968)       22

Content: young executive found to have typical symptoms of diabetes; nature of disease; effectiveness of treatment

14 minutes, free loan: National Medical Audiovisual Center (# 11)

25. "Quiet Victory" (1967)        22

Content: nurse's responsibility to four persons with diabetes, teaching and guidance in detection center, outpatient center, hospital, home

32 minutes, free loan: National Medical Audiovisual Center (# 11)

26. "Understanding Diabetes" (1967)     22

Content: basic scientific concepts, epidemiology, management, prevention of acute problems. Live photography, animated drawings

35 minutes, free loan: National Medical Audiovisual Center (# 11)

27. "Better Odds for a Longer Life" (1966)   24

Content: cartoon animation; functions of heart; atherosclerosis; ways to reduce risks

20 minutes, rental: American Heart Association Film Library, 267 W. 25th St., New York, N.Y. 10001

28. "Eat to Your Heart's Content"      24

Content: case study of typical American family and dietary faults; some ways to correct diet

13 minutes, rental: American Heart Association (# 27)

**FILMSTRIPS, SLIDES**
**(35 mm, color, record or script)**

29. "How Food Affects You" (1969)     1, 2

Content: cartoon type illustrations of functions of nutrition; names nutrients; examples of function; 4 food groups

Filmstrip, $5.50: Photo Lab, Inc., 3825 Georgia Ave. N.W., Washington, D.C. 20011

48 slides, $8.00: Office of Communication, Photography Division, U.S. Department of Agriculture, Washington, D.C., 20250

|  | Chapter<br>Correlation |
|---|---|

30. "Natural Foods—Good, Bad, Different" (1973) — **2, 16, 17**
   29 slides, cassette, script, $12.00: Visual Communications Office, 412 Roberts Hall, Cornell University, Ithaca, N.Y. 14850
31. "The 130 Billion Dollar Food Assembly Line" (1972) — **2, 17**
   Content: movement of food from producer to consumer; emphasis on productivity, dollar values
   Filmstrip, 47 frames, $5.50: Photo Lab, Inc. (# 29)
   Slides, $13.00: Office of Communication (# 29)
   Narrative cassette, $3.00: either source
32. "Nutrition" (1969) — **2, 4**
   Content: how food is used by body; nutrient functions and sources; 4 food groups
   20 multicolor transparencies for overhead projector, teacher supplement, $48.50: DCA Educational Products, Inc., 4865 Stenton Ave., Philadelphia, Pa. 19144
33. "Gastric Function" (September 1971) * — **3, 28**
   25 slides, 12 syllabi, $28.50: Educational Services, Nutrition Today, 101 Ridgely Ave., Annapolis, Md. 21404
34. "Gastrointestinal Absorption" (March 1967) — **3, 28**
   9 slides, 12 syllabi, $15.25: Nutrition Today (# 33)
35. "The Esophagus" (January 1973) — **3**
   19 slides, 12 syllabi, $23.50: Nutrition Today (# 33)
36. "Nutrition Series" (1972)
   1. Science of nutrition — **1**
   2. Social aspects of nutrition — **15**
   3. Energy and the carbohydrates — **7, 8**
   4. The fats — **6**
   5. Proteins, the building blocks — **5**
   6. Fat-soluble vitamins — **11**
   7. Water-soluble vitamins — **12**
   8. Water and minerals — **9, 10**
   9. Nutrition in the home — **13**
   10. Nutrition in the hospital — **18**
   Self-teaching units—filmstrip, audiotape cassette, work sheet, post test, each unit $14, set, $140: Multi Media Office, Mt. San Jacinto College, 21400 Highway 79, Gilman Hot Springs, Calif. 92340
37. "Protein/Iron" (1973) — **5, 9**
   Content: protein role, amino acids, protein synthesis, costs from various sources; iron, needs for high intake, iron absorption, role

---

* The dates for slides from *Nutrition Today* refer to articles appearing in the journal. The articles, slides, and syllabi have been developed by internationally recognized authorities, and are highly recommended for nursing programs.

35 slides, leader's guide, $6.00 for set: Visual Communications Office (# 30)

38. "Iron Metabolism" (Summer 1969)         9
10 slides, 12 syllabi, $16.00: Nutrition Today (# 33)

39. "How the Body Uses Water" (Spring 1970)       10
9 slides, 12 syllabi, $15.80: Nutrition Today (# 33)

40. "Vitamins and You"       11
Content: importance of vitamins for childhood
Filmstrip, $4.00: Vitamin Information Bureau, Inc., 575 Lexington Ave., Dept. JN, New York, N.Y. 10022

41. "Vitamin E" (July, 1973)       11
14 slides, 12 syllabi, $24.30: Nutrition Today (# 33)

42. "Nutrition (Scope ® Manual)"       11, 12
Content: nutrition, deficiency diseases
49 slides, color, black and white, $20.00: The Upjohn Company, Unit 9435, Kalamazoo, Mich. 49001

43. "Vitamin C Makes the Difference" (1972)       12
Content: vitamin C sources, four food groups, buying and storage of fruits and vegetables; meal planning, 6 citrus recipes
Filmstrip, 50 frames, narrative guide, $2.50; slides, $5.00: Sunkist Growers, Inc., Consumer Service, Box 7888, Valley Annex, Van Nuys, Calif. 91409

44. "Straight Talk About Pregnancy and Prenatal Care"       13
(1972)
Content: wide range income and ethnic groups; parent education; food needs, shopping, weight gain
Part 1, Straight talk about pregnancy, 80 slides; part 2, What to eat, 21 slides; part 3, Labor and delivery, 31 slides; teacher guide, scripts, record or cassettes, $15; National Foundation—March of Dimes, 1275 Mamaroneck Ave., White Plains, N.Y. 10605

45. "What Should a Pregnant Woman Eat" (Summer,       13
1970)
16 slides, 12 syllabi, $20.90: Nutrition Today (# 33)

46. "The Beginnings of Life"       13
Content: development of embryo, fetus; vitamins and minerals
Filmstrip, wall chart, 25 student leaflets, $6.00: Vitamin Information Bureau, Inc. (# 40)

47. "Prenatal Diet Counseling"       13
Set of 12 cards or slides, suggested narrative, $12.00: Creative Teaching Aids, 4161 Carmichael Ave., Suite 210, Jacksonville, Fla. 32207

48. "Food During Pregnancy" (1970)       13
Content: importance of eating right foods during preg-

nancy and throughout life; needs for calcium, iron, vitamins; adjustments for breast feeding; 4 food groups

11 minutes, filmstrip, record, $42.50; slides, record, $63.50: National Health Films, Box 13973, Station "K," Atlanta, Ga. 30324

49. "Where Old Age Begins" (December 1967)      13
11 slides, 12 syllabi, $17.25: Nutrition Today (# 33)

50. "Breakfast and the Bright Life"      13
Content: social aspects of food; role of breakfast in weight control
Filmstrip, 96 frames, teacher's guide: Educational Director, Cereal Institute, 135 S. La Salle St., Chicago, Ill. 60603

51. "Feeding Your Young Children"      14
Content: child's development needs; building positive attitudes toward food; children 2–6
Filmstrip, 60 frames, leader guide, $2.00: National Dairy Council, Inc., 111 North Canal St., Chicago, Ill. 60606

52. "What Nutrients Do Our Infants Really Get?"      14
(September 1973)
15 slides, 12 syllabi, $19.75: Educational Services, Nutrition Today (# 33)      14

53. "Your Baby's Food" (1970)      14
Content: nutritional and psychological adjustments
11 minutes, filmstrip, record, $42.50; slides, $63.50: National Health Films (# 11)

54. "Your Food—Chance or Choice" (1966)
Content: teen-agers food choices; disc-jockey type narrative; rock music; awareness of food, principles nutrition, decision making
Filmstrip, 106 frames, teacher's guide, record, $5.00 National Dairy Council (# 1)

55. "Puerto Rican Food Habits" (1971)      15
Content: culture, food habits, favorite foods, change within framework of culture
45 slides, script, $8.75: Visual Communications Office (# 30)

56. "Food Additives" (July, 1973)      16, 17
14 slides, 12 syllabi, $19.95: Nutrition Today (# 33)

57. "Ann's Additive Story" (Its Meaning to Your Food and      16, 17
Health)
36 frames, filmstrip, $5.50: Photo Lab, Inc. (# 29)
slides, $11.00, Photography Division (# 29)

58. "Spending Your Food Dollar"      17
77 frames, study guide, free loan: Money Management

Institute, Household Finance Corporation, Prudential Plaza, Chicago, Ill. 60601

59. "Stress: On Just Being Sick" (Spring, 1970)                                          18
    13 slides, 12 syllabi, $19.25: Nutrition Today (# 33)

60. "Just One in a Crowd" (1965)                                                         22
    1. It's up to you (basic information)—10 min.
    2. Watching what you eat—11 min.
    3. Living with a diet—9 min.
    4. Taking care of yourself—14 min.
    5. Learning rules of health—9 min.
    6. Joining the crowd—9 min.
    Six filmstrips, tapes or record, $100: Creative Arts Studio, Inc., 814 H Street, N.W., Washington, D.C. 20201

61. "Planning Diabetic Diets"                                                           22
    Content: foods on exchange lists, flexibility of meal planning; sample prescription, meals
    16 minutes, filmstrip, guide, $47.50; slides, $85.00: National Health Films (# 11)

62. "Diabetes for Diabetics"                                                            22
    Content: the pancreas; identification insignia; measuring equipment; exchange lists; insulin; glucagon; urine testing
    203 slides: Diabetes Press of America, Inc., 30 S. E. 8th St., Miami, Fla. 33131

63. "The Child with Diabetes" (March, 1971)                                             22
    11 slides, 12 syllabi, $18.45: Nutrition Today (# 33)

64. "Diet and Arthritis" (1967)                                                         23
    Content: susceptibility to faddism, basic food needs, equipment helpful to patient
    Filmstrip, 26 frames, narrative guide, free loan: Diabetes and Arthritis Control Program, Public Health Service, 4040 N. Fairfax Drive, Arlington, Va. 22203

65. "Phenylketonuria" (1964)                                                            23
    Content: biochemical, clinical, diagnostic, genetic, and diet aspects
    Filmstrip, 116 frames, free loan: Audio Visual Division, Mead Johnson and Company, 2404 Pennsylvania Ave., Evansville, Ind. 47721

66. "Treatment in Phenylketonuria" (1965)                                               23
    Content: details of diet; role of physician, nutritionist, nurse
    Filmstrip, 89 frames, free loan: Mead Johnson and Company (# 65)

67. "Planning Sodium Restricted Diets"                                                  25
    Content: basic information on sodium, sources; food lists for planning diets; 500 mg diet and how to modify; seasonings

Filmstrip, 19½ minutes, record, guide, $47.50; slides,
$85.00: National Health Films ( # 11)
68. "Intestinal Malabsorption" (September 1968)                    28
10 slides, 12 syllabi, $17.80: Nutrition Today ( # 33)

# Appendix C

# GLOSSARY

The first step in the study of any subject is gaining an understanding of the vocabulary. Every student should have a standard dictionary and should form the habit of using it whenever he comes across a word he does not know.

This glossary includes words frequently used in medicine and nutrition and that are not, for the most part, defined fully in the text. Many terms directly related to nutrition are defined in the text, and the student should refer to the chapters in which these terms are discussed. Consult the index for page references to such terms.

**absorption.** In physiology, the uptake of nutrients by the walls of the small intestine for transfer to the circulation.

**acetone bodies.** Intermediate products in the oxidation of fatty acids; acetone, acetoacetic acid, and beta-hydroxy-butric acid.

**acidosis.** Abnormal accumulation of acids in the body, or loss of base.

**ACTH** (adrenocorticotropic hormone). A hormone produced by the pituitary gland that controls the action of the adrenal cortex; sodium metabolism, for example.

**acute.** Sudden, severe symptoms of short duration.

**adipose.** Fatty tissue; body stores of fat.

**adrenal.** Organ near the kidney that secretes several hormones.

**amylase** (amylopsin). An enzyme in saliva or pancreatic juice that digests starch.

**anemia.** A decrease in the number of red blood cells or hemoglobin or both.

**anion.** Chemical substance that carries a negative electrical charge.

**anorexia.** Loss of appetite.

**antibiotic.** A substance that checks the growth of microorganisms.

**antibody.** A protein substance produced within the body that destroys bacteria.

**antioxidant.** A substance that prevents oxidation; often added to foods to prevent rancidity.

**anuria.** Absence of urinary output.

**ascites.** Accumulation of fluid in the abdominal cavity.

**atherosclerosis.** Thickening of inside wall of arteries by fat-cholesterol containing deposits.

**avitaminosis.** Deficiency or lack of vitamins in the diet, or failure to absorb them; specific symptoms result from each vitamin deficiency.

**bile.** Secretion of the liver that aids in fat digestion and absorption.

**blanch.** To preheat in boiling water or steam; used to inactivate enzymes before freezing food, or to remove the skins of fruits.

**bland.** Mild in flavor.

**braise.** To cook food in a tightly covered pan with a small amount of liquid.

**buffer.** A substance that lessens the change in pH that otherwise would occur with the addition of acids or alkalies.

**calcification.** Hardening of tissue by deposits of calcium salts; bone, for example.

**calculi.** Hard substances formed in the body; kidney stones.

**caliper.** An instrument for measuring the thickness of an object; used in medicine to measure thickness of fat layers.

**calorimeter.** An instrument for measuring heat change. A bomb calorimeter measures calories in food; a respiration calorimeter measures oxygen and carbon dioxide exchange of an individual.

**carboxylase.** An enzyme necessary for the metabolism of glucose; thiamine is a component.

**catalyst.** A substance that speeds up a chemical reaction.

**cation.** Chemical substance that carries a positive electrical charge.

**cecum.** The large blind pouch in which the large intestine begins.

**cellular.** Pertaining to the function of cells that make up the tissues.

**chlorophyll.** The green coloring matter in plants that is responsible for the process of photosynthesis.

**cholecystokinin.** A hormone secreted in the wall of the duodenum when fat is present; causes contraction of the gallbladder and flow of bile.

**chronic.** Of long duration; opposed to acute.

**chyme.** The liquid food mass that has been digested in the stomach and is ready for passage through the duodenum.

**coagulation.** Change from a fluid to a semisolid or solid state; curd; clot.

**coenzyme.** A substance such as a vitamin that is a part of an enzyme.

**colitis.** Inflammation of the colon.

**colon.** The large intestine, beginning at the cecum.

**coma.** Unconsciousness; may result from accumulation of acids as in diabetes mellitus.

**congenital.** Present at birth.

**consistency.** Refers to the texture of a diet; liquid, soft, low-fiber, etc.

**convulsion.** Involuntary contraction of the muscles; may occur in eclampsia, uremic poisoning, and many other conditions.

**cortisone.** A hormone of the adrenal gland.

**cretin.** An individual who has inadequate physical and mental development because of insufficient thyroid secretion.

**cultural.** In study of food habits, refers to social, religious, national habits of a group of people.

**decompensation, heart.** Failure of the heart to adequately pump blood through the circulation.

**dehydration.** Abnormal loss of water from the body. Also, removal of water from food.

**delirium.** Mental disturbance characterized by physical restlessness, excitement, confusion, and delusions.

**denaturation.** The change of the physical state of a substance; for example, the coagulation of a protein.

**dentine.** The major calcified portion of the tooth; covered by enamel over the crown, and by cementum on the root portion of the tooth.

**dermatitis.** Inflammation of the skin.

**dextrose.** A single sugar; also called glucose.

**dietetic food.** A food prepared for specific uses in modified diets; for example, low-sodium, or packed without sugar.

**distention.** The state of stretching or enlarging; often refers to the accumulation of gases in the intestinal tract and the resultant feeling of fullness.

**diuretic.** Any substance that increases the volume of the urine.

**DNA** (deoxyribonucleic acid). A protein substance in nucleus that carries genetic information.

**duodenum.** The first part of the small intestine beginning at the pylorus.

**dysentery.** An inflammation of the colon; often caused by bacterial or parasitic infection.

**edema.** Accumulation of fluid in the body.

**electrolyte.** Chemical substance in body fluids that can carry an electrical charge, for example, sodium ($Na^+$) or chlorine ($Cl^-$).

**embryo.** Early stage of development of the fetus.

**emulsification.** The breaking up of large particles into much smaller particles and suspending them in another liquid; for example, bile breaks up fat into minute droplets for digestion.

**endemic.** Refers to a disease being prevalent in a particular area.

**endocrine.** Any of the ductless glands such as the thyroid, adrenal, pituitary that secrete hormones into the blood circulation.

**endosperm.** The starchy portion of the cereal grain.

**enzyme.** A substance formed by living cells that speeds up chemical reactions; a living catalyst.

**epithelium.** Outer layer of the skin; includes the linings of the hollow organs, the respiratory, gastrointestinal, and genitourinary tracts.

**erepsin.** A group of protein-splitting enzymes secreted by the small intestine.

**esophageal varices.** Varicose veins of the esophagus.

**extracellular.** Around the cells.

**extractive, meat.** Nonprotein, nitrogen-containing, water-soluble substances in meat.

**fallout.** The radioactive dust that settles following explosion of a nuclear bomb.

**feces.** Excretion from the bowels.

**fetus.** Unborn young, especially in the later stages of development.

**fibrinogen.** A protein in blood necessary for clotting.

**flatulence.** Gas in the intestinal tract.

**gastrectomy.** Operation for removal of part or all of the stomach.

**gastritis.** Inflammation of the stomach.

**genetic.** Dealing with heredity.

**genitourinary.** Pertaining to the organs of reproduction and the urinary tract.

**geriatrics.** Branch of medicine concerned with diseases of older people.

**gluten.** Protein substance in cereal grains, especially wheat, that gives elastic quality to doughs.

**glycerol.** The organic compound to which fatty acids are attached to form a fat.

**gristle.** The tough connective-tissue fibers of meat.

**hemicellulose.** A complex, indigestible carbohydrate found in cell walls of plants.

**hemoglobin.** Red pigment in blood cells that carries oxygen.

**hemorrhage.** Loss of blood.

**hepatic.** Refers to the liver.

**herbs.** Group of plants having odors and flavors useful in the seasoning of foods; for example, sage, marjoram, thyme, and many others.

**hormone.** Chemical substance produced by a gland of the body and transported by the blood for activity in other tissues; thyroxine, insulin, and others.

**hydrolysis.** The splitting of a substance into simpler compounds by the addition of water.

**hyper-.** A prefix meaning increased, or greater than normal.

**hyperalimentation.** Intravenous feedings of solutions that are more concentrated than substances in blood.

**hyperglycemia.** Increased level of glucose in the blood.

**hyperlipidemia.** Elevation of one or more fatty components of blood, such as triglycerides, cholesterol, or lipoproteins.

**hypertension.** High blood pressure.

**hypervitaminosis.** Excess of vitamin storage in the body; for example, an overdosage of vitamin A or D.

**hypo-.** A prefix meaning below normal.

**hypochromic.** Less color than normal; for example, hypochromic anemia.
**hypothyroidism.** Inadequate secretion of thyroid gland.

**ileum.** Lower part of the small intestine.
**insulin.** Hormone secreted by the islands of Langerhans in the pancreas; changes blood glucose to glycogen, increases uptake of glucose by the cell, and facilitates the formation of fat.
**intracellular.** Within the cell.
**intravenous.** Within the veins.
**irradiation.** Expose to rays such as ultraviolet rays, x-rays.

**jejunum.** Middle part of the small intestine, beginning at the duodenum and extending to the ileum.

**ketosis.** Condition resulting from the accumulation of ketones (acetone bodies) as a result of incomplete oxidation of fatty acids.

**labile.** Easily destroyed.
**lactase.** Enzyme produced by the small intestine; splits lactose to glucose and galactose.
**lacteal.** A small lymphatic vessel that takes up fatty substances from the intestinal wall.
**legumes.** Class of plant foods including beans, lentils, peas, peanuts.
**lignin.** Indigestible carbohydrate found in the cell wall of plants.
**lipase.** Enzyme produced by the pancreas that digests fats.

**macrocyte.** Giant red blood cell.
**malabsorption.** Failure to absorb the various nutrients from the intestinal tract; occurs in celiac disease, sprue, dysentery, diarrhea.
**maltase.** Enzyme that splits maltose to two molecules of glucose.
**marbled.** Referring to meat, fine streaks of fat appearing throughout the lean portion of meat.
**marinate.** To soak meat, fish, or salad ingredients in a seasoned mixture such as wine, vinegar, French dressing.
**median.** The middle point; half of the values in a series of measurements will be above and half below this point.
**micro-.** Prefix meaning small; for example, *microcyte* is a very small cell; *microorganisms* include bacteria, yeasts, molds.
**myo-.** Refers to muscle; *myocardium* is the heart muscle; *myoglobin* is the iron-containing pigment in muscle.

**nausea.** Sick at the stomach with tendency to vomit.
**nephritis.** Inflammation of the kidney.
**nyctalopia.** Night blindness.

**osmosis.** Passage of fluid through membranes from weaker to stronger solution.

**ossification.** Hardening of the bone.

**oxidase.** A class of enzymes that brings about oxidation of products in metabolism.

**oxidation.** Combination of a substance with oxygen; an increase in the positive valence of an atom through the loss of electrons.

**parathyroid.** Gland located near the thyroid that secretes hormone for control of calcium metabolism.

**parenteral.** Outside the gastrointestinal tract; for example, injection into vein, under the skin.

**pasta.** Spaghetti, macaroni, noodles, and the like made from durum wheat flour.

**pathogenic.** Disease-producing.

**pectin.** A complex, indigestible carbohydrate that has the capacity to hold water; found in many fruits such as apples.

**pepsin.** Enzyme secreted by the stomach for digestion of proteins.

**peptidases.** Class of enzymes that split peptides to amino acids.

**peptones.** Intermediate products in protein digestion.

**peristalsis.** Waves of contraction of muscle fibers in the intestinal tract that cause food to move through the tract.

**photosynthesis.** The process by which plants synthesize carbohydrates from carbon dioxide and water in the presence of light.

**placenta.** Organ attached to the wall of the uterus through which the fetus receives nourishment.

**plasma.** Fluid portion of the blood.

**poly-.** Prefix meaning much or many.

**polydipsia.** Excessive thirst.

**polyneuritis.** Inflammation of the nerves as in thiamine deficiency.

**polypeptide.** Groups of amino acids; intermediate stage in protein digestion.

**polyphagia.** Excessive appetite.

**polyuria.** Excessive amount of urine.

**protease.** Group of enzymes that digest proteins.

**ptyalin.** Starch-splitting enzyme in the saliva; also known as amylase.

**purée.** The pulp obtained by pressing food through a sieve to remove the fiber.

**purines.** Nitrogen-containing substances of a nonprotein nature occurring especially in meats; metabolized to uric acid.

**pylorus.** Circular opening of the stomach into the duodenum.

**rancid.** Having a disagreeable flavor or odor; usually affects foods high in fat content.

**rectum.** The lower part of the large intestine extending to the anal canal.

**regimen.** Dietary program.

**rehabilitation.** Restoration of health and efficiency as much as possible by physical, dietary, or other therapy.

**renal.** Referring to the kidney.

**rennin.** Enzyme secreted by the stomach that brings about coagulation of milk.

**retina.** The layer of the eye that receives the image and is connected to the brain by the optic nerve.

**secretin.** Hormone produced by the duodenum; stimulates pancreatic activity.
**sedentary.** Occupied in quiet activities; sitting, for example.
**serum.** Clear liquid that separates from clotted blood.
**sphincter.** A muscle surrounding and closing an opening;.for example, pyloric sphincter.
**spore.** Reproductive part of a microorganism; very resistant to heat.
**stabilizer.** A substance added to food to help maintain quality over a period of time.
**steapsin.** Enzyme in the small intestine that digests fat; also called lipase.
**steatorrhea.** Excessive amount of fat in the feces.
**subcutaneous.** Beneath the skin.
**sucrase.** Enzyme produced by the small intestine that splits sucrose to glucose and fructose.
**supplementary.** Additional.
**syndrome.** A number of symptoms occurring together that are typical of a certain disease; for example, malabsorption syndrome.
**synthesis.** Formation of complex substances from simpler substances.

**tenderizer.** An enzyme preparation that partially breaks down meat fibers, thereby making the meat more tender.
**thrombosis.** Formation of clot in blood vessel, as in heart (coronary thrombosis) or brain (cerebral thrombosis).
**toxemia.** Condition in which the blood contains poisonous substances; for example, excess of nitrogenous wastes.
**toxin.** Poisonous product produced by cells; for example, botulin.
**trauma.** Injury.
**trypsin.** Protein-splitting enzyme produced by the pancreas.

**ultraviolet rays.** Light rays of shorter wave length than visible rays.
**urea.** The chief nitrogenous waste product in the urine.
**uremia.** Elevation of nitrogenous constituents in blood because of failure of kidney to remove them; renal failure.
**uric acid.** Nitrogenous product resulting from the breakdown of purines.
**uterus.** The womb.

**vascular.** Refers to the blood and lymph vessels in the body.
**villus.** Tiny fingerlike projection on the mucous lining of the small intestine; supplied with blood and lymph vessels.
**viosterol.** Activated ergosterol; vitamin D.
**visual purple.** Organic compound in retina of the eye that is changed to yellow by light; vitamin A is required for its synthesis.

# INDEX

Illustrations are indicated by numbers that appear in **boldface** type.

Vitamin A (*cont.*)
  storage in liver, 98, 99
  summary, 104
  toxicity, 99–100
Vitamin B₁, 108
Vitamin B₆, 112–13, 116
  dietary allowances, 32, 112
    Canadian, 334
Vitamin B₁₂, 113, 116
  cobalt, 85, 113
  dietary allowances, 32, 112
    Canadian, 334
Vitamin C, 106–108. *See also* Ascorbic
  acid
Vitamin D, 100–102
  calcium utilization, 78, 100
  deficiency, 100, 101
  dietary allowances, 32, 101
    Canadian, 335
  functions, 100
  nomenclature, 100
  precursors, 100
  sources, 101–102
  summary, 104
  toxicity, 102
Vitamin E, 102
  dietary allowances, 32, 102
    Canadian, 335
  summary, 104
Vitamin K, 102–103
  summary, 104

Water, 87–90
  balance, 77, 89–90
  body, 87

Water (*cont.*)
  dehydration, 89
  edema, 90
  fluoridation, 84–85
  food sources, 89, 306–28
  functions, 88
  loss from body, 88
  of oxidation, 89
  requirement, 88
  sources to body, 89
Weight, control, 72, 206–15
  desirable, table, 333
  gain, and aging, 128
    plans, 214–15
    pregnancy, 130
    rate, infants, 136
  loss, plans, 209–13
  maintenance, 206–207
  standards, 29–30
Weight-height table, 333
Women, dietary allowances, 32
  "reference," 31
  weight-height table, 333
World Health Organization, 17
World nutrition problems, 16–17

Xerophthalmia, 99

Yogurt, 272

Zinc, 84
  dietary allowances, 32
    Canadian, 335
  summary, 94